GUIDE TO INTERPRETING 12-LEAD ECGs

J. Marcus Wharton, M.D.

Clinical Instructor in Medicine
University of California, San Francisco, School of Medicine

Chief Medical Resident
San Francisco General Hospital Medical Center

Nora Goldschlager, M.D.

Clinical Professor of Medicine
University of California, San Francisco, School of Medicine

Director, Coronary Care Unit and
Electrocardiographic Laboratory
San Francisco General Hospital Medical Center

Medical Economics Books
Oradell, New Jersey 07649

Library of Congress Cataloging in Publication Data

Wharton, J. Marcus.
Guide to interpreting 12-lead ECGs.

Bibliography: p.
1. Electrocardiography. 2. Heart—Diseases—Diagnosis. I. Goldschlager, Nora. II. Title. III. Title: Interpreting 12-lead ECGs. [DNLM: 1. Electrocardiography—Methods. WG 140 W553g]
RC683.5.E5W435 1983 616.1'207547 83-13214
ISBN 0-87489-314-3

Cover design by Tom Darnsteadt
Interior design by Penny Seldin

ISBN 0-87489-314-3

Medical Economics Company Inc.
Oradell, New Jersey 07649

Printed in the United States of America

To Bill and Ruby,
and to Simone

Contents

Abbreviations

ASD: atrial septal defect
ASH: asymmetric septal hypertrophy
AV: atrioventricular
BBB: bundle branch block
COPD: chronic obstructive pulmonary disease
IVCD: intraventricular conduction delay
LAA: left atrial abnormality
LAD: left axis deviation
LAFB: left anterior fascicular block
LBBB: left bundle branch block
LGL: Lown-Ganong-Levine (syndrome)
LPFB: left posterior fascicular block
LV: left ventricle; left ventricular
LVH: left ventricular hypertrophy
MI: myocardial infarction
PE: pulmonary embolism
PVC: premature ventricular contraction
RAA: right atrial abnormality
RAD: right axis deviation
RBBB: right bundle branch block
RV: right ventricle; right ventricular
RVH: right ventricular hypertrophy
SA: sinoatrial
WPW: Wolff-Parkinson-White (syndrome)

Acknowledgments

We are very grateful to Mr. Richard Aho of the Department of Electrocardiography, San Francisco General Hospital Medical Center, for his cheerful perseverance in the location and retrieval of many of the electrocardiograms presented in this book. Our thanks are also due to Drs. Melvin M. Scheinman, James Marks, Frederick Renold, and Lynn Morris for their helpful contributions of interesting cases.

J. Marcus Wharton, M.D.
Nora Goldschlager, M.D.

Publisher's Notes

As *Guide to Interpreting 12-Lead ECGs* went to press, the co-authors were already well along in their work on a companion volume, tentatively entitled *Quick Reference to Cardiac Arrhythmias,* to be published in the spring of 1985 by Medical Economics Books.

J. Marcus Wharton, M.D., is Clinical Instructor in Medicine at the University of California, San Francisco, School of Medicine, and Chief Resident in Medicine at San Francisco General Hospital Medical Center. He plans to begin a Fellowship in Cardiology at Duke University School of Medicine, Durham, N.C., in the fall of 1984.

Nora Goldschlager, M.D., is Clinical Professor of Medicine at the University of California, San Francisco, School of Medicine. At San Francisco General Hospital Medical Center, she is Director of the Coronary Care Unit and the Electrocardiographic Laboratory. She is an editorial consultant and contributor to a number of cardiology journals, and co-author of *Arrhythmias Case Studies* and *Cardiac Pacing: Principles and Case Studies,* published by Medical Examination Publishing Company.

The publisher gratefully acknowledges the painstaking work of artist Janet Kroenke, who worked on each of the more than 1,000 ECG tracings in this book to make them suitable for publication.

SECTION I

An Approach to the Interpretation of 12-Lead ECGs

An Approach to the Interpretation of 12-Lead ECGs

Electrocardiography is a tool of great practical importance to physicians of all specialties—from general internal medicine and family practice to surgical subspecialties, obstetrics, and even psychiatry. It is also, of course, one of the basic building blocks of cardiology and cardiovascular surgery.

The ECG is essential to the diagnosis of a number of major cardiac disorders, including myocardial ischemia and infarction, hypertrophy, and rhythm disturbances. Since the 12-lead ECG is so often used in clinical practice and is of significant diagnostic power, everyone involved in patient care should have a firm grasp of the subject.

ECG interpretation involves recognition not only of classic abnormal patterns, but also of disorders that can mimic them. This recognition is best accomplished by understanding *how* patterns are generated, and not simply by rote memory. Whenever possible, this book provides descriptions of both ECG patterns and their underlying electrophysiology.

Accurate interpretation of 12-lead ECGs also requires careful attention to both the obvious and the subtle, ideally by way of a methodical approach. We have found the following sequence helpful and have used it in this book: (1) assessment of rhythm; (2) measurement of the PR, QRS, and QT intervals; (3) determination of the mean frontal plane QRS axis; and (4) morphologic description of the (a) P wave, (b) PR segment, (c) QRS complex, (d) ST segment, (e) T wave, and (f) U wave.

At first, this approach may seem tedious, but with practice it can be used with facility to yield more information and satisfaction from 12-lead ECG interpretation. A brief description of the major ECG configurations follows:

The P wave represents atrial depolarization. The activating impulse is normally generated in the sinoatrial (SA) node in the right atrium, then spreads through both atria. Since the wave front starts at or near the SA node, the right atrium is depolarized before the left. Consequently, the initial portion of the P wave is generated by right atrial forces; the terminal portion by left atrial forces. The normal duration of the P wave is 0.08-0.11 second. The normal range of the mean frontal plane P wave axis is from 0° to +75°; actual values usually fall between +45° and +60°.

The PR segment is the portion of the tracing from the end of the P wave to the beginning of the QRS complex. During this period, atrial repolarization occurs. The PR segment is normally isoelectric (on the baseline).

The PR interval is measured from the onset of the P wave (atrial activation) to the onset of the QRS complex (ventricular activation). It includes the time required for the sinus impulse to spread through the atria, atrioventricular (AV) node, and His-Purkinje system. It does not include the sinoatrial conduction time—the interval between impulse formation in the sinus node and the onset of atrial activation. The normal PR interval is 0.12-0.20 second.

The QRS complex is generated by ventricular depolarization. Initial activation normally spreads from left to right across the interventricular septum, followed by virtually simultaneous activation of both ventricles. Because of the left ventricle's greater thickness, its lateral epicardial surface is depolarized last. The initial portion of the QRS complex (the first 0.04 second) represents the septal forces, normally directed anteriorly, superiorly, and to the right; the terminal portion represents the left ventricular forces, directed laterally and to the left.

The QRS interval is the distance between the onset of the Q (or R) wave and the end of the S wave. It reflects the total duration of ventricular depolarization. It is best measured in the lead (limb or precordial) where it is longest (assuming adequate demarcation). The normal interval is 0.04-0.12 second.

The mean frontal plane QRS axis represents the direction of the mean (or net) vector of the QRS complexes (and of the ventricular depolarization waves) from the perspective of the frontal plane. The axis is easily estimated using the hexaxial reference system (see Fig. 1 in the Appendix) derived from adding the augmented limb leads (aVR, aVL, and aVF) to a triaxial modification of Einthoven's triangle (a diagram of the spatial orientation of limb leads I, II, and III).

To calculate the approximate axis: Find the limb lead with the most isoelectric or biphasic (equally positive and negative) QRS complexes. The axis will be perpendicular to this lead, and will point toward the leads with tall R waves. For example, if the QRS complex is isoelectric in lead aVL, upright in leads II and aVF, and predominantly negative in lead aVR, the approximate mean frontal plane QRS axis is +60° (−30° plus +90° = +60°).

The isoelectric line often falls between two leads and must be estimated. (Set it closer to the more isoelectric lead.) More elaborate methods for determining the mean frontal plane QRS axis have been devised (e.g., algebraic sums of R and S waves from two leads plotted on a graph derived from the hexaxial reference system); however, the simpler method just described should be suitable for analyzing the cases in this book.

The mean frontal plane QRS axis is normally between −30° and +90° in adults over the age of 30, and between 0° and +110° in younger persons. An axis between −30° and −90° (or 0° and −90° in the young) constitutes left axis deviation; an axis between +90° and ± 180° (or +110° and ± 180° in the young) is right axis deviation. An axis between −90° and ± 180° is considered superior axis deviation.

The ST segment extends from the end of the QRS complex (the J point) to the beginning of the T wave. It represents the interval between ventricular depolarization and repolarization. The ST segment is classically isoelectric in the normal ECG, but has many normal variations.

The T wave is generated by ventricular repolarization. Since its mean frontal plane axis is usually similar to the QRS axis, it is expected to be upright in leads I, II, and V5-6. In leads III, aVL, and aVF, it may be upright or inverted depending on the heart's electrical position. In the anterior precordial leads, the T wave is normally upright in the adult, due to the anterior direction of its vector; however, an inverted T wave confined to lead V1 is frequently encountered in normal individuals. In children, the T wave vector is often directed posteriorly, and T wave inversion occurs normally across the right anterior precordium; this pattern may persist into adulthood.

The U wave is a small deflection sometimes occurring immediately after the T wave and often superimposed upon it. It is usually best seen in the precordial leads. The precise etiology is uncertain, but it may reflect late repolarization of Purkinje fibers or afterpotentials of ventricular depolarization. Its direction is generally the same as the T wave.

The QT interval (or QTU interval, where QT cannot be precisely discerned) is measured from the onset of the QRS complex to the end of the T (or U) wave. It reflects the time required for complete depolarization and repolarization of the ventricles. The QT interval varies with heart rate (see Table 12 in the Appendix) and must be compared with established values to ascertain normality. In general, its duration should be less than half of the RR interval (the distance between consecutive QRS complexes). Formulas have been derived to "correct" the QT interval for heart rate; the most frequently used is: $QT_c = QT/\sqrt{RR}$. The normal QT_c (corrected QT interval) is 0.40 second or less.

These are the major ECG features to keep in mind while following the analyses in this book. The cases included here have been chosen for their applicability to daily clinical practice. Perhaps the most important message of this book is: *Clinical correlation with observed ECG patterns is essential.*

SECTION II Ventricular and Atrial Hypertrophy

CASE 1

Left Ventricular Hypertrophy With ST-T Abnormalities

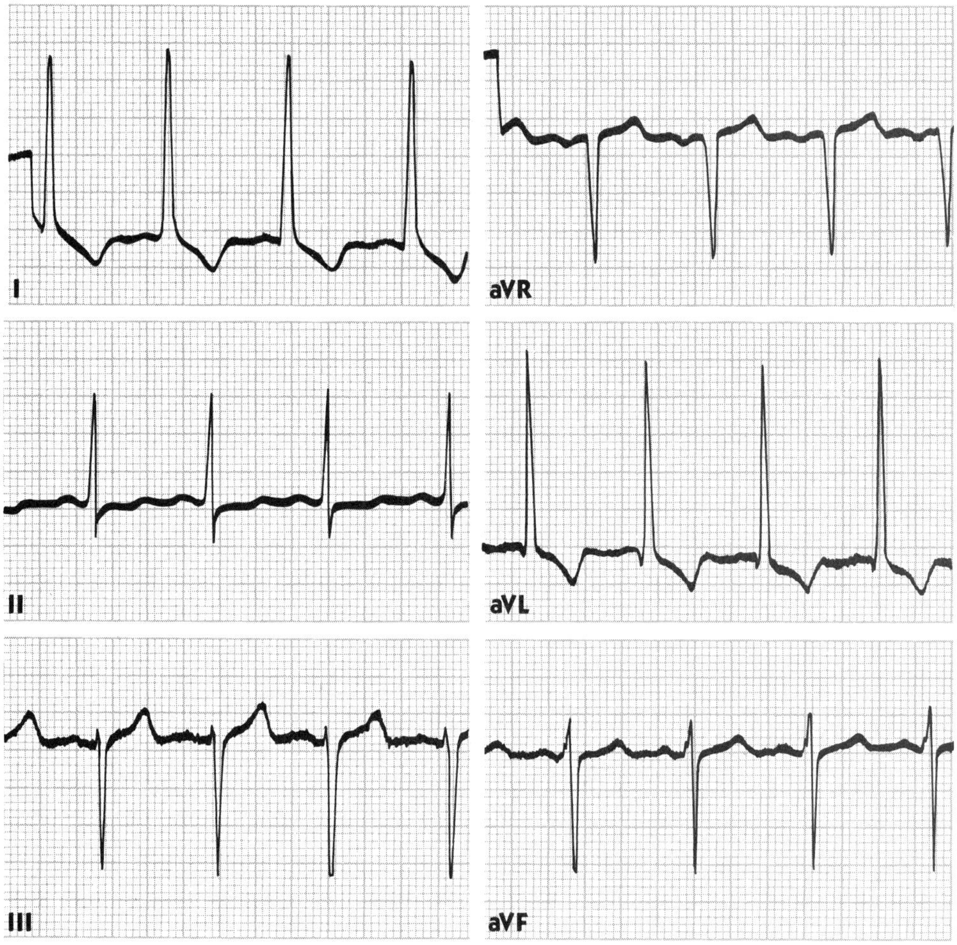

This ECG was recorded from a 74-year-old woman with long-standing untreated hypertension. The rhythm is sinus, and the PR and QRS intervals are normal. The QT interval is prolonged at 0.36 second ($QT_c = 0.45$). The mean frontal plane QRS axis is $-15°$.

There are tall R waves and T wave inversion in leads I, aVL, and V3-6. The R wave in lead aVL is 26 mm, and the sum of the S wave in lead V1 and the R wave in lead V5 is 46 mm. (SV1 or V2 + RV5 or V6 > 35 mm suggests left ventricular hypertrophy.) The intrinsicoid deflection (the interval from the onset of the QRS complex to the beginning of the downstroke of the R wave) is slightly prolonged (0.04 second) in left ventricular leads. This is a measure of the time required for the ventricular depolarization wave to travel from the endocardial surface through the myocardium to the epicardial surface.

This ECG has classic features of left ventricular hypertrophy (LVH), scoring 6 of 13 possible points (for amplitude and ST-T changes) under the point score system in Table 1 (see Appendix). As the left ventricle hypertrophies, its increased mass and size create increased depolarization forces directed leftward, laterally, and posteriorly. The increased thickness prolongs the time required for an electrical impulse to pass through the ventricle, thus increasing the QRS duration (although not in this case) and the intrinsicoid deflection. The prolonged QT interval, often seen in LVH, represents the delay in repolarization of the hypertrophied myocardium.

The T wave inversion in the lateral leads reflects hypertrophy-induced alterations in repolarization of the left ventricle. This pattern can also be produced by digitalis; thus its specificity for LVH is reduced in digitalized patients. In some cases, lateral nontrans-

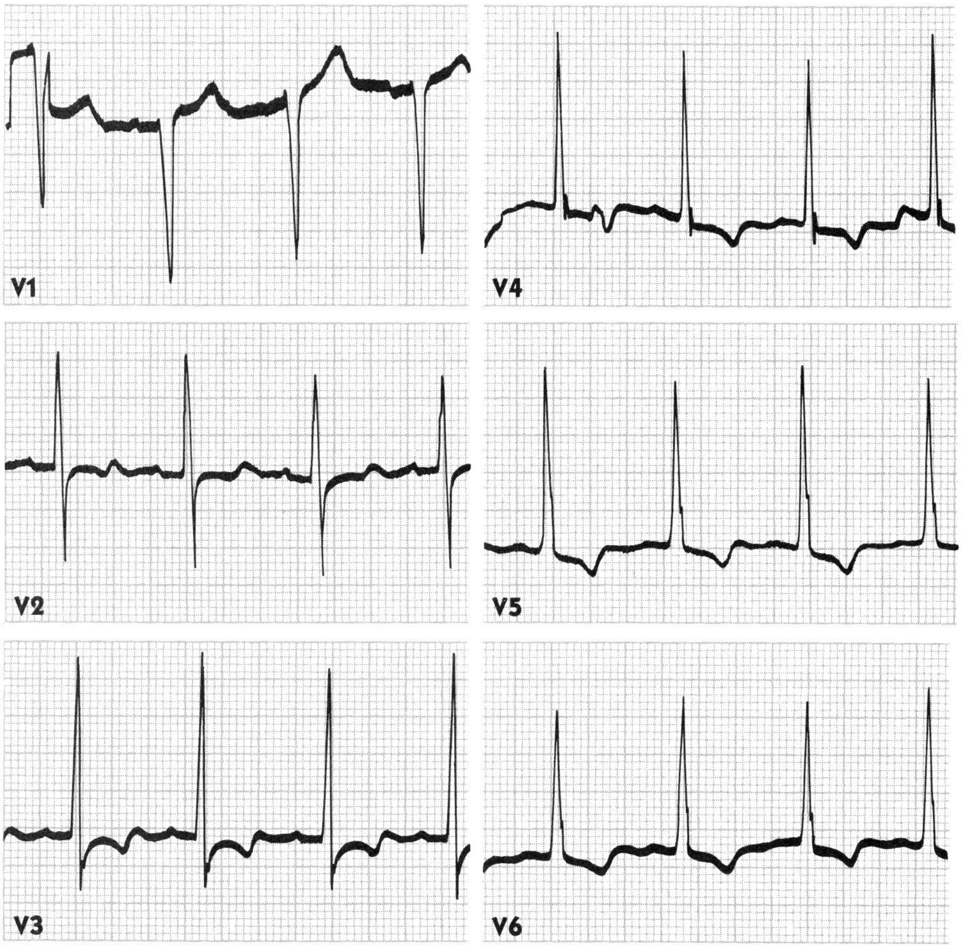

mural ischemia or myocardial infarction may be present in association with this pattern. However, these conditions cannot be diagnosed from a single ECG and must be excluded by clinical and enzymatic data.

CASE 2

Left Ventricular Hypertrophy Without ST-T Abnormalities

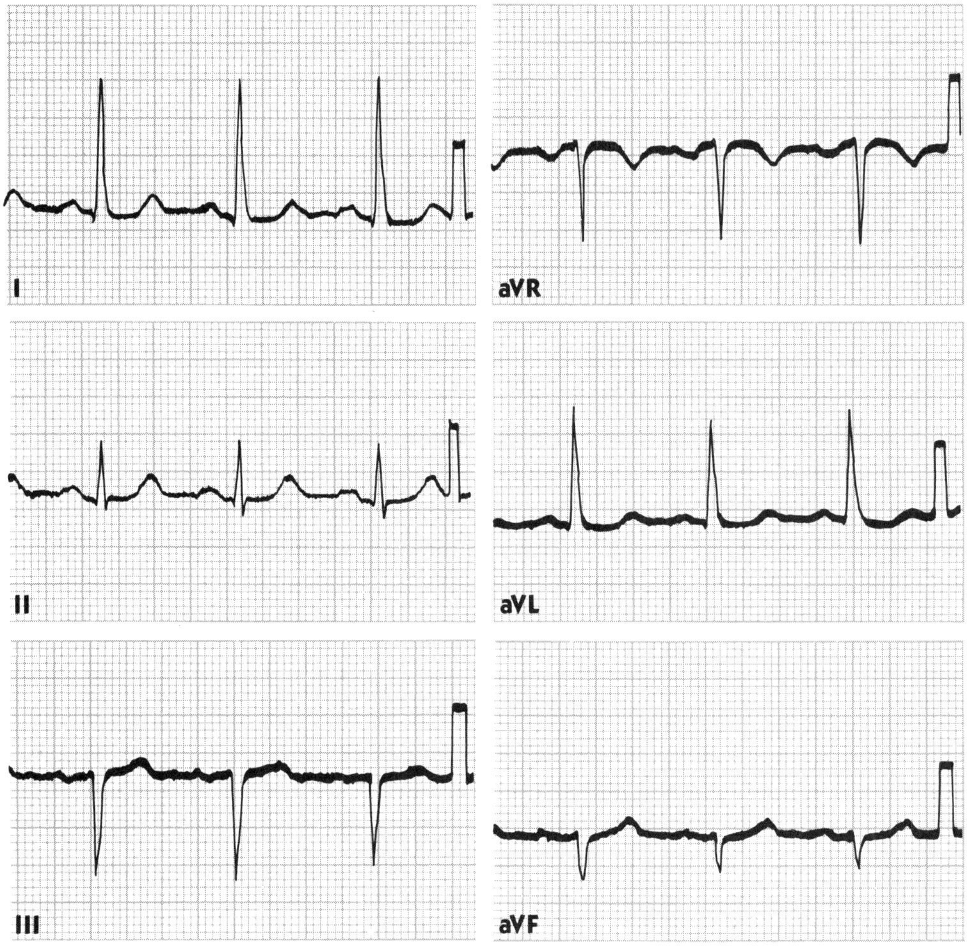

This 56-year-old man has asymmetric septal hypertrophy (ASH). His ECG reveals sinus rhythm, normal PR and QRS intervals, and a QT interval of 0.40 second, prolonged for the rate ($QT_c = 0.45$). The mean frontal plane QRS axis is $-15°$. The P wave duration in lead II is 0.14 second, and the intrinsicoid deflection in the lateral leads (I, aVL, V5-6) is 0.04 second. The R wave in lead aVL is 16 mm, and the S wave in lead V2 plus the R wave in lead V5 equals 45 mm. There is slight J point elevation in leads V1-3.

This patient has left ventricular hypertrophy (LVH), although there are no associated ST-T abnormalities (see Case 1). When precordial lead voltage criteria for LVH are present without the associated ST-T abnormalities, the ECG only *suggests* LVH. The diagnosis must then be confirmed by other means. However, an R wave in lead aVL exceeding 12 mm

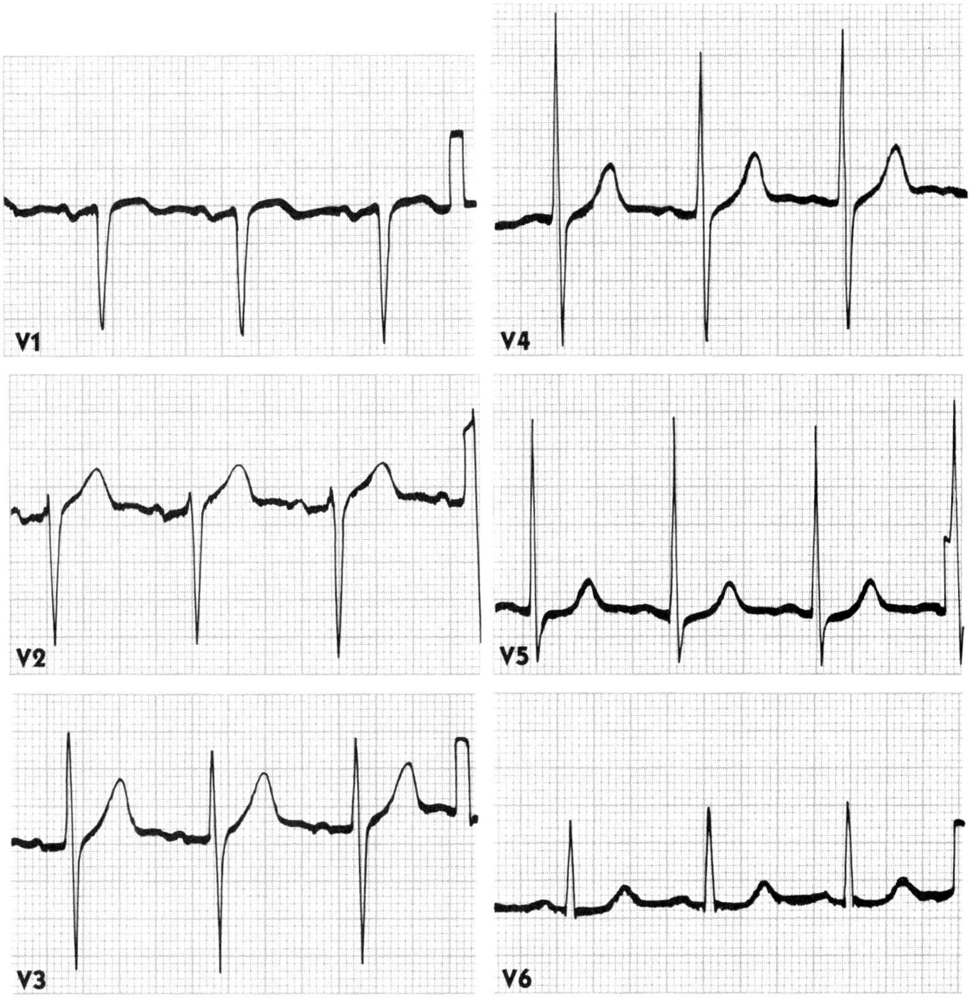

is virtually 100% specific (though only moderately sensitive) for this diagnosis.

Other indications of LVH in this case are: leftward axis deviation, slight prolongation of the intrinsicoid deflection, and broad, notched P waves in lead II suggestive of left atrial abnormality (see Case 9).

CASE 3

Left Ventricular Hypertrophy Mimicking Anterior Wall Myocardial Infarction

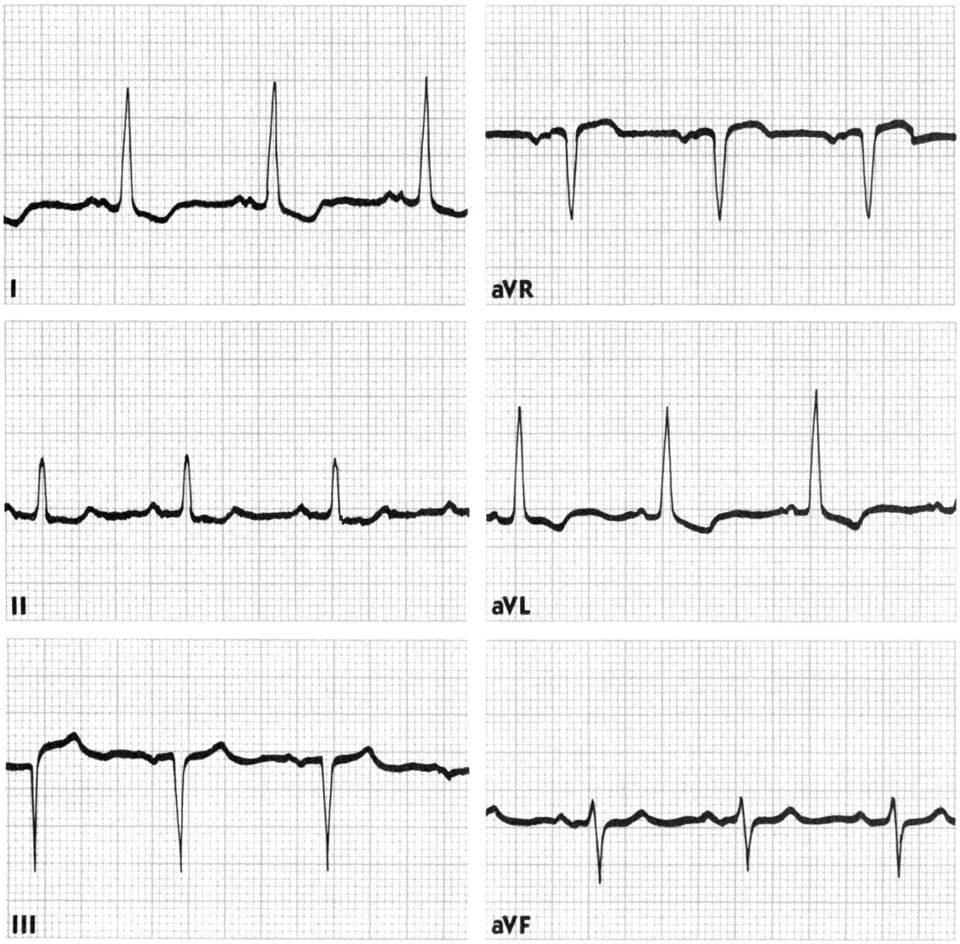

This 67-year-old man has long-standing hypertension and ischemic heart disease. His ECG shows sinus rhythm; normal PR, QRS, and QT intervals; and a mean frontal plane QRS axis of − 20°. The intrinsicoid deflection in lead V5 is 0.05 second. The P waves are broad and notched (seen best in leads I and aVL) in the pattern of left atrial abnormality (LAA). There are QS complexes in leads V1-3. The R wave measures 14 mm in lead aVL and 30 mm in lead V5. ST-T abnormalities are present in the lateral leads. Mild J point elevation can be seen in leads V1-3.

This patient clearly has left ventricular hypertrophy (LVH). His ECG meets the criteria for 11 of the 13 points listed in Table 1 (Appendix). In view of the patient's history of ischemic heart disease, the lack of R waves in the anterior leads raises the possibility of previous anterior wall myocardial infarction (MI). However, LVH per se can also produce this

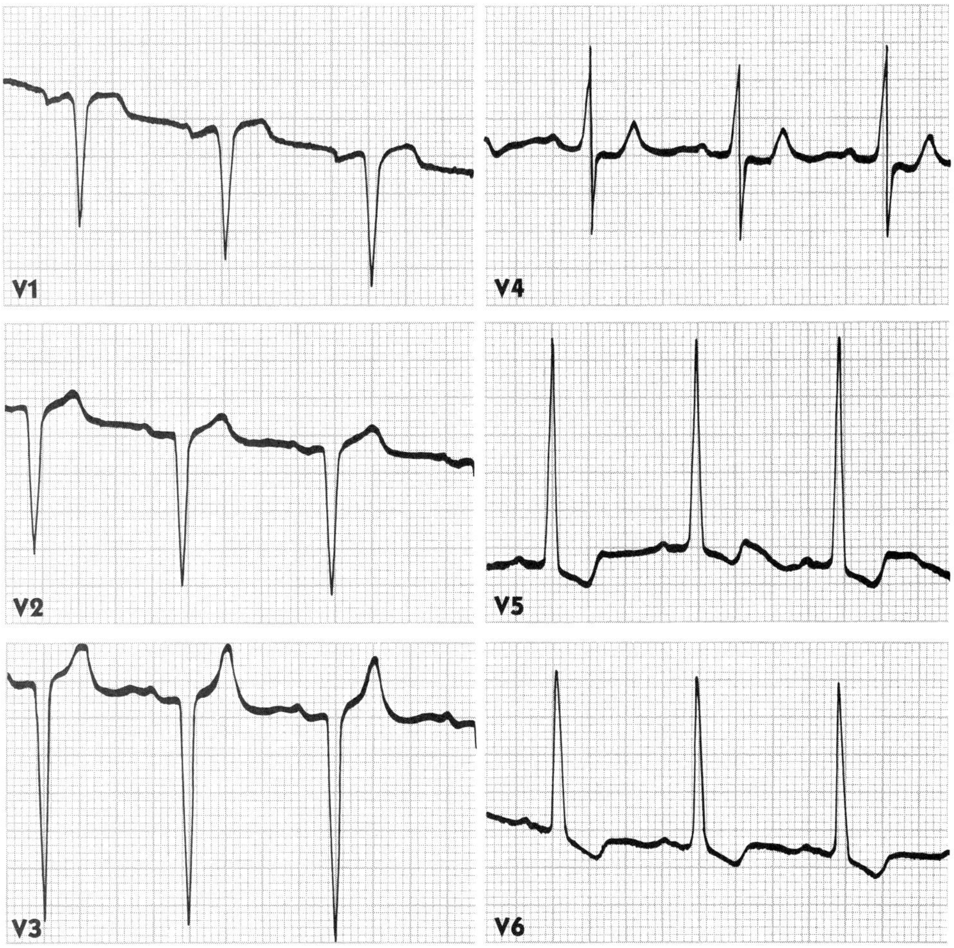

pattern. As the left ventricle hypertrophies, it rotates leftward and posteriorly (as does the mean frontal plane QRS vector). This causes a decrease in anterior forces, reflected by poor R wave progression or absent R waves in the anterior precordial leads. This can progress to the point where QS complexes indistinguishable from those in anterior wall MI are seen in the anterior leads.

A number of other conditions (in addition to LVH and anterior wall MI) can cause poor R wave progression or absent R waves anteriorly. They include chronic obstructive pulmonary disease, right ventricular hypertrophy, and left anterior fascicular block (see Table 2 in the Appendix). Poor R wave progression *alone,* without any accompanying ECG abnormalities, is a nonspecific finding that should not be considered abnormal.

CASE 4

Asymmetric Septal Hypertrophy Mimicking Inferoposterolateral Wall Myocardial Infarction

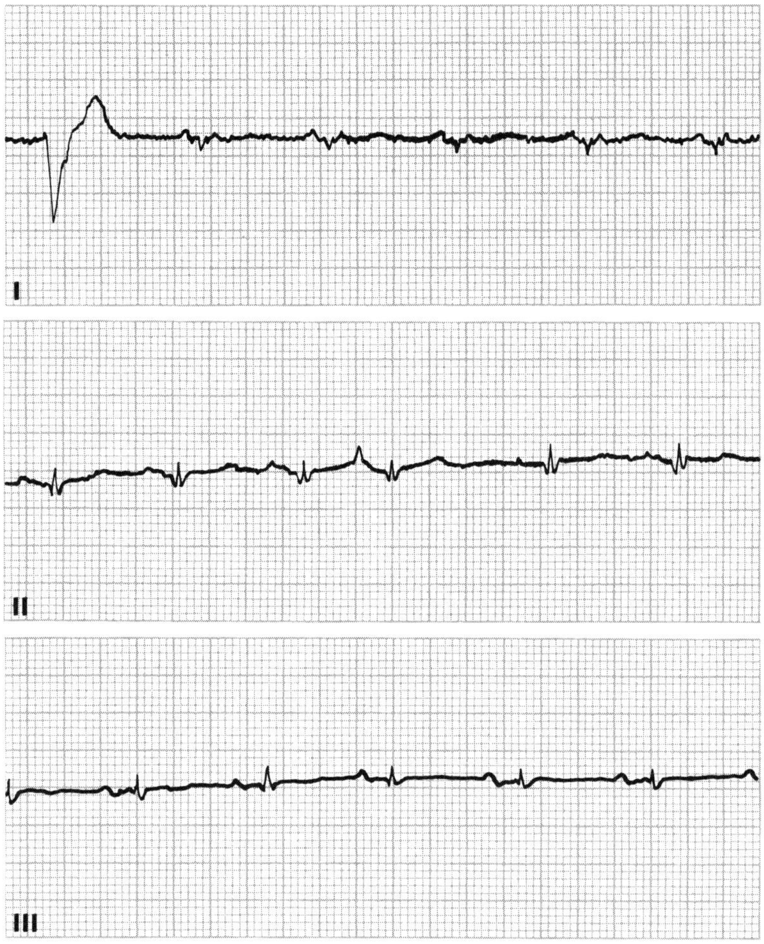

This 63-year-old man has asymmetric septal hypertrophy (ASH), documented by echocardiography. He was admitted for exacerbation of congestive heart failure. His ECG shows sinus rhythm with occasional premature ventricular complexes, normal PR and QRS intervals, and a QT interval that is slightly prolonged (0.38 second) for the rate. The mean frontal plane QRS axis is rightward at +110°. The P waves are normal.

Significant Q waves exceeding 25% of the height of the QRS complex can be seen in leads I, II, aVL, aVF, and V5-6. Tall initial R waves are followed by deep S waves in lead V1, with an R:S ratio approaching unity. The R waves progressively diminish across the precordium: qrS complexes appear in lead V4 and QrS complexes in leads V5-6.

The inferolateral Q waves are suggestive of inferolateral wall myocardial infarction (MI). However, ASH can generate similar Q waves laterally or, more commonly, inferiorly. The normal initial septal depolarization, directed anterosuperiorly and to the right, is accentuated in septal hypertrophy. This produces Q waves in the inferior and/or lateral leads and R waves anteriorly in leads V1-2 mimicking posterior wall MI (see Case 28). Even the mean QRS vector may be redirected superiorly and rightward, so

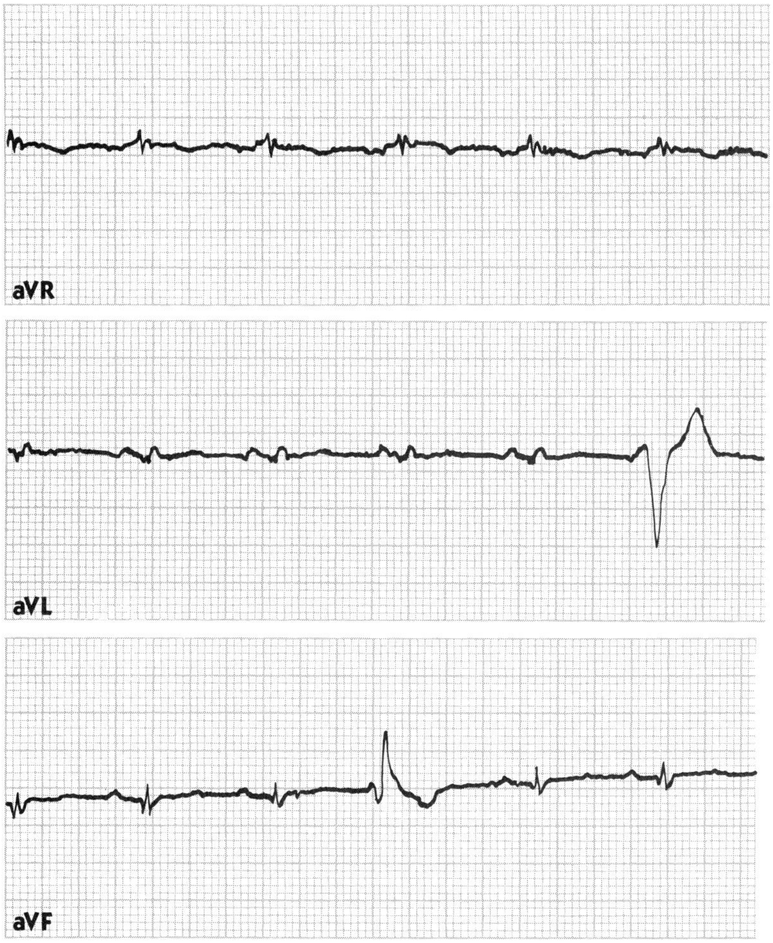

continued

that poor R wave development in the lateral limb and precordial leads and right axis deviation may be seen, as in this patient.

The most common ECG finding in cases of ASH is left ventricular hypertrophy (see Case 2). In these patients, the septal hypertrophy is counterbalanced by hypertrophy of the left ventricular free wall, so that prominent, but insignificant, Q waves (<25% of the R wave height and/or <0.04 second in duration) are inscribed in the lateral leads. Bundle branch block patterns and pre-excitation syndromes may also occur in ASH.

CASE 4 *(continued)*

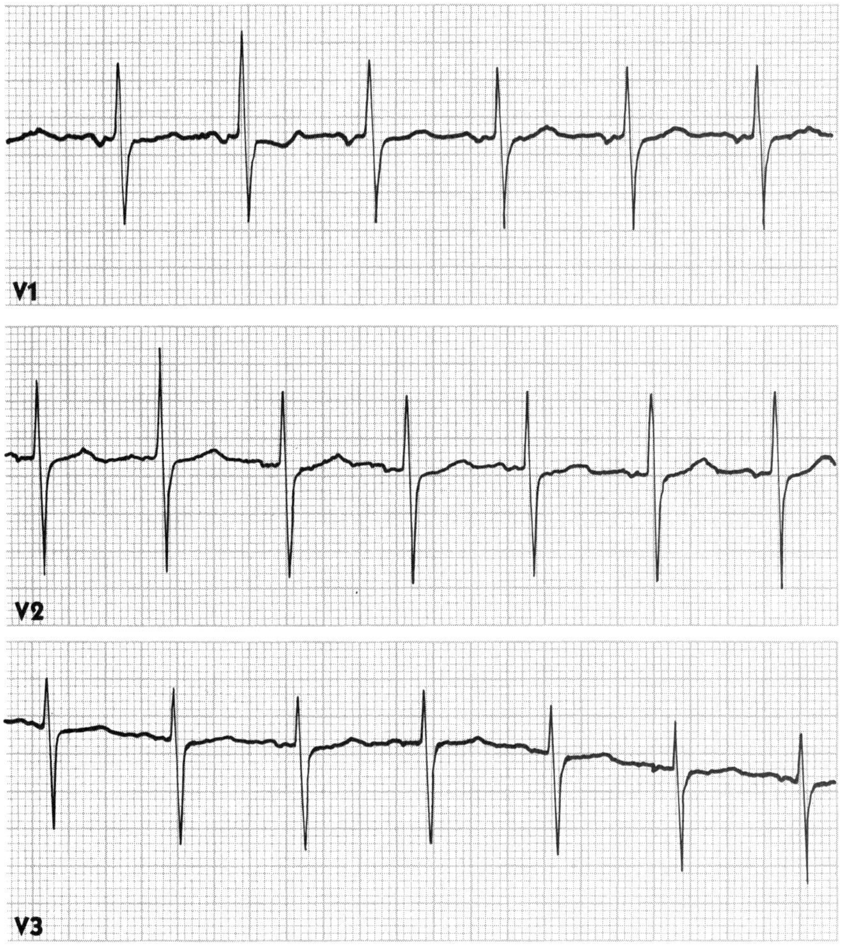

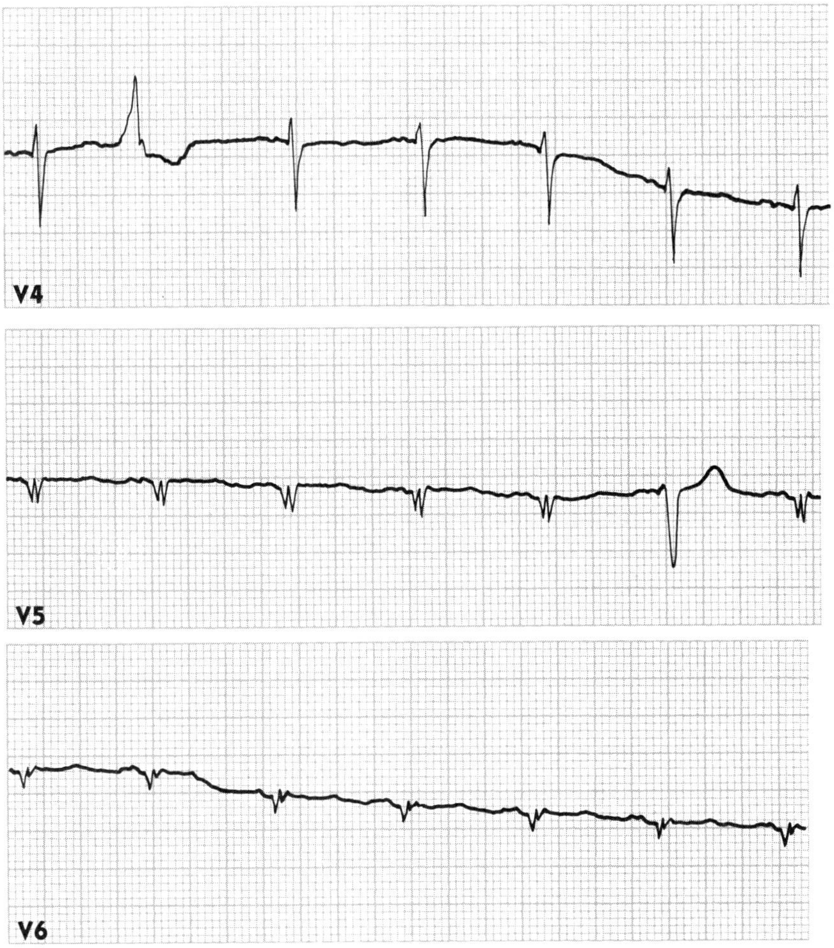
V4
V5
V6

CASE 5

Right Ventricular Hypertrophy

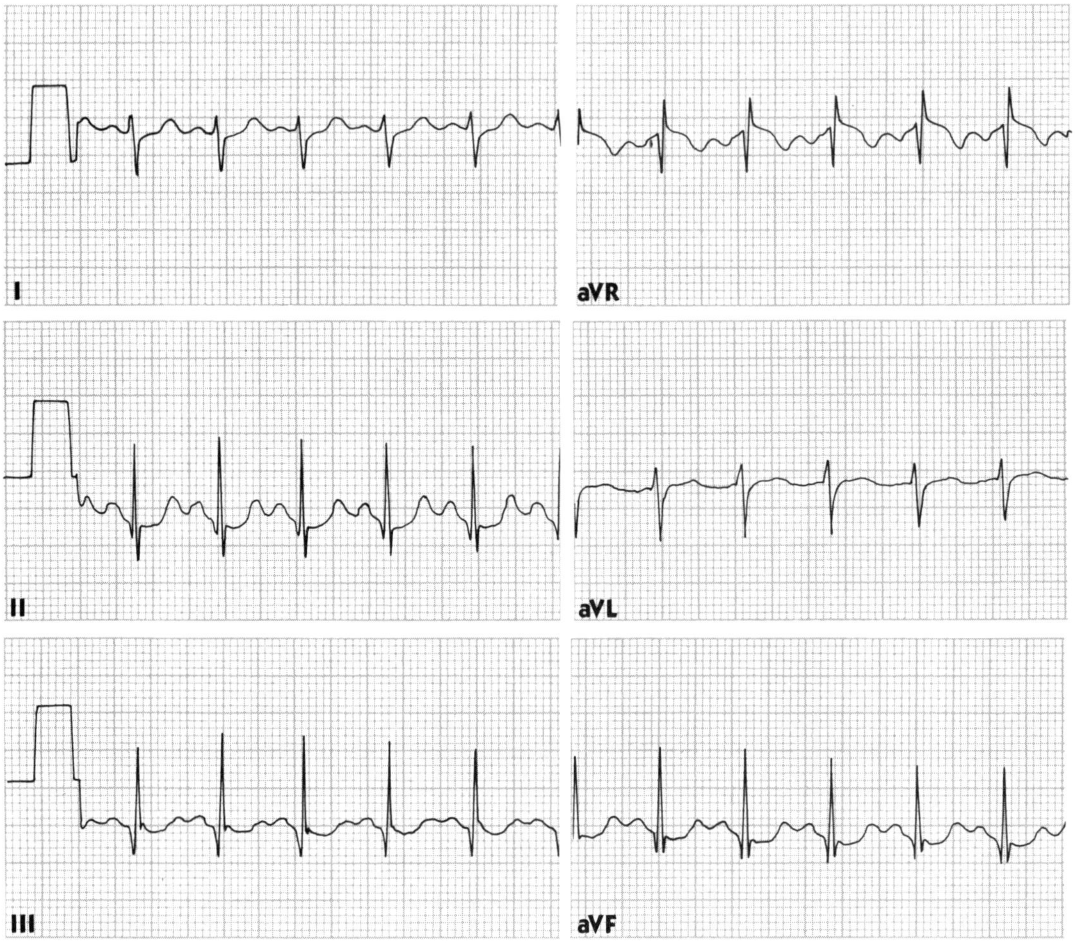

This ECG was recorded from a 23-year-old woman with systemic lupus erythematosus who presented with severe dyspnea and hypoxemia at rest. Her chest X-ray was normal. Cardiac catheterization revealed moderate pulmonary hypertension and normal coronary arteries.

The rhythm is sinus tachycardia. The PR and QRS intervals are normal, and the QT interval (0.32 second) is prolonged for the rate. The mean frontal plane QRS axis is directed rightward and is outside the normal limit (+110°) for the patient's age. The R:S ratio in lead V1 approaches 1.0, and S waves are present in the lateral leads. There are no ST-T abnormalities. Prominent q waves unassociated with ST-T abnormalities are present in leads II, III, and aVF.

This ECG represents right ventricular hypertrophy (RVH). The right ventricle is positioned anteriorly, directly beneath the sternum. As the mass and/or size of the right ventricle increase, the ECG displays increasing forces of depolarization anteriorly (in leads V1-2) and rightward, resulting in rightward deviation of the mean frontal plane QRS axis. Rightward axis deviation is requisite to the ECG diagnosis of RVH, though the axis need not be outside the limits of normal. A documented rightward axis *shift* is often sufficient to suggest RVH.

Since the normal QRS contour in lead V1 is rS (reflecting the predominating lateral and posterior forces of the left ventricle), an R:S ratio of 1.0 or more in V1 suggests RVH. A pure R or qR wave in lead V1, as well as notching of the ascent of the R wave, is also characteristic of RVH. (See Table 3 in the Appendix.) The large anterior forces in RVH, recorded as positive deflections (R waves) in the anterior leads, are recorded as negative deflections (S waves) in the left lateral leads (I, aVL, V4-6). In analo-

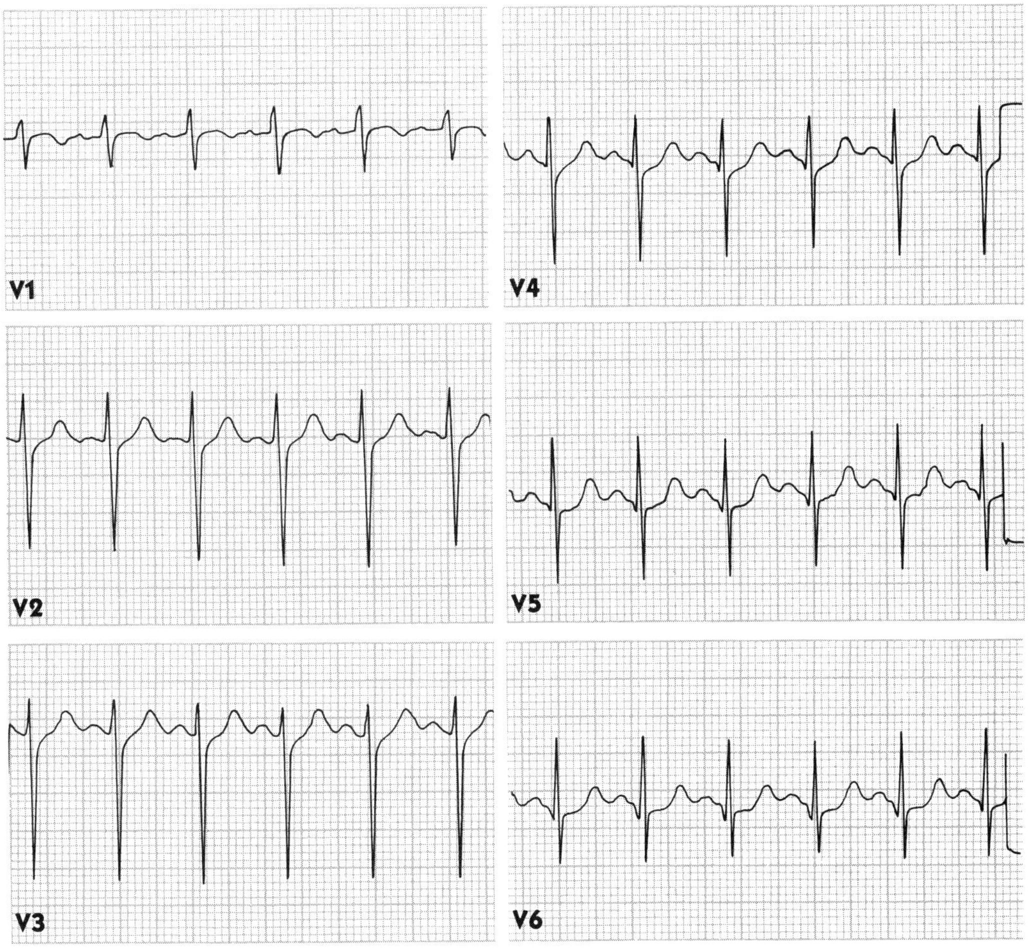

gous manner to the ST-T changes in LVH, altered repolarization in RVH is reflected in anterior and/or inferior T wave inversions.

The possibility of posterior wall myocardial infarction (MI) must be considered if a prominent R wave and associated ST-T abnormalities are present in lead V1 (see Case 28 and Table 4 in the Appendix). Inferoposterolateral wall MI might be suggested by prominent inferior Q waves, anterior R waves, and lateral S waves. Either diagnosis requires confirmation by independent clinical means.

The key factors in the ECG diagnosis of RVH in this patient are the right axis deviation and the increased amplitude of the R wave and abnormal R:S ratio in lead V1. The prominent q waves in leads II, III, and aVF may result from accentuation of the superiorly directed septal vector (see Case 4). As normal coronary arteries and left ventriculogram were documented angiographically, this ECG represents an example of a pseudoinfarction pattern (see Table 7).

Finally, the right axis deviation and qR complexes in leads II, III, and aVF could suggest left posterior fascicular block (LPFB). However, LPFB (see Case 19) usually occurs concomitantly with right bundle branch block and is not expected in this clinical entity.

CASE 6

Right Ventricular Hypertrophy and Right Atrial Abnormality

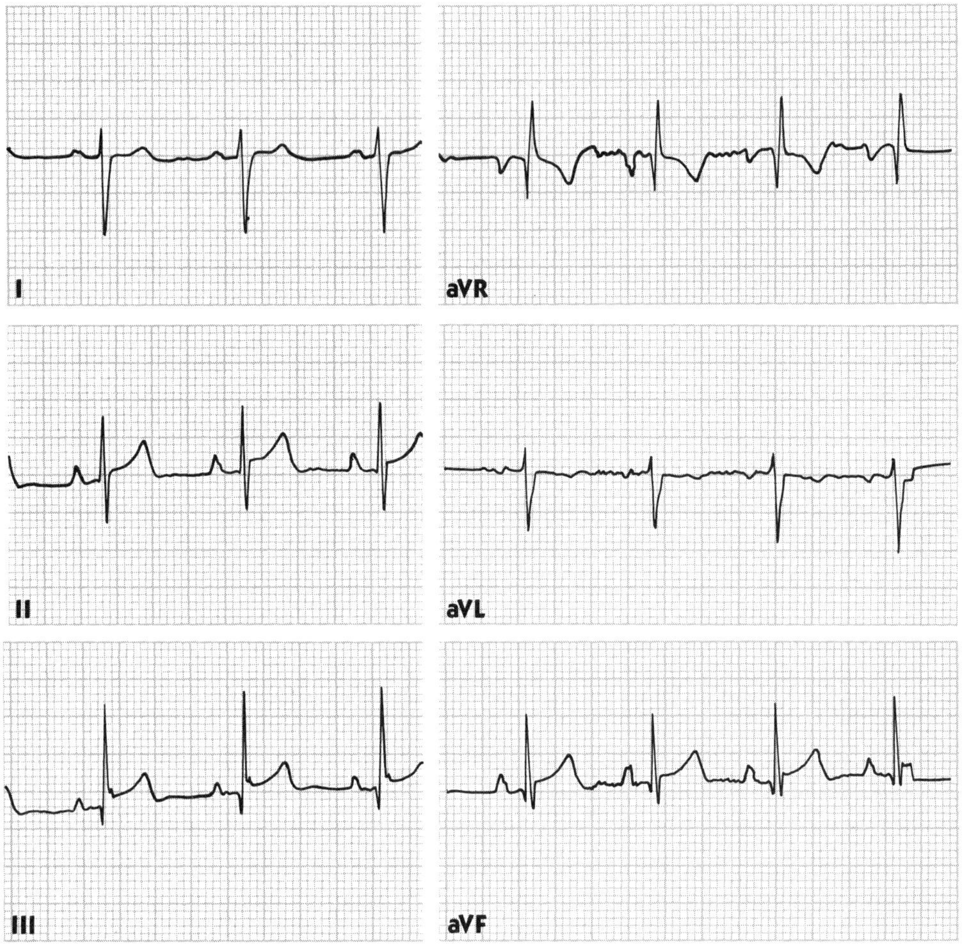

This 20-year-old man has congenital myopathy resembling muscular dystrophy and a long history of respiratory failure due to his muscle disorder. The cardiac rhythm is sinus, and the intervals are normal. The mean frontal plane QRS axis is deviated markedly to the right at +135°. In lead II, the P wave is peaked and about 2.8 mm in height. In lead V1, the P wave has an initial positive deflection and then a deep negative deflection; it is peaked and upright in leads V2-4. There is a QR pattern in leads aVR and V1, and there are deep S waves in the lateral precordial leads (I, aVL, V5-6). Q waves are present in leads II, III, aVR, aVF, and V1. The T waves are deeply inverted in the anterior precordial leads, and there is J point and ST segment elevation in leads II, III, aVF, and V5-6.

This ECG illustrates some of the abnormalities of right ventricular hypertrophy (RVH) and concomitant right atrial abnormality (RAA). In contrast to Case 5, in which an R:S ratio in lead V1 can be calculated, a QR pattern is present here in addition to marked right axis deviation (a finding strongly suggestive of RVH). The QR pattern in V1 most likely reflects initial posteriorly directed septal activation followed by the accentuated anterior forces of right ventricular depolarization. The tall, peaked P waves in lead II are diagnostic of RAA (the so-called "P pulmonale" pattern). The peaked but inverted P waves in lead V1 might suggest left atrial enlargement or hypertrophy (see Case 9), but this pattern is observed in profound right atrial enlargement and hypertrophy as well; the peaked, upright P waves in leads V2-3 and the normal P wave duration confirm that right, rather than left, atrial abnormality is present. These patterns result from progressive displacement—anteriorly and to the left—of forces

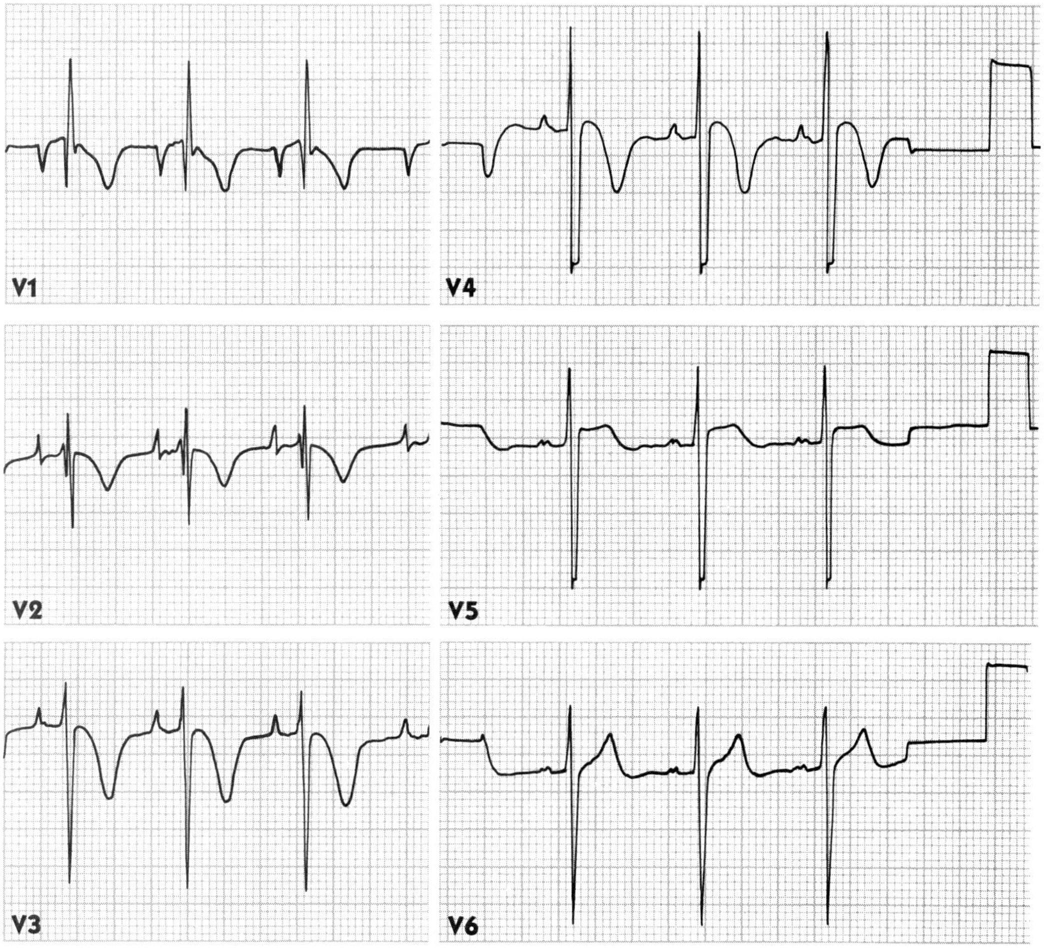

generated by the enlarged right atrium, which are directed toward the middle precordium and away from the right precordium.

The Q waves in the inferior leads are not significantly deep (≥25% of the R wave height) and/or wide (≥0.04 second), but the J point and ST segment elevations in the inferolateral leads might suggest myocardial injury. This possibility requires confirmation by other means. Similarly, the deep T wave inversions in the anterior leads, which probably reflect altered repolarization due to RVH, might suggest anterior wall ischemia. This diagnosis also requires independent confirmation.

CASE 7

Right Atrial Abnormality

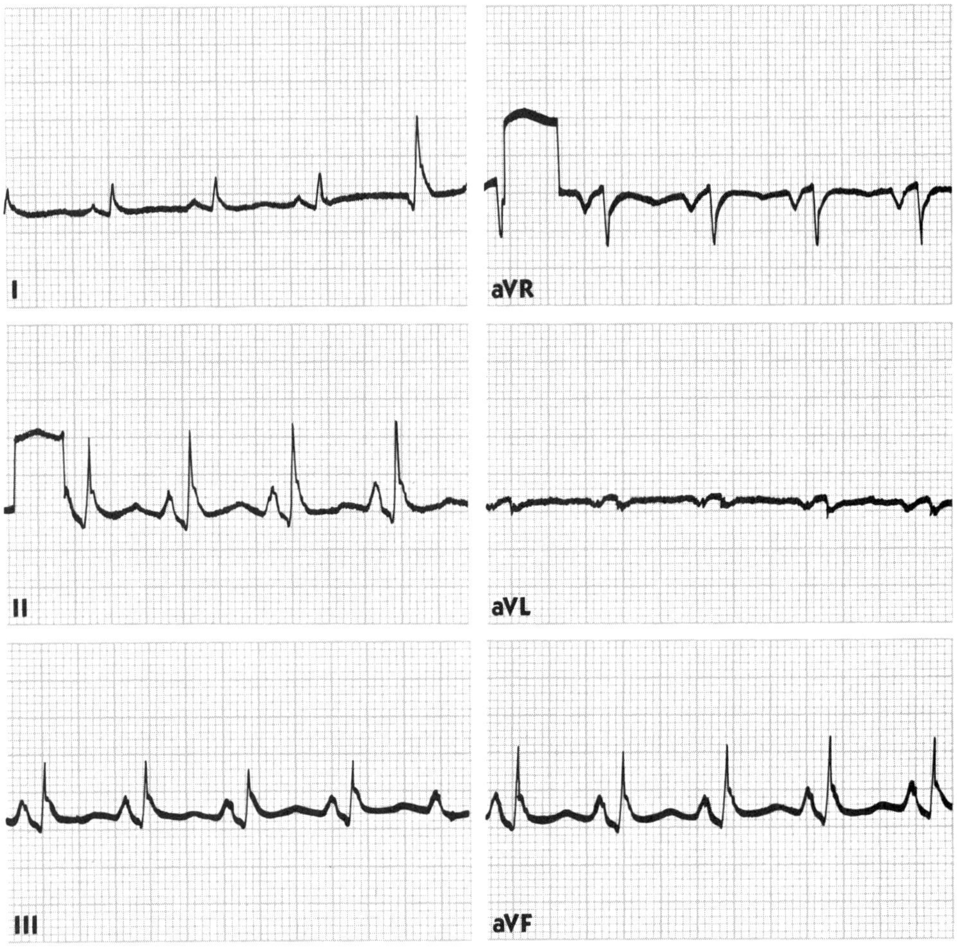

This ECG was recorded from a 73-year-old woman with a long history of cigarette smoking, asthma, and chronic obstructive pulmonary disease (COPD), who was admitted for exacerbation of asthma.

Her ECG reveals mild sinus tachycardia, a mean frontal plane QRS axis of $+60°$ (somewhat rightward for this age group), and moderate prolongation of the QT interval to about 0.40 second due to quinidine therapy for supraventricular arrhythmias. The P wave is 4 mm in height and notably peaked in lead II; it is also peaked and upright in lead V1. The PR segment (the portion of the tracing between the end of the P wave and the onset of the QRS complex, appearing during atrial repolarization) is depressed. This is especially noticeable in the inferior leads. The QRS complexes, ST segments, and T waves are of normal morphology.

These ECG findings indicate right atrial abnormality (RAA), most likely hypertrophy in view of the

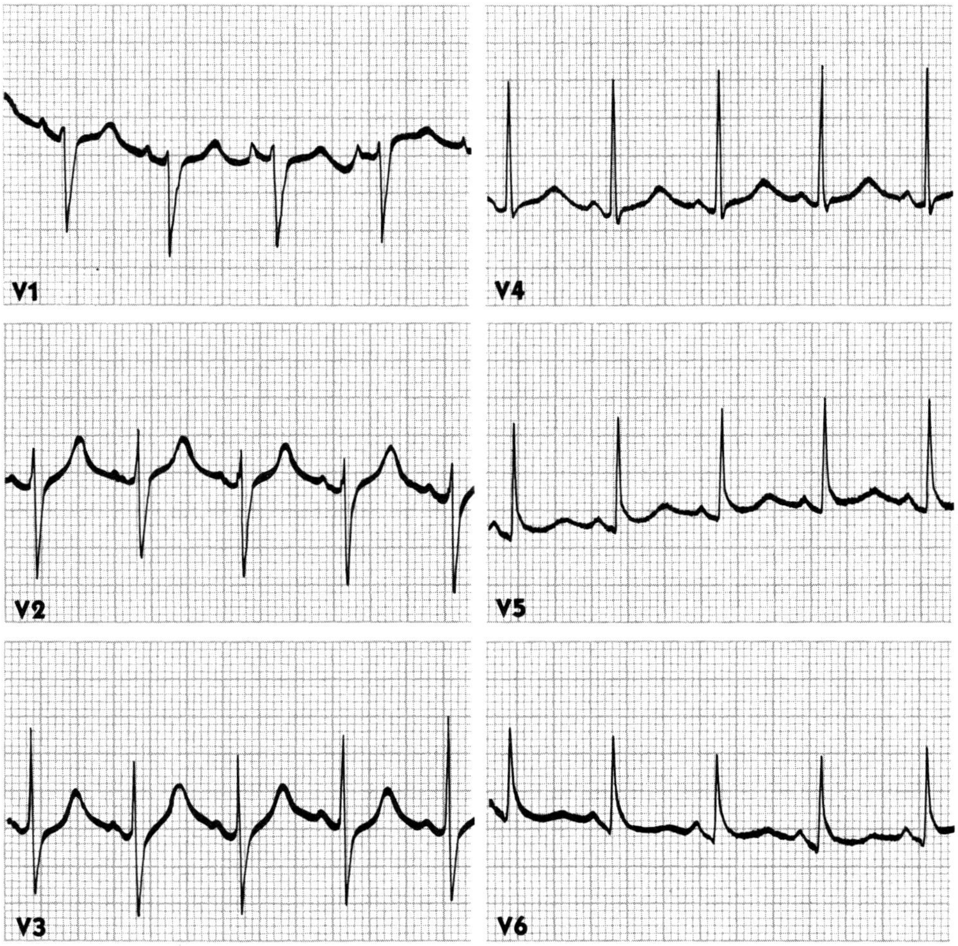

patient's history. But there is no ECG evidence of right ventricular hypertrophy. The ECG pattern of RAA may be seen in any disorder that results in increased right-sided pressure and/or volume. It is most frequently seen in COPD. Depression of the PR segment, frequently seen in RAA, reflects accentuated atrial repolarization forces. PR segment depression may also be seen in atrial infarction and pericarditis, but without the associated abnormalities of P wave contour. Marked depression of the PR segment can mimic Q waves in the leads in which it is best seen and can lead to the erroneous diagnosis of myocardial infarction.

CASE 8

Biventricular Hypertrophy

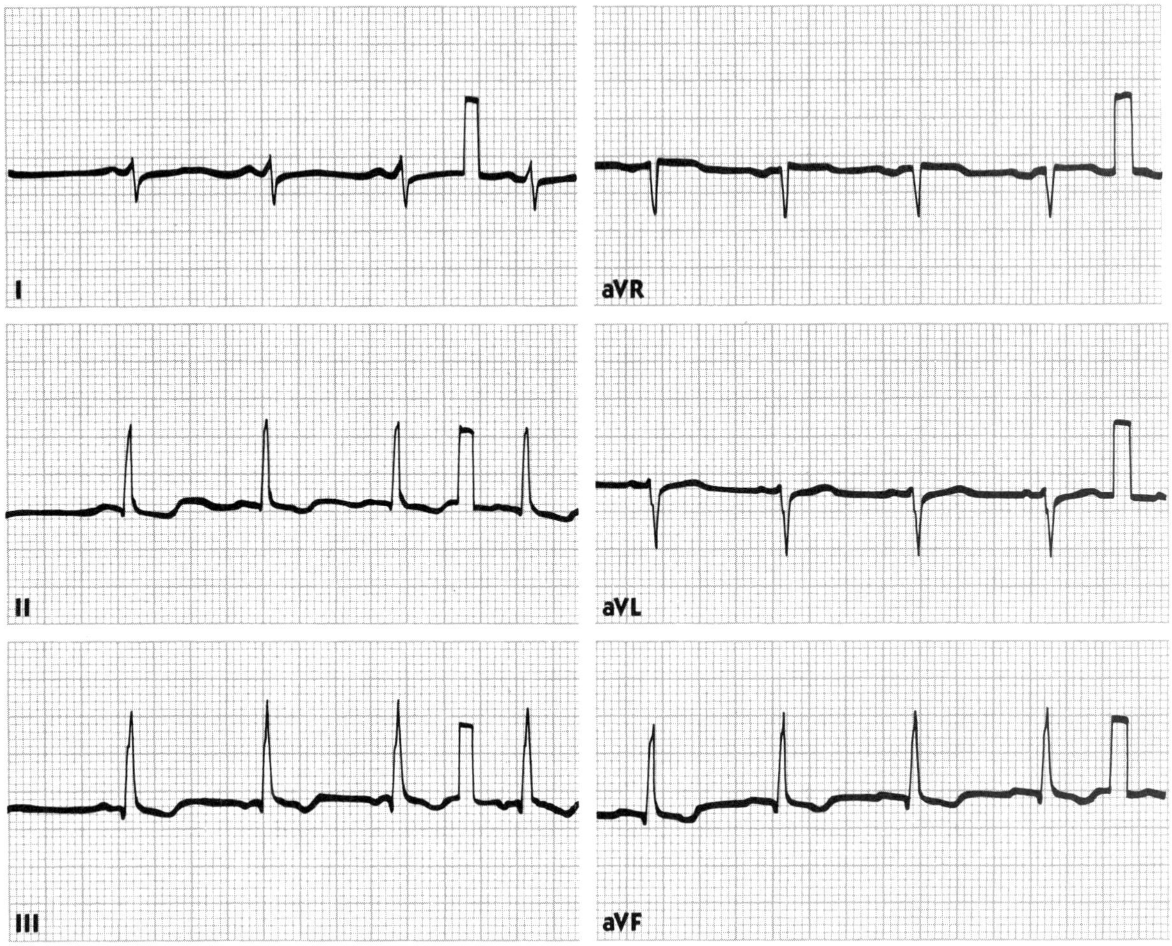

This ECG was recorded from a 66-year-old woman admitted for congestive heart failure and chest pain. It shows sinus rhythm with frequent premature atrial complexes and normal intervals. There is rightward deviation of the mean frontal plane QRS axis to +110°. The P wave in lead V1 has a prominent terminal negative deflection. There is an rS pattern in lead I and a qR pattern in leads II, III, and aVF. In the precordial leads, deep S waves appear anteriorly and tall R waves laterally; the S wave in V2 plus the R wave in V5 equals 51 mm. The T waves are inverted in the inferolateral leads.

At first inspection it would appear that this ECG shows left ventricular hypertrophy (LVH) alone. Voltage criteria are met, and the typical associated ST-T abnormalities are present in the lateral leads. Left atrial abnormality consistent with hypertrophy is also suggested. But in LVH, left axis deviation is expected, and this ECG shows abnormal deviation to the right.

There are two possible explanations for the right axis deviation. First, right ventricular hypertrophy may be present in addition to the LVH. Because the mass of the left ventricle so outweighs that of the right and because the forces of the left ventricle are directed leftward and posteriorly, the prominent anterior forces (R waves) expected in RVH are partially or completely nullified when LVH is present. In such cases, the precordial leads show the typical features of LVH (see Cases 1-3), while the mean QRS vector often remains rightward. The diagnosis of biventricular hypertrophy is suggested

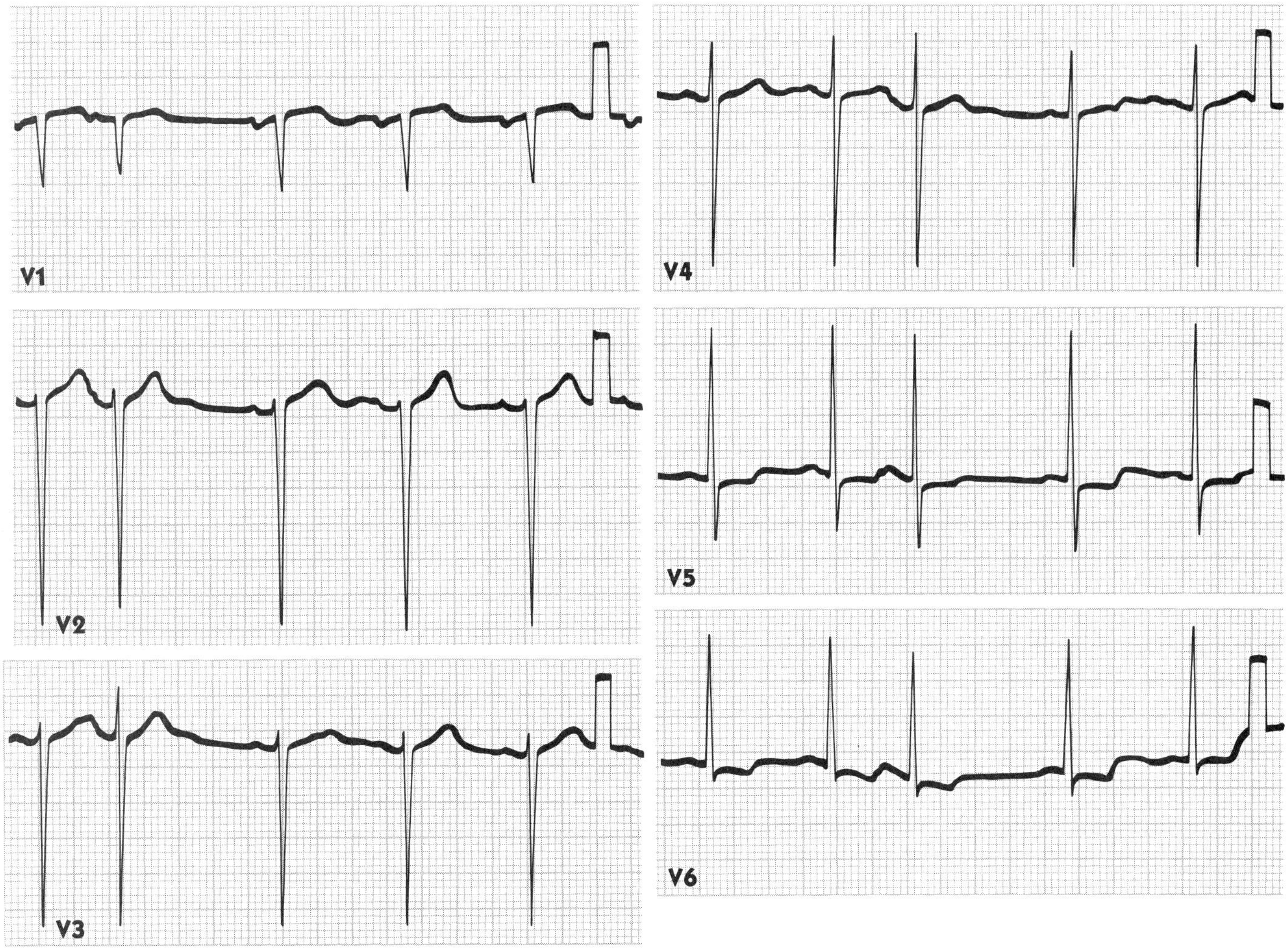

when the precordial leads have an LVH pattern (with or without prominent anterior forces) but the mean frontal plane QRS axis is directed rightward.

The other possible explanation for the right axis deviation is left posterior fascicular block (LPFB). In LPFB (see Case 19), rS complexes are seen in leads I and aVL and qR complexes in leads II, III, and aVF, as in this case. However, isolated LPFB is uncommon. Concomitant right bundle branch block is usually present.

The ST-T abnormalities in the inferolateral leads are nonspecific and could represent ischemia, nontransmural myocardial infarction, or ventricular hypertrophy. The correct diagnosis requires independent confirmation.

CASE 9

Left Atrial Abnormality and Right Axis Deviation

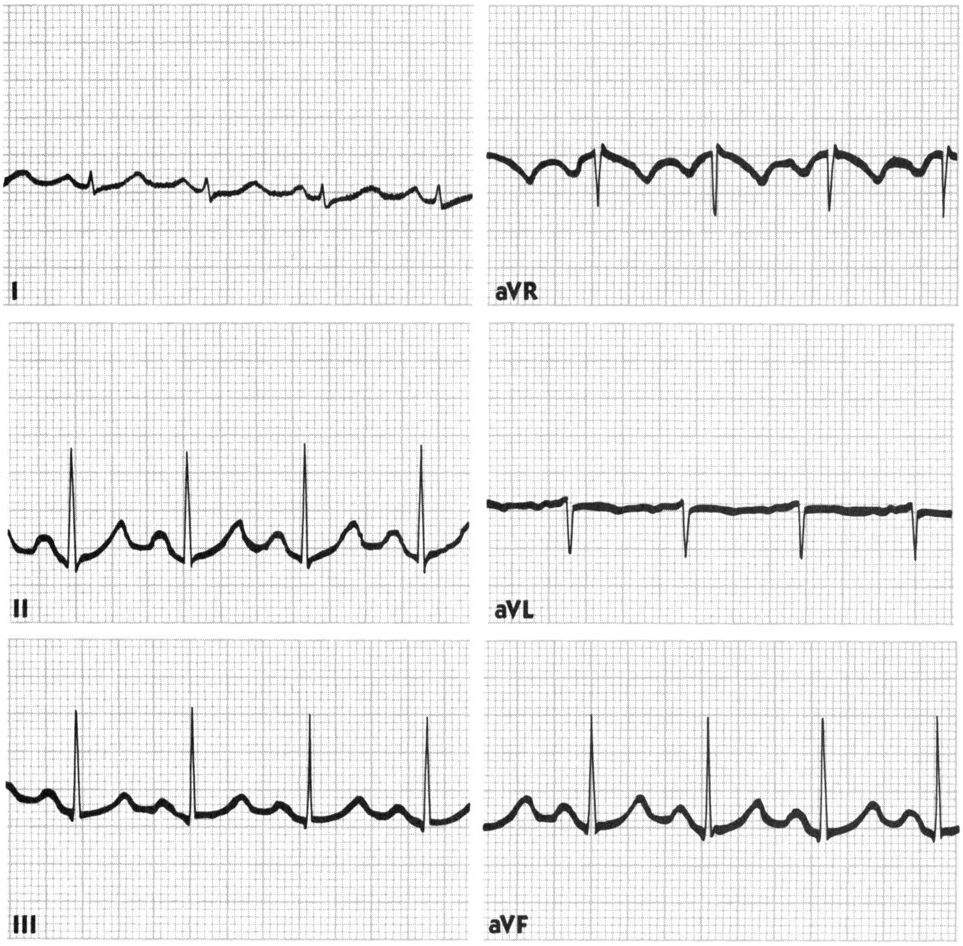

This ECG was recorded from a 30-year-old woman with rheumatic mitral stenosis. It shows sinus rhythm, normal intervals, and a mean frontal plane QRS axis of about +90°. In lead II the P wave is 0.12 second wide, and in lead V1 it has a terminal negative component exceeding 1 mm^2, consistent with left atrial abnormality (LAA). The PR segment is depressed. There are notched R waves in lead V1 and tall R waves in leads V2-3, but no prolongation of the QRS duration to suggest right intraventricular conduction delay. The differential diagnosis of notched R waves in V1 includes posterior wall myocardial infarction (clinically unlikely in this case) and Wolff-Parkinson-White conduction (criteria not met in this ECG).

This patient has LAA, and the right axis deviation (RAD) and notched R waves in lead V1 suggest

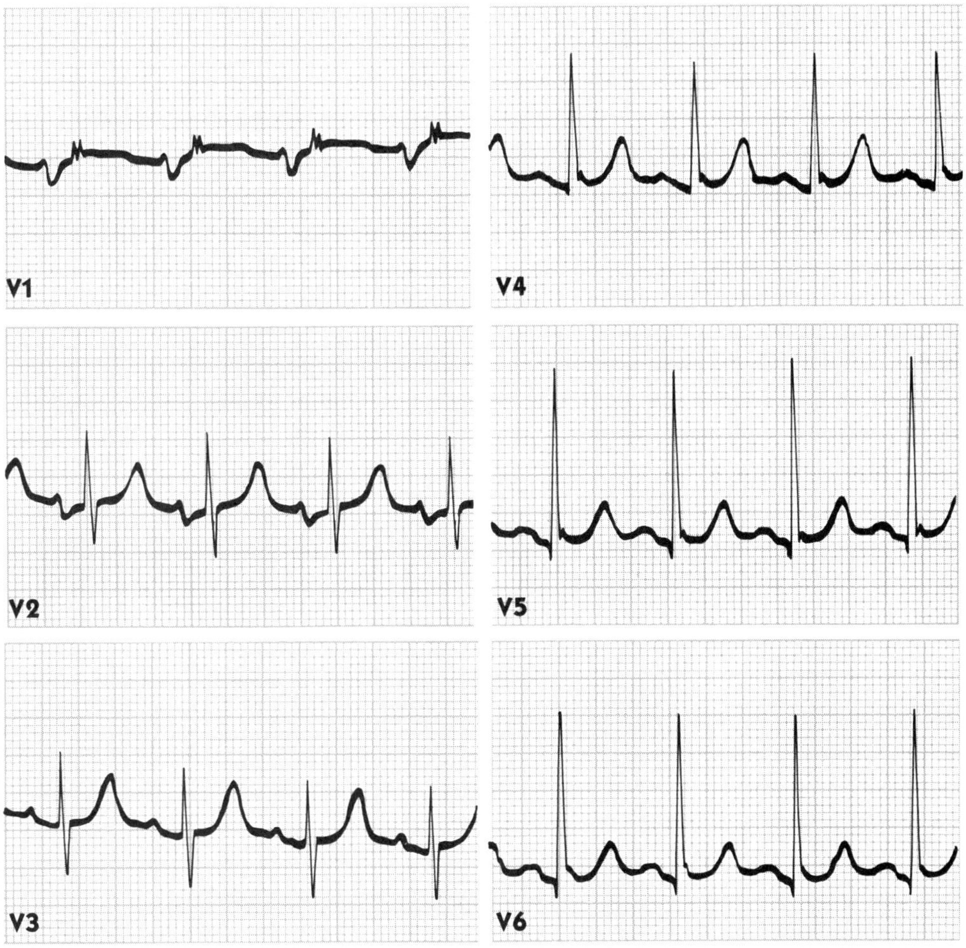

right ventricular hypertrophy (RVH). In the presence of rheumatic heart disease, this combination strongly suggests mitral stenosis with left atrial enlargement and/or hypertrophy and pulmonary hypertension.

The ECG pattern of LAA (so-called "P mitrale") consists of a prolonged P wave of 0.12 second or more, generally notched in lead I or II, inverted terminally in lead V1, and often having a leftward axis. The terminal negative deflection in the anterior precordial leads is due to posteriorly directed forces generated by the enlarged left atrium. RVH, manifested as RAD with prominent R waves or abnormal R:S ratio in the anterior precordial leads, occurs as pulmonary hypertension develops. If a patient has atrial fibrillation with RAD, mitral stenosis should also be suspected, particularly in a female patient under 45 years of age.

CASE 10

Pseudo-P Pulmonale

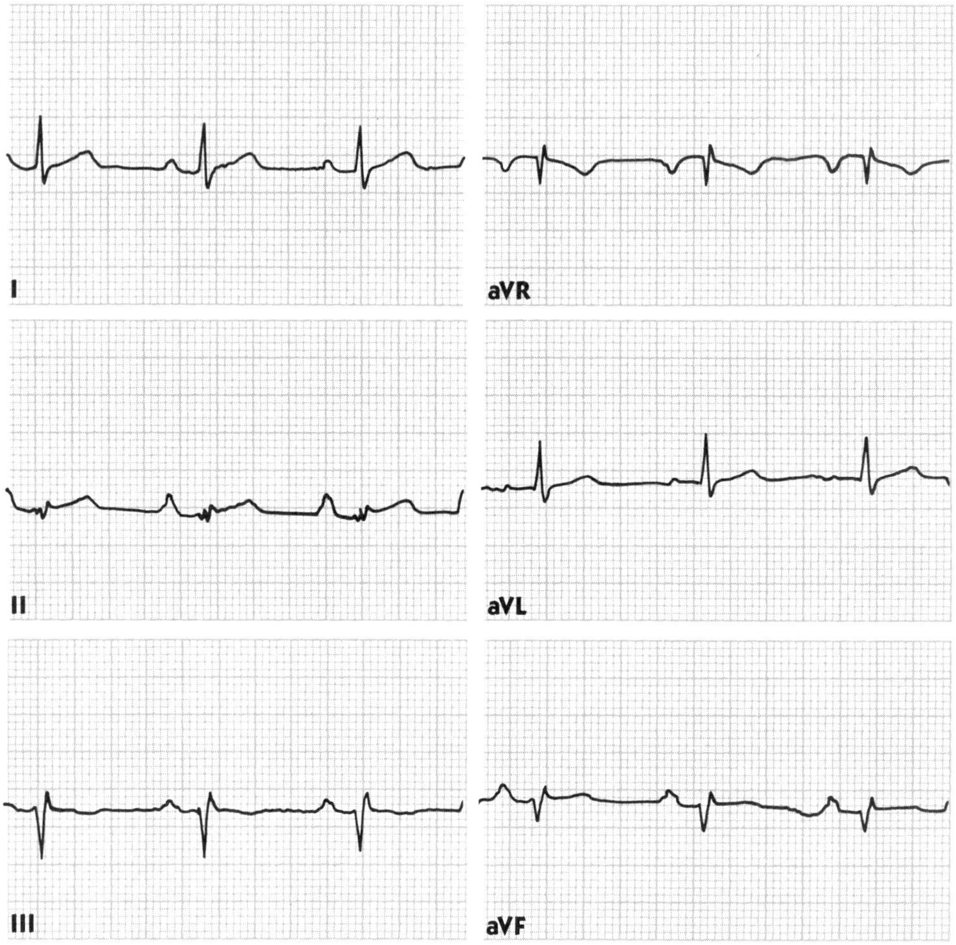

This ECG, recorded from a 72-year-old man with recent anterior wall myocardial infarction (MI), shows a mean frontal plane QRS axis of about −30°, a borderline long PR interval, and normal QRS and QT intervals. The anterior wall MI is reflected in the QS complexes in leads V2-3 and the ST segment elevation and T wave abnormalities in leads V2-5 (see Case 24).

The P waves have a normal duration but are quite tall in the inferior leads, reaching 2.5 mm in lead II. In lead V1, they have a broad, deep terminal deflection. Thus, the limb leads suggest right atrial abnormality (RAA), whereas lead V1 suggests left atrial abnormality (LAA). Careful scrutiny of the P wave configuration in the inferior leads reveals that its ascending slope is slower than its descending slope. Since right atrial depolarization is responsible for the initial portion of the P wave and left atrial depolarization for the latter portion, it is left atrial depolarization that is causing the pronounced P wave amplitude. This pattern, in which LAA mimics RAA, is termed "pseudo-P pulmonale." The pattern results from the large posteriorly and inferiorly directed forces generated by the hypertrophied and/or dilated left atrium.

Pseudo-P pulmonale is associated with left ventricular disease, including left ventricular hypertrophy and infarction, and with mitral valve disease. It reflects increased left atrial pressure. Isolated right atrial hypertrophy patterns do occur (see Case 7), but the absence of ECG evidence of right ventricular hypertrophy (see Table 3 in the Appendix) should raise the suspicion of pseudo-P pulmonale. The pattern in lead V1 is confirmatory of the correct atrial chamber enlargement.

Pseudo-P pulmonale must be distinguished from biatrial enlargement, in which criteria for both RAA and LAA are met. In biatrial enlargement the ini-

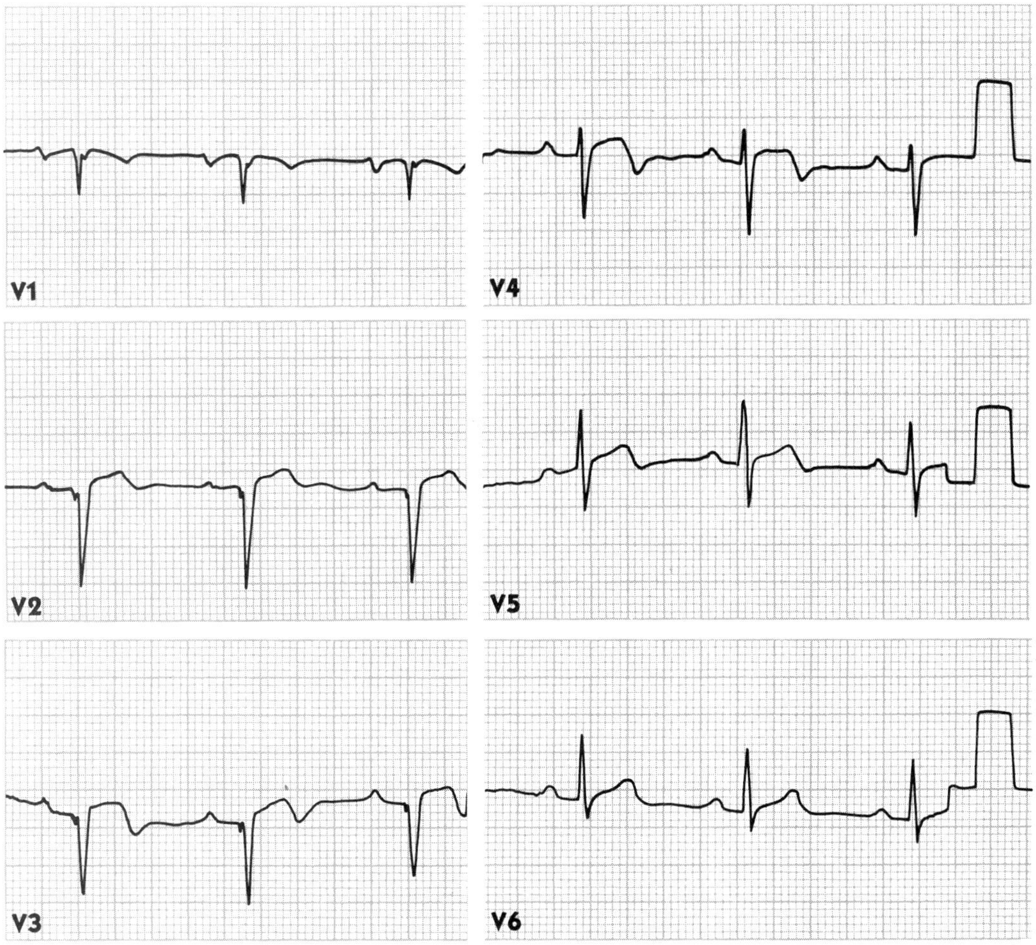

tial portion of the P wave (representing forces generated by the right atrium) is peaked and tall (≥ 2.5 mm in lead II), whereas in pseudo-P pulmonale the terminal portion is tall in lead II (as in this case). The presence in lead V1 of more than 1.5 mm of positive initial P wave deflection, together with criteria for LAA, also suggests biatrial enlargement.

SECTION III

Bundle Branch Blocks

CASE 11

Right Bundle Branch Block

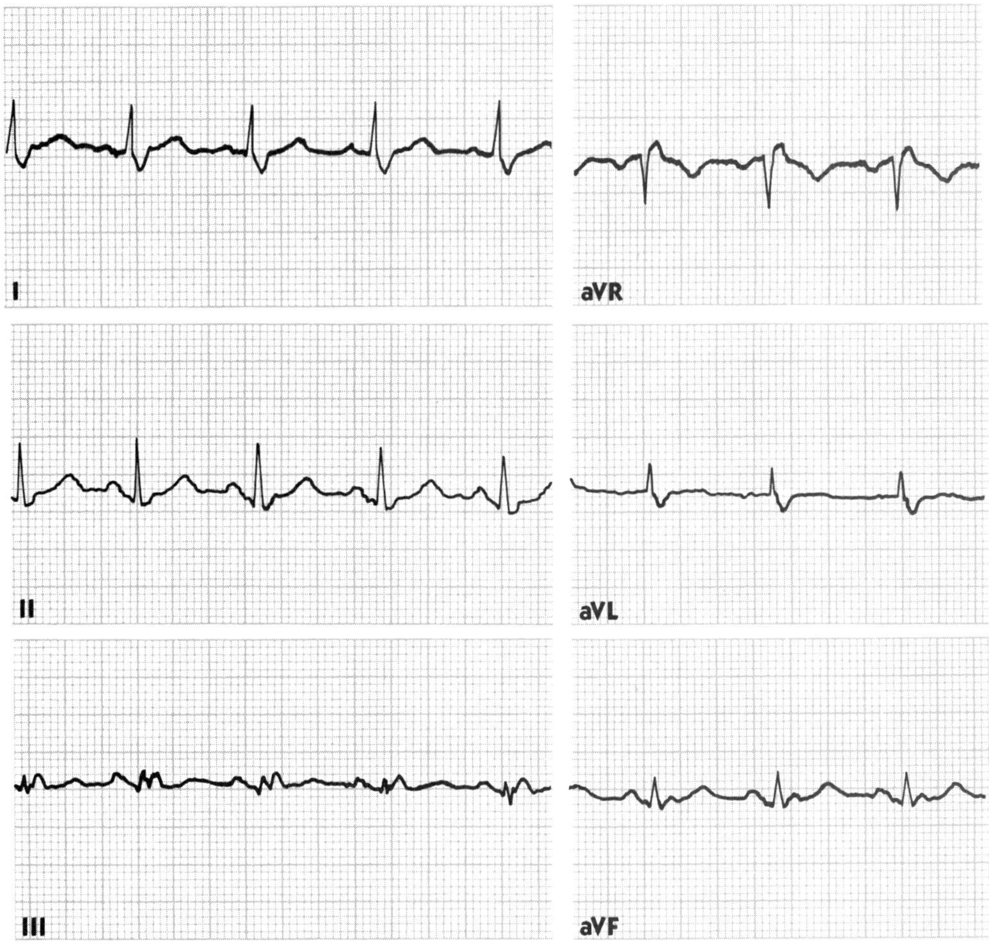

This ECG was recorded from a 56-year-old man admitted for resection of lung carcinoma. It shows sinus rhythm, a mean frontal plane QRS axis of about +40°, and normal intervals except for the QRS duration, which is prolonged to 0.12 second. In leads aVR and V1, the QRS complexes show an rSR′ configuration; the broad R′ wave represents terminal conduction delay over the right ventricle. There are broad S waves in leads I, II, aVL, and V4-6, representing the right-sided conduction delay as seen from left-sided leads. In the anterior precordial leads that reflect right ventricular activity (V1-2), the T waves are inverted.

QRS prolongation to 0.12 second or more reflects conduction delay in the bundle branches and/or ventricular myocardium. When conduction delay involves bundle branches, the specific QRS patterns indicate which bundle branch is involved. This ECG shows the classic signs of right bundle branch block (RBBB): an rSR′ pattern with a wide R′ in lead V1 and broad (but not necessarily deep) S waves in I, aVL, and V5-6.

In RBBB, left ventricular activation is normal. Thus, as the initial depolarization begins on the left side of the interventricular septum, the initial 0.04-second vector remains unchanged and is directed anterosuperiorly and rightward. Next, the left ventricle is depolarized, inscribing the S wave in lead V1 and the R wave in lead V6. Finally, the right ventricle is depolarized. In RBBB, impulse transmission leading to right ventricular depolarization is delayed, since it occurs through muscle rather than down the right bundle branch. Thus, the terminal 0.04 second or so of the QRS complex represents anteriorly directed right ventricular depolarization, inscribing an R′ in lead V1 and an S wave in

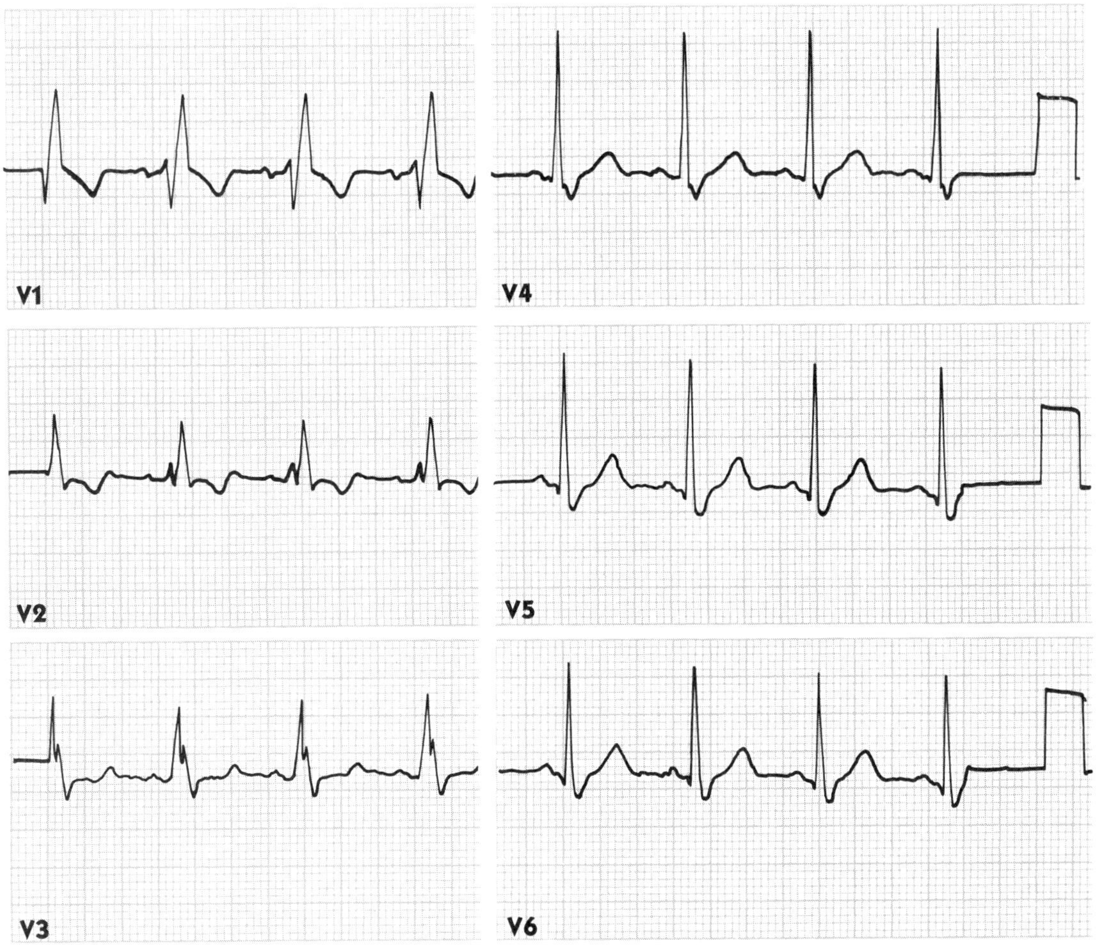

lead V6. The S waves, although broad, are not usually deep because the distance between the lateral leads and the right ventricle attenuates the registered potential and because right ventricular mass is normal.

When ventricular depolarization is altered, as in bundle branch block, repolarization will also be altered. As a general rule, with "secondary" T wave changes, the T wave vector will be opposite to the terminal QRS vector. In RBBB, where the terminal portion of the QRS complex is directed anteriorly and rightward, the T wave vector is expected to be directed posteriorly and leftward. In the anterior leads, the terminal portion of the QRS complex is upright (R′) and the T waves are inverted; in the lateral leads, the terminal QRS is negative and the T waves are upright. These secondary changes reflect altered repolarization due to delayed ventricular activation. Secondary T wave changes can themselves be altered by additional processes such as ischemia or infarction; they are then called "primary" changes (see Case 14).

Occasionally the S wave in leads I and aVL is so prominent that it is mistakenly included in the calculation of the mean frontal plane QRS axis. This can make the axis seem more rightward than it actually is. In RBBB, the QRS axis should be calculated from only the "unblocked" portion of the complex, i.e., the portion *before* the inscription of the waves reflecting the terminal conduction delay. RBBB per se does not cause right axis deviation.

CASE 12

Right Bundle Branch Block With Right Axis Deviation

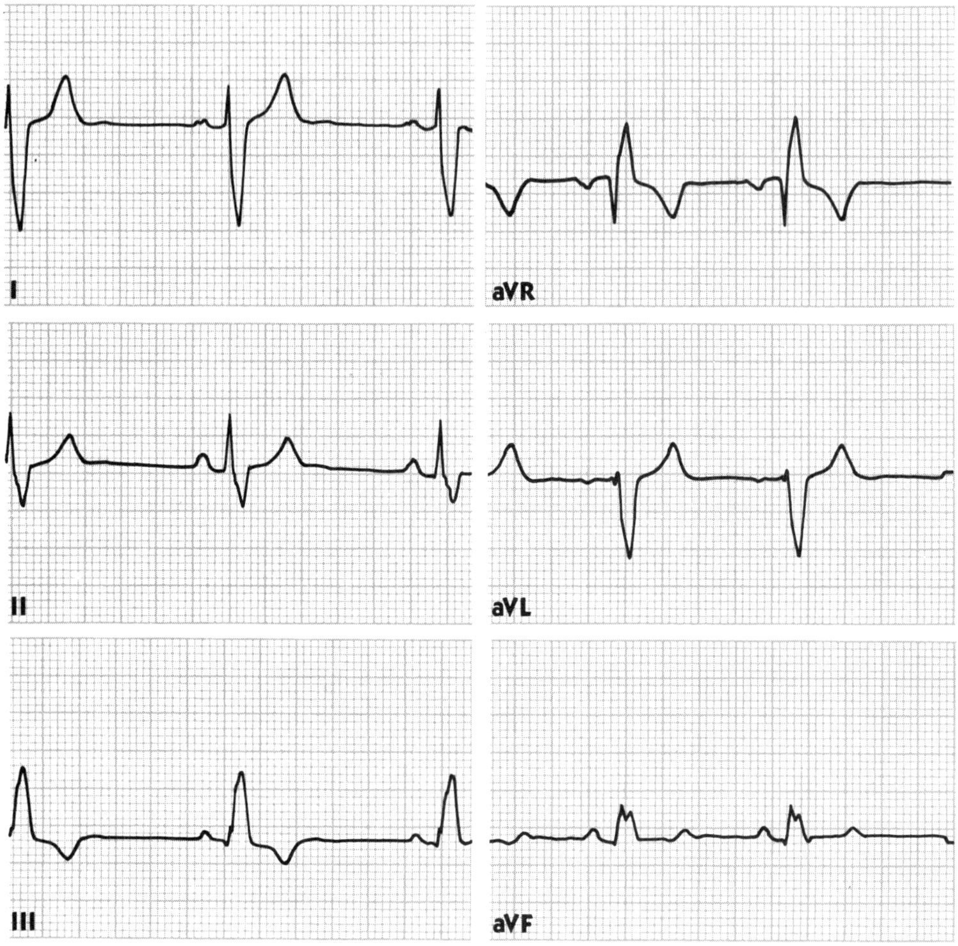

This ECG was recorded from a 22-year-old woman with primary pulmonary hypertension. Sinus arrhythmia—a rhythmic variation in sinus rate and a normal finding in young adults—is present. The QRS duration is prolonged to 0.14 second, and the QT interval is slightly prolonged to 0.44 second. The P waves are normal. There is an rsR′ pattern in lead V1 and deep, broad S waves in the lateral leads, consistent with right bundle branch block (RBBB). (See Case 11.) The R′ wave in lead V1 is 30 mm in amplitude, and there is rightward deviation of the mean frontal plane QRS axis to +120°.

QRS axis in BBB should be determined from the initial 0.04-0.06 second of the QRS complex, *before* the onset of the waves generated by delayed right (or left) ventricular depolarization. In this case, the point of change in the downslope of the S wave in lead I and the onset of the R′ in lead III signal the

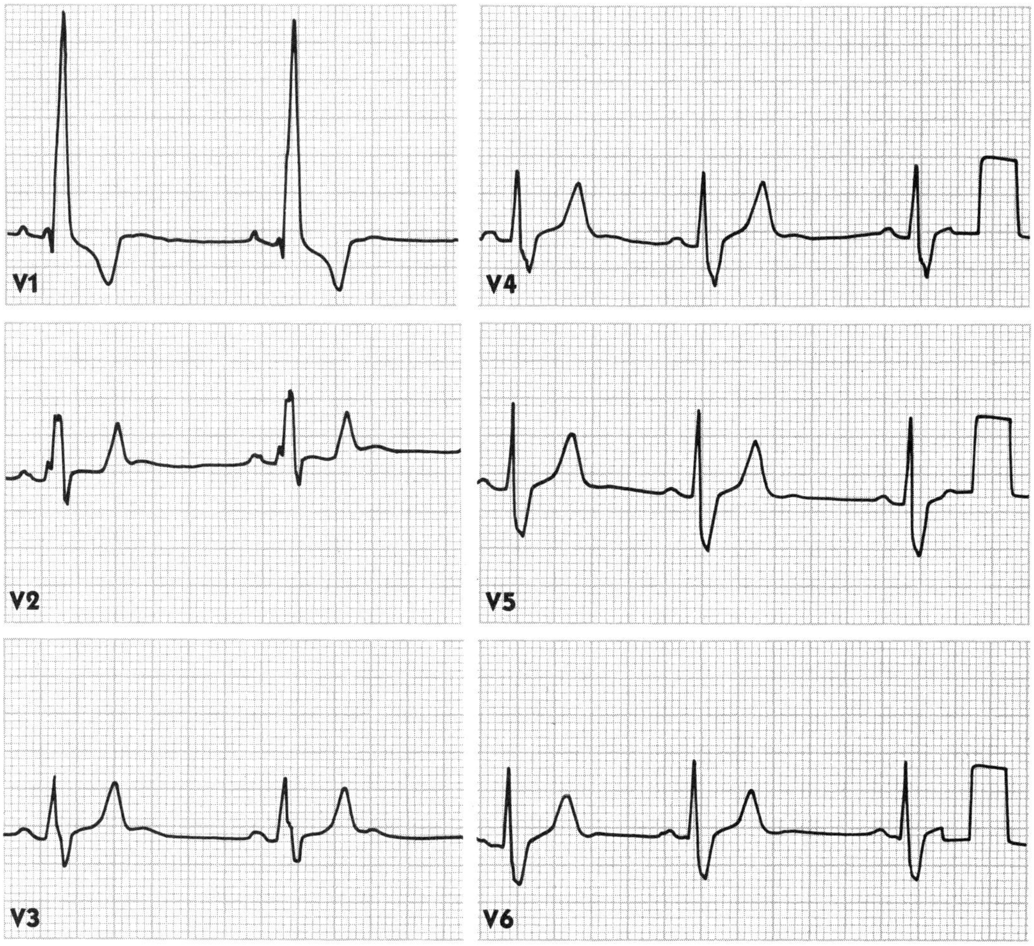

beginning of delayed right ventricular depolarization. The mean frontal plane QRS axis should therefore be determined from the initial 0.06 second of the complex, before these deflections.

This patient has RBBB; however, BBB per se does not cause axis deviation. Thus, right axis deviation (RAD) is not expected in RBBB alone. In this case, RAD suggests concomitant right ventricular hypertrophy (RVH) or left posterior fascicular block (see Case 19). RVH is more likely in view of the patient's clinical diagnosis. The markedly tall R′ wave in lead V1, although compatible with RVH, is not diagnostic, since the altered right ventricular activation in RBBB can itself be associated with prominent anterior voltage. In the presence of BBB, ventricular hypertrophy cannot generally be diagnosed from the ECG.

CASE 13

Left Bundle Branch Block

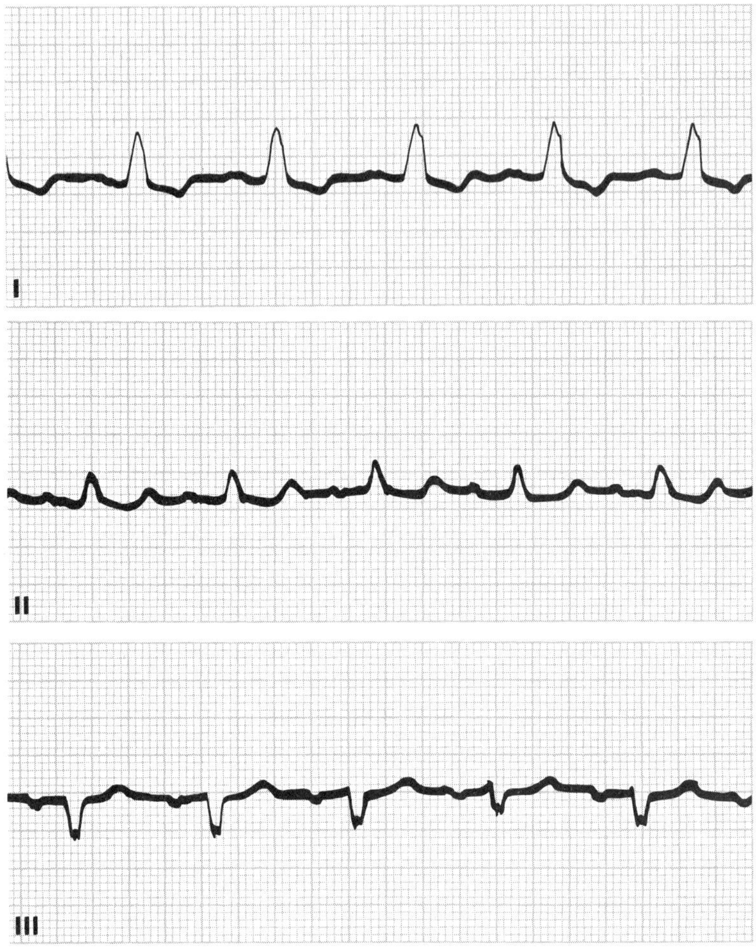

This ECG was recorded from a healthy 84-year-old man. The rhythm is sinus, the PR interval is prolonged to 0.22 second, and the QRS duration is prolonged to 0.13 second. The mean frontal plane QRS axis is 0°. The broad QRS complex consists of a monophasic R wave without a septal q wave in leads I, aVL, and V5-6. The T waves are upright anteriorly and inverted laterally, representing secondary T wave changes. QS complexes appear in leads V1-2.

This ECG shows the classic pattern of left bundle branch block (LBBB), with an associated first degree AV block. The morphologic criteria for LBBB are a broad QRS complex of 0.12 second or more; a broad, monophasic R wave in the lateral leads I, aVL, and V6; and a deep terminal S or QS deflection anteriorly in lead V1.

When impulse transmission is delayed in the left bundle branch, depolarization of the left ventricle occurs by contiguous spread of the electrical wave front through the myocardium from the normally depolarized right ventricle. As a result, initial septal depolarization occurs from right to left (the normal sequence is left to right), the septal vector may point posteriorly rather than anteriorly, and no initial q waves are inscribed in the lateral leads. Another frequent finding is absence of r waves in the anterior leads; however, when initial right ventricular septal depolarization occurs in a posteroanterior direction, a small r wave will be present.

After the initial septal depolarization, the right ventricle is activated in normal fashion. Delayed depolarization of the left ventricle follows. Because the left ventricle has much greater mass than the right, the forces it generates obscure those of the right ventricle. Consequently, the ECG shows a broad, monophasic, upright QRS complex in leads I, aVL, and V5-6 and a broad QS or rS complex anteriorly in leads V1-2. Since ventricular depolarization is abnor-

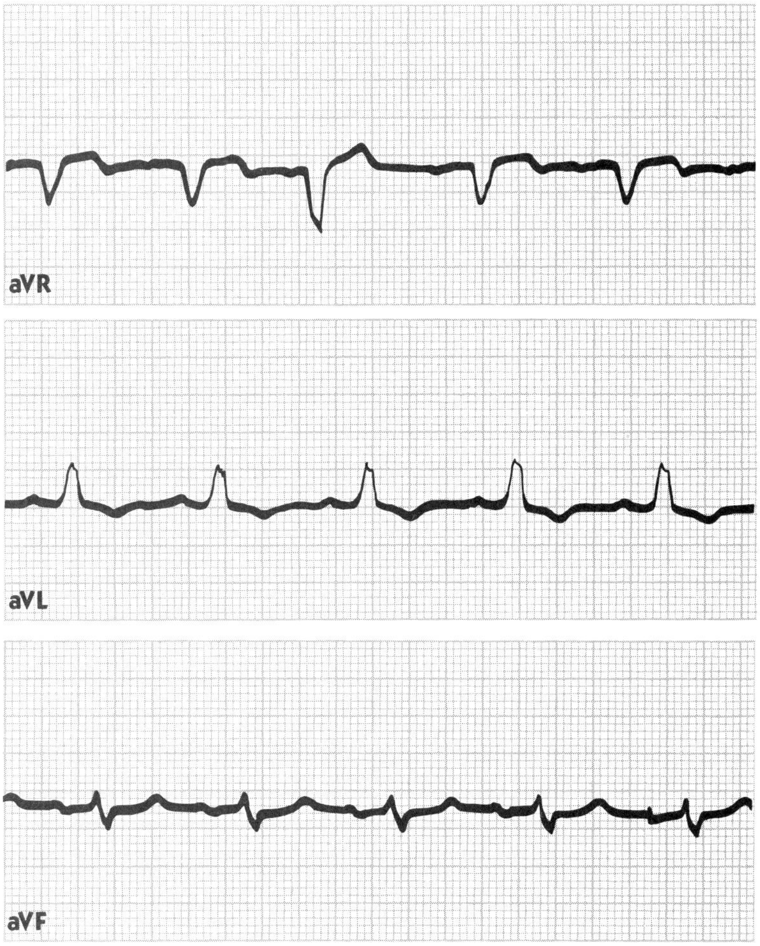

continued

mal in LBBB, repolarization is also altered, resulting in the secondary T wave changes.

The QS complexes seen in the anterior leads in LBBB raise the possibility of anterior wall myocardial infarction. This diagnosis cannot be excluded without further knowledge of the patient's medical history. If the secondary T wave abnormalities expected in LBBB do not appear, the possibility of ongoing or recent myocardial ischemia or infarction must be seriously entertained. The presence of a q wave in leads I, aVL, and V5-6 is not an expected finding in LBBB (see Case 15), and it implies septal muscle damage.

Despite the frequently observed prominent voltages, left ventricular hypertrophy cannot be determined with certainty from the ECG when LBBB is present. Clinical correlation with the ECG findings is necessary.

CASE 13 *(continued)*

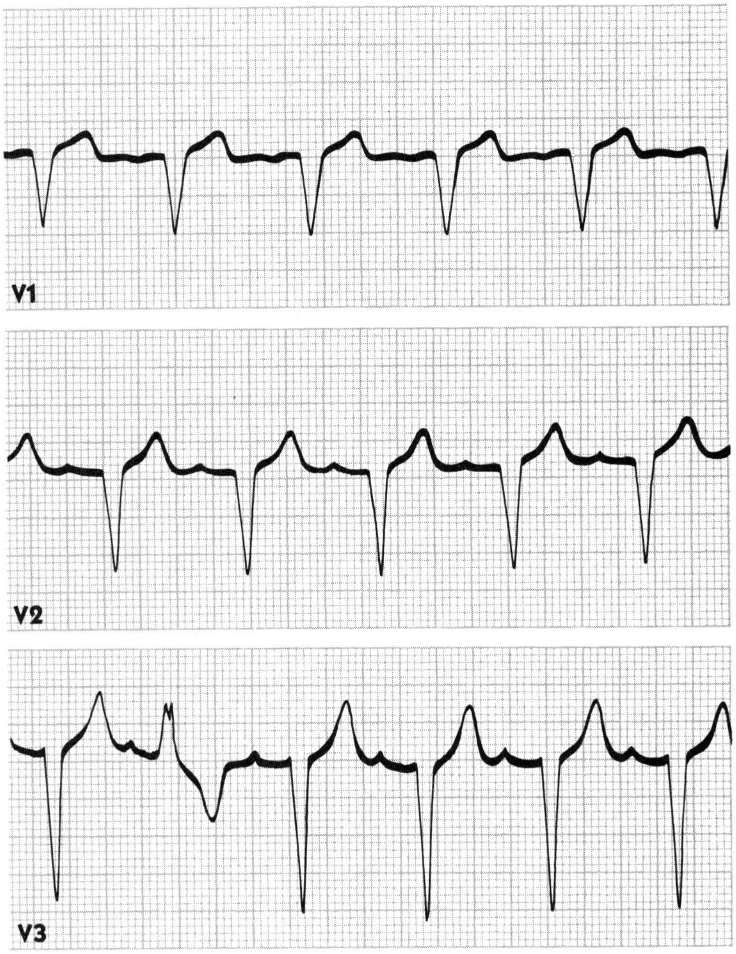

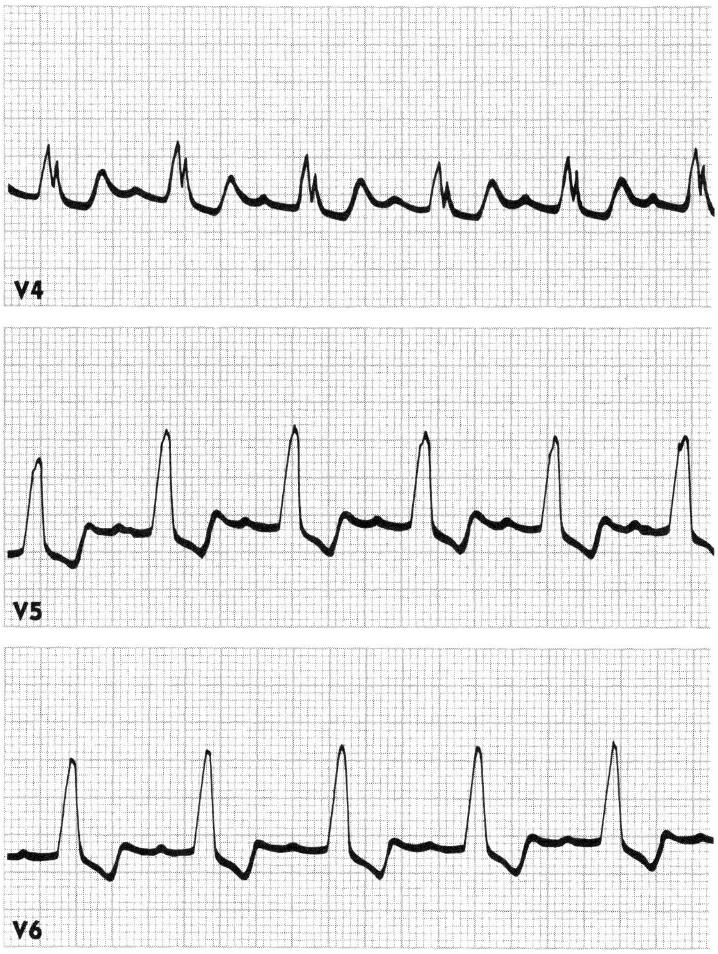
V4
V5
V6

CASE 14

Left Bundle Branch Block With Primary ST-T Changes

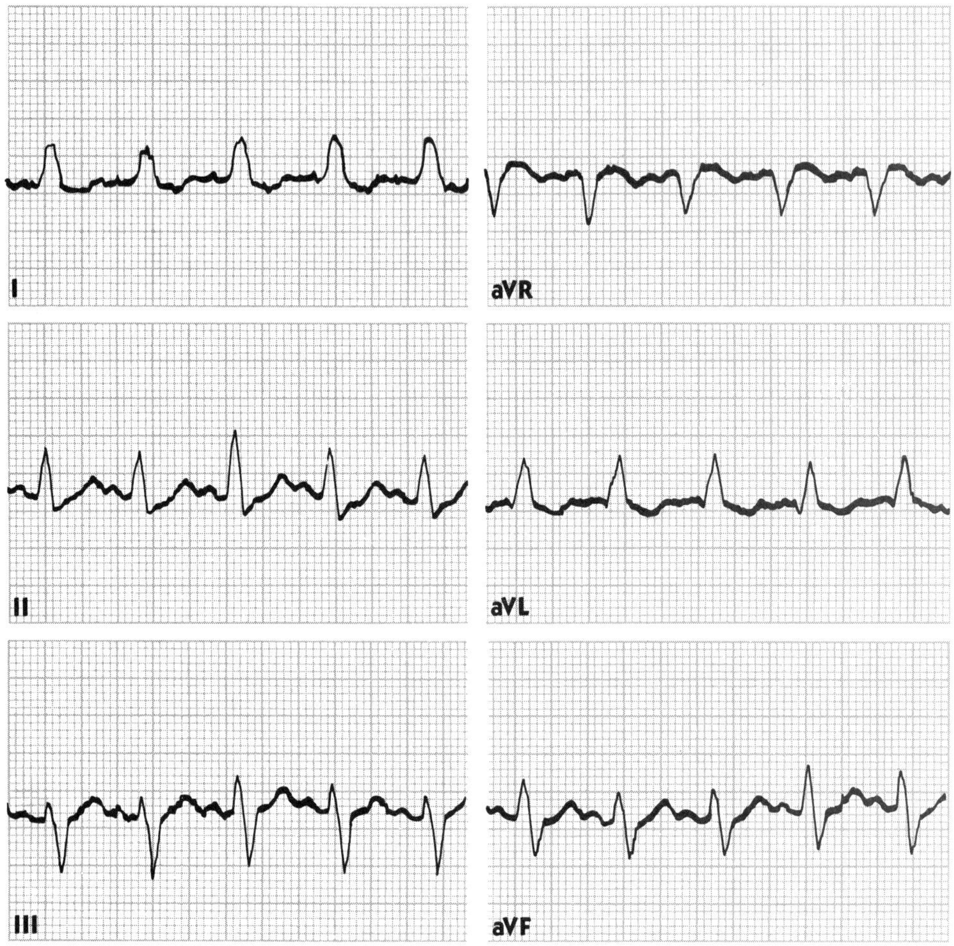

This ECG was recorded from a 61-year-old man who came to the Emergency Room complaining of severe chest pain. The rhythm is sinus tachycardia. The PR interval is normal, and the mean frontal plane QRS axis is 0°. The QRS complexes show a left bundle branch block (LBBB) pattern with an associated long QT interval. The ST segment is elevated in leads V1-4. The T waves are inverted in leads I and aVL and are upright across the precordium and inferiorly in leads III and aVF.

This patient's history suggests angina or myocardial infarction. But because of the LBBB pattern, ischemia or infarction cannot be diagnosed with certainty from the ECG alone. Nevertheless, in the appropriate clinical setting, certain ECG changes may *suggest* myocardial ischemia or infarction.

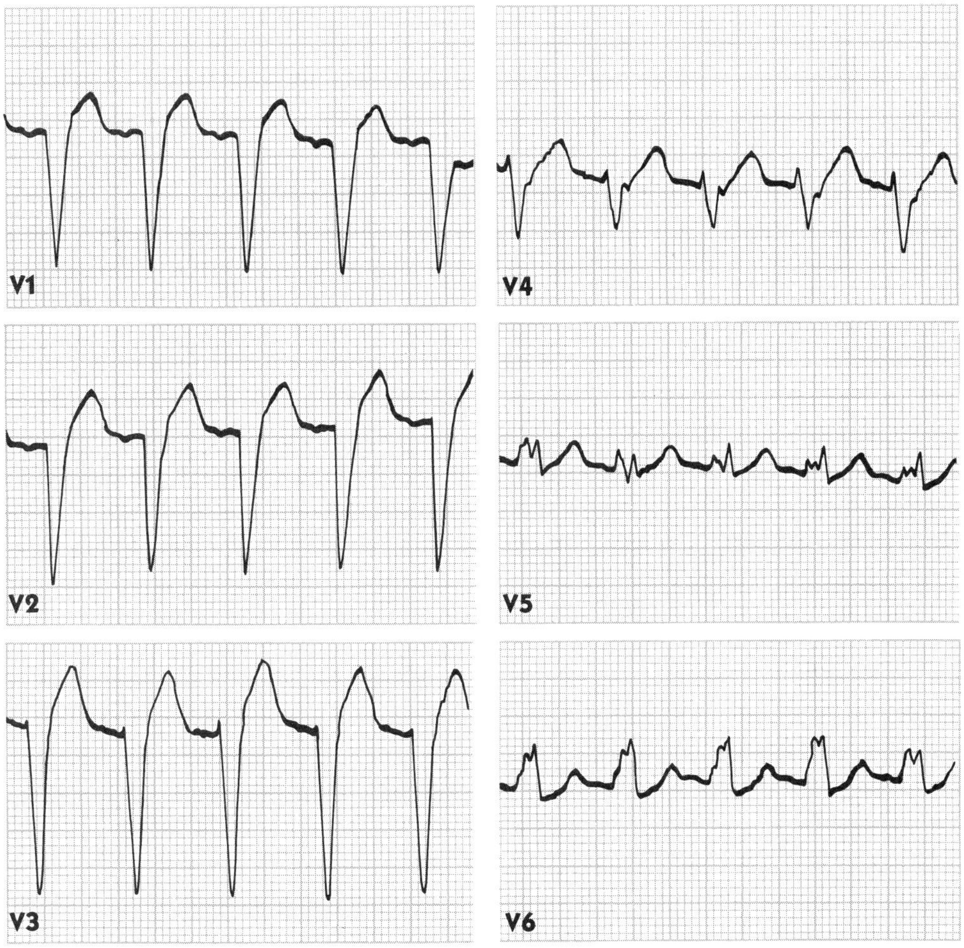

In LBBB, *secondary* T wave changes, that is, T wave vectors opposite to the terminal QRS vectors, are expected. Thus, the terminal S waves anteriorly and R waves laterally are associated with upright and inverted T waves, respectively. In this ECG, the upright T waves laterally (leads V5-6) are not the expected secondary T wave changes. They are *primary* alterations generated by processes other than delayed intraventricular conduction. When the clinical situation supports it, primary T wave abnormalities can suggest a diagnosis of ischemia, infarction, or any other process that causes T wave alterations (see Table 5 in the Appendix).

CASE 15

Left Bundle Branch Block With Septal Myocardial Infarction

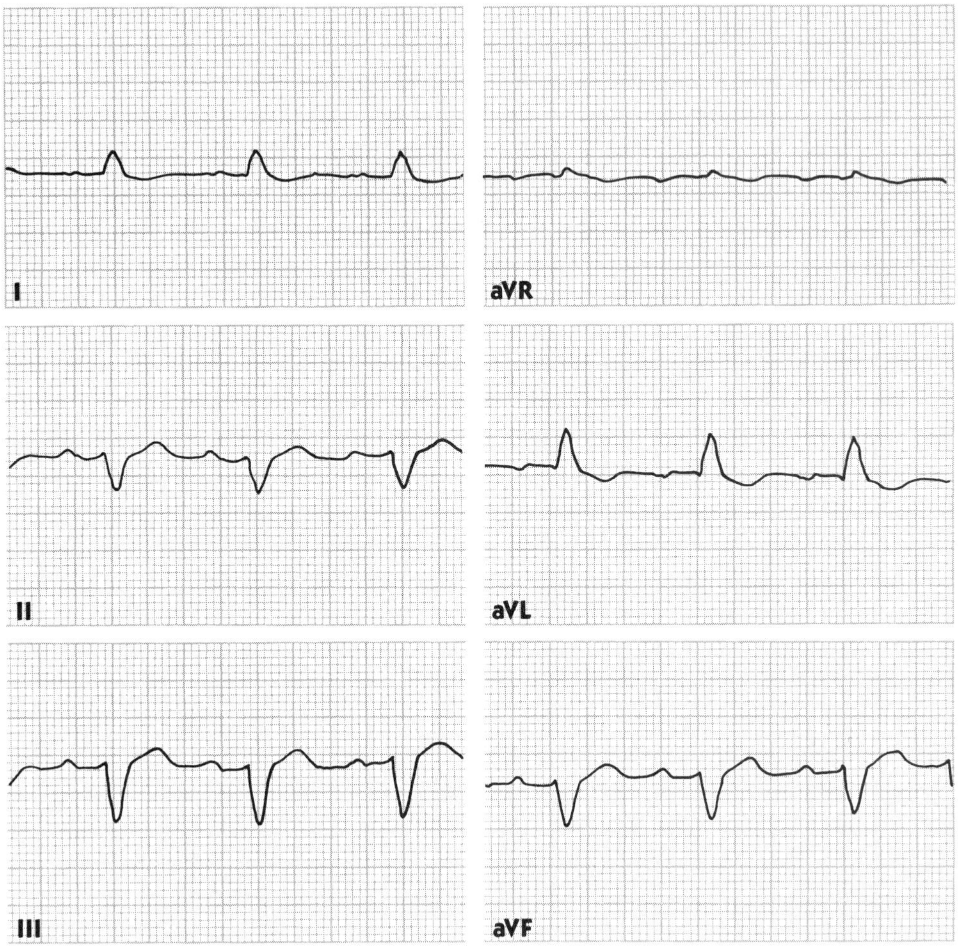

This ECG was recorded from a 57-year-old man with known left bundle branch block (LBBB) and past myocardial infarction (MI) documented enzymatically. It shows sinus rhythm, first degree AV block (PR interval = 0.24 second), a prolonged QRS interval (0.16 second), and a slightly prolonged QT interval (0.42 second). The mean frontal plane QRS axis is abnormally leftward at $-60°$. The P wave in lead V1 shows an initial peak of 2 mm, followed by a terminal negative deflection greater than 1 mm^2, consistent with left atrial abnormality and possible biatrial enlargement (see Cases 9 and 10).

The QRS morphology is notable for a broad S wave in lead V1 and a primarily monophasic R wave in lead V6, both in the pattern of LBBB. Close inspection reveals very small q waves in leads aVL and V5-6 (best seen in aVL), as well as small s waves in V5-6.

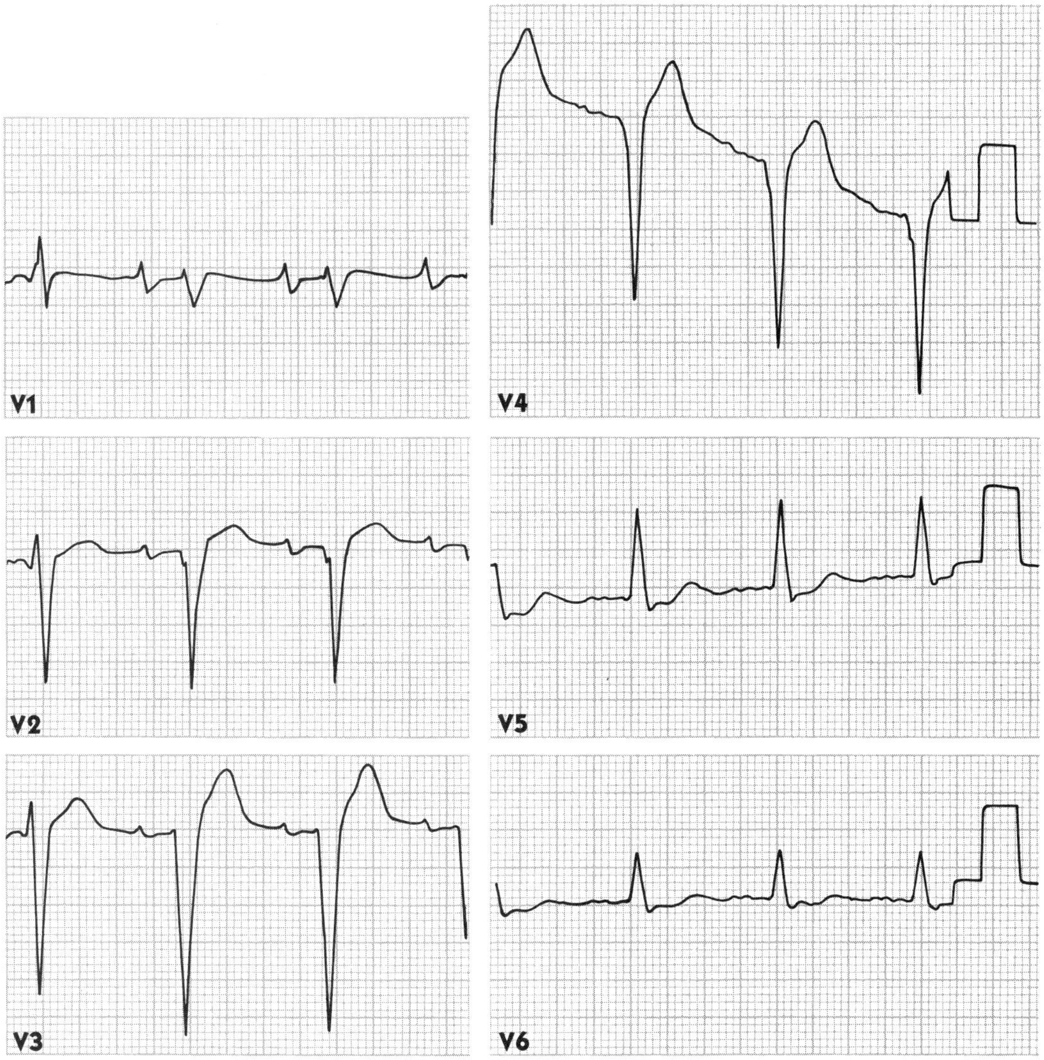

The T waves show secondary changes consistent with LBBB—except in leads V5-6, where the T waves are upright. This finding is compatible with the patient's past MI.

Septal q waves in the lateral leads are not expected in LBBB. This abnormal pattern suggests septal MI. Normal left-to-right septal depolarization does not occur in LBBB; the septum is activated from right to left, with a consequent leftward initial septal vector. Septal q waves will not be inscribed unless loss of septal myocardium has occurred, allowing initial right ventricular forces to be "seen." In the presence of LBBB, a Q (or q) wave in lead aVL alone is sufficient to suggest the diagnosis of septal MI.

CASE 16

Left Anterior Fascicular Block Mimicking Anterior Wall Myocardial Infarction

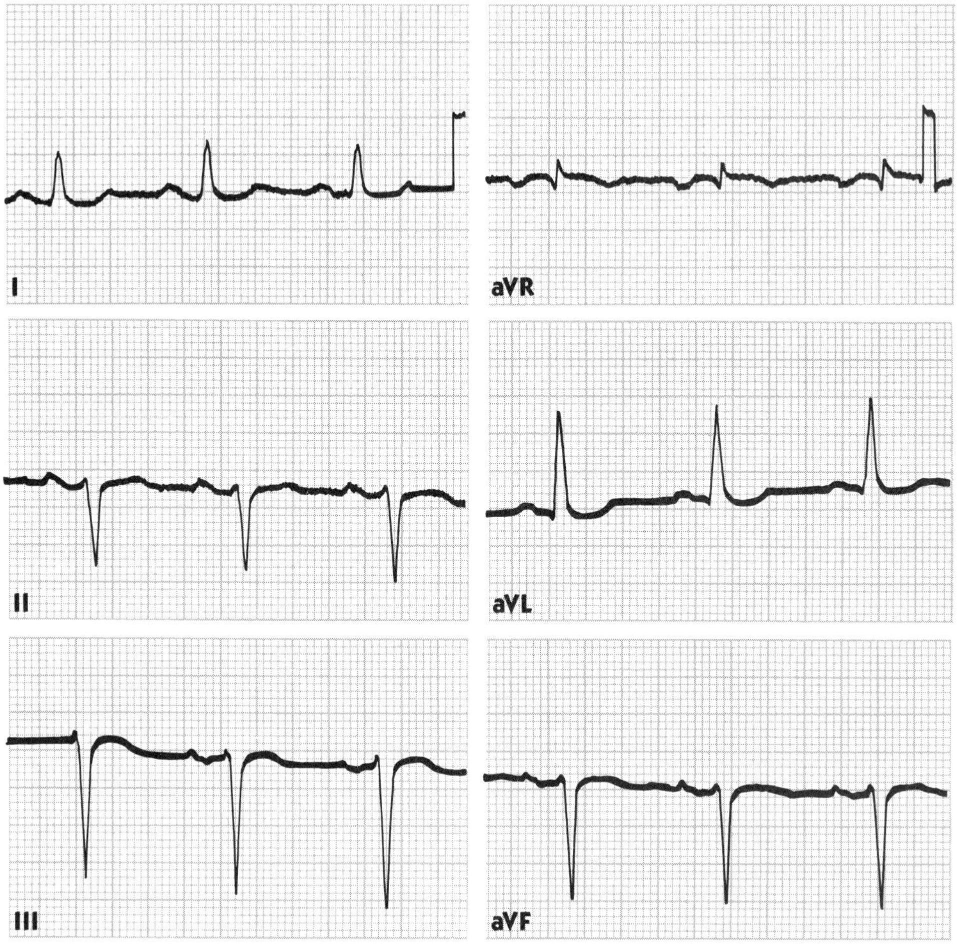

This 57-year-old man has stable angina pectoris and hypertension. His ECG shows sinus rhythm, a prolonged PR interval of 0.22 second, slight prolongation of the QRS duration to 0.11 second, and a normal QT interval. The mean frontal plane QRS axis is abnormally leftward at $-60°$, and the limb leads show a pattern characteristic of left anterior fascicular block (LAFB): qR complexes in leads I and aVL and rS complexes in leads II, III, and aVF. The P wave is notched and prolonged to 0.13 second in lead II, suggesting left atrial abnormality (see Case 9). The R wave in lead aVL is 13 mm in amplitude. There are QS complexes in leads V1-2 and rS complexes across the rest of the precordium.

The QRS vector in LAFB is generated by an altered sequence of left ventricular depolarization: The inferior and posterior areas are depolarized (via the left posterior fascicle) in advance of the anterosuperior areas. The initial QRS vector thus points inferiorly and posteriorly. This produces q waves in the anterior and/or lateral leads and poor R wave progression in the precordial leads. Although LAFB causes q waves, in most cases they are not pathological per se (≥ 0.04 second long and/or $\geq 25\%$ of the R wave height), an important factor in distinguishing LAFB from anterior wall myocardial infarction (see Case 17). In this case, the QS complexes in leads V1-2 are not caused by the LAFB and must be explained by another process, such as anterior wall MI or left ventricular hypertrophy (LVH).

R wave voltage in lead aVL is not useful in assessing LVH in patients with LAFB. It reflects the mean

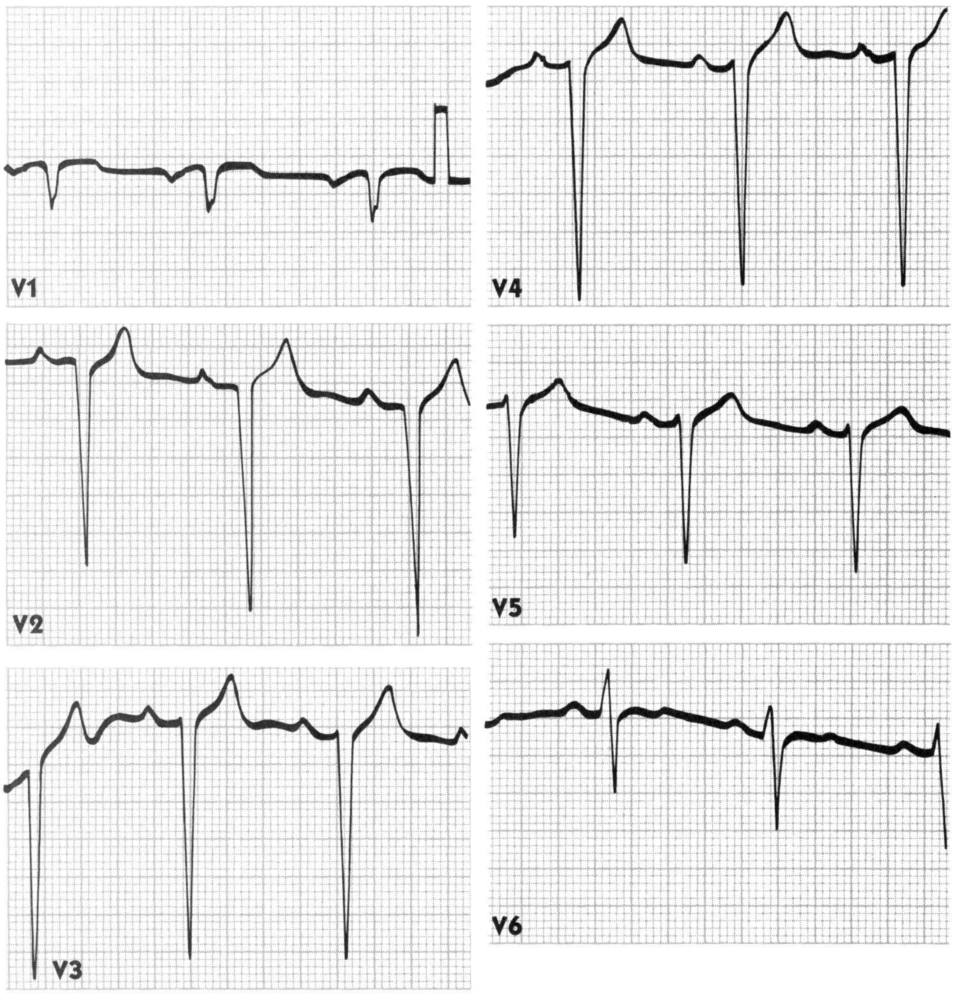

QRS vector, which points directly toward aVL. Precordial lead voltage criteria for LVH, however, probably can be applied. This ECG shows a 30-mm S wave in lead V2, suggesting the possibility of LVH. In addition, LVH would explain the QS complexes in the early precordial leads (see Case 3). Past anterior wall MI is another possible explanation. Either diagnosis requires verification by independent means. (See Table 2 in the Appendix.)

CASE 17

Right Bundle Branch Block and Left Anterior Fascicular Block

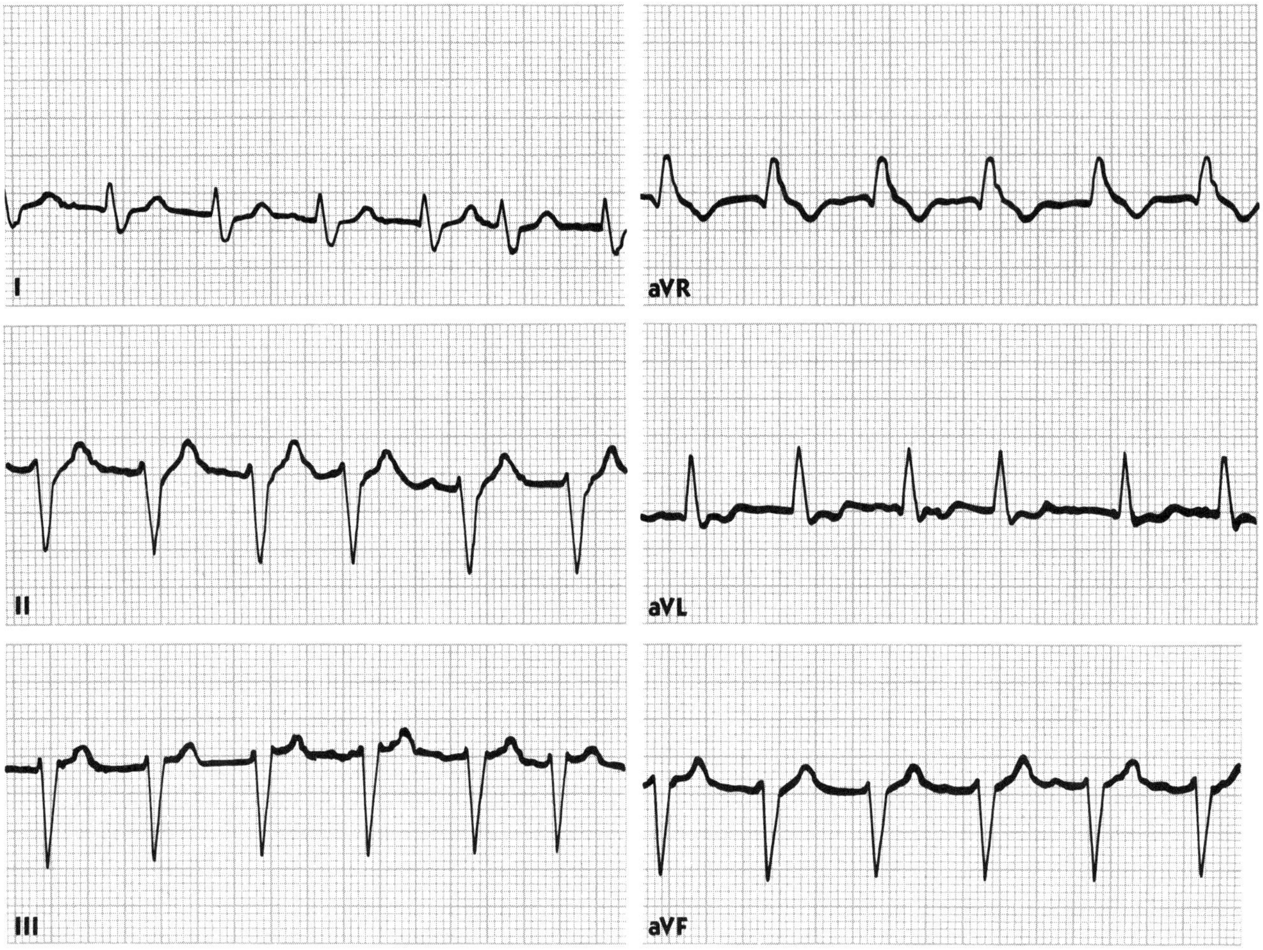

This 76-year-old man claimed to have had a "heart attack" several years previously. His ECG shows sinus rhythm, first degree AV block, and frequent atrial premature beats. The P waves appear normal, although they are not easily discerned. The QRS duration is widened to 0.14 second, and the mean frontal plane QRS axis is abnormally leftward, approaching −90°. There is an rR′ complex with terminal delay in lead V1 and deep, wide terminal S waves laterally. Small q waves appear in leads aVL and V2-3. Secondary T wave changes are present, i.e., the T waves are inverted anteriorly and upright laterally.

This patient has right bundle branch block (RBBB) and marked left axis deviation. This combination represents bifascicular block involving the right bundle branch and the left anterior fascicle of the left bundle branch. The prolonged PR interval reflects additional conduction delay either in the AV node or left posterior fascicle.

In left anterior fascicular block (LAFB), initial depolarization of the left ventricle occurs inferiorly and posteriorly and later depolarization anteriorly and superiorly. If the anterior precordial leads are recorded high on the chest wall relative to initial depolarization, the wave front is directed away from the surface leads, producing a small initial q wave that could be mistaken for anterior wall myocardial infarction (MI). Recording the precordial leads one interspace or more lower on the chest wall will eliminate the q waves due to LAFB.

The initial wave front may also be directed somewhat rightward as well as inferoposteriorly, producing small q waves in the lateral leads that

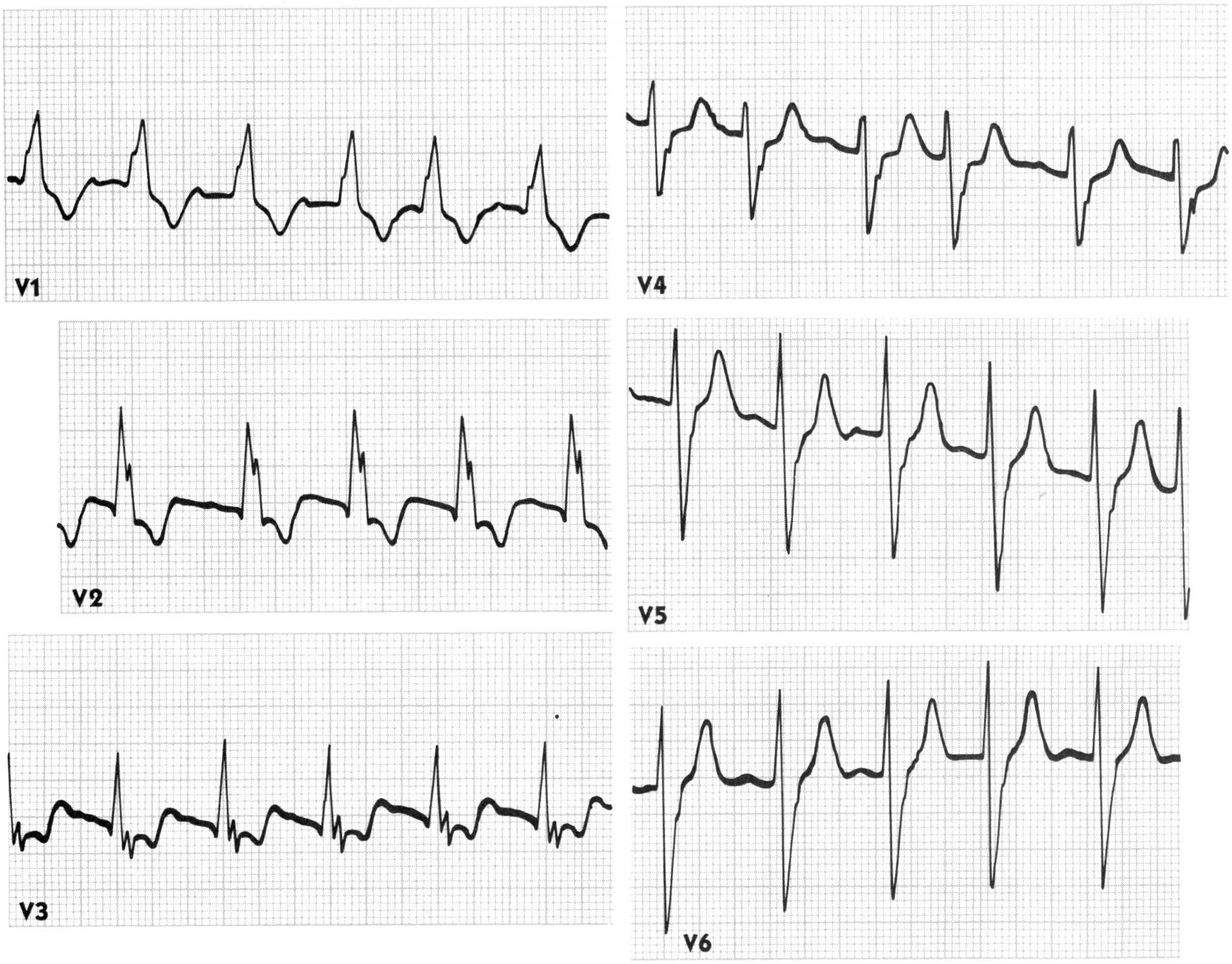

could be mistaken for lateral wall MI. Thus, in LAFB, small q waves in the anterior and/or lateral leads reflect altered depolarization rather than myocardial damage.

LAFB can also generate S waves across the precordial leads, with absence of expected R wave progression. This pattern, too, could appear to reflect lateral wall MI. It results when the terminal mean QRS vector points superiorly and posteriorly enough to be directed away from precordial leads V5 and V6.

CASE 18

Right Bundle Branch Block and Left Anterior Fascicular Block With Ischemia/Infarction

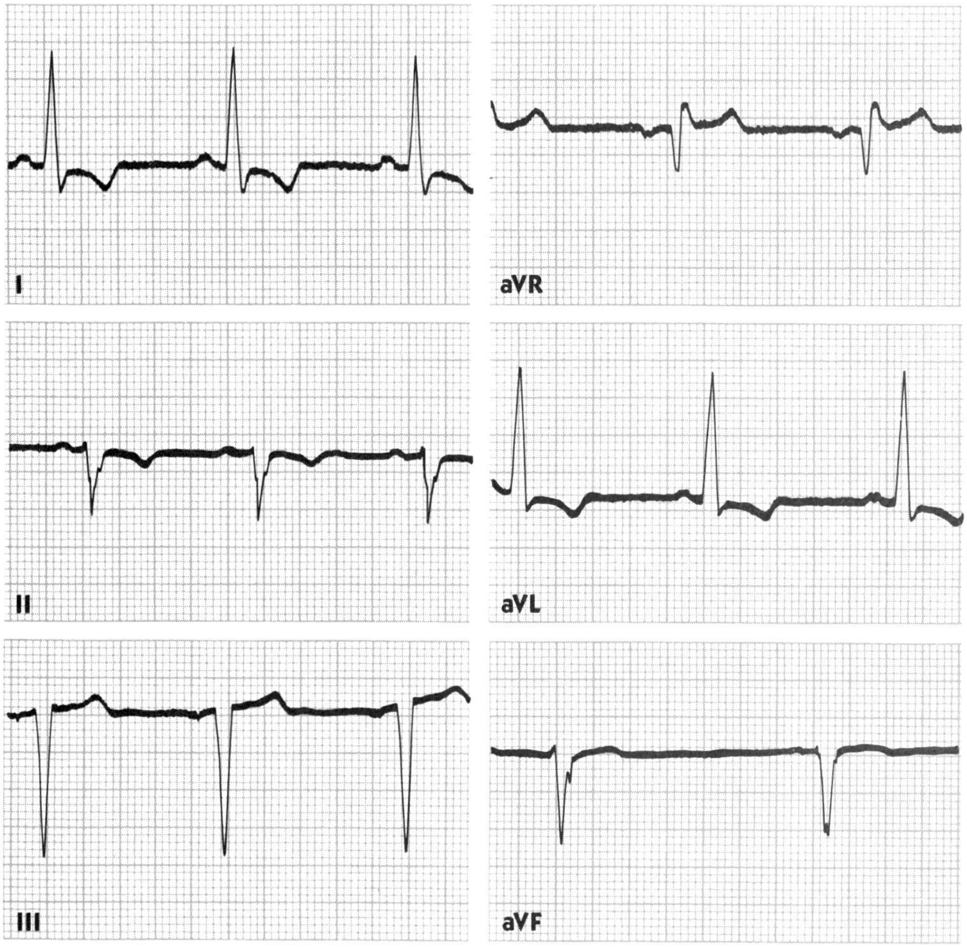

This 54-year-old woman was admitted with severe substernal chest pain of acute onset. Her ECG shows sinus rhythm and occasional premature ventricular complexes. The intervals are normal, except for a prolonged QRS duration of about 0.12 second. The P waves have normal contour. There are small r waves in leads II, III, and aVF; rSR′ complexes in lead V1; and deep terminal S waves laterally. The R wave in lead aVL exceeds 12 mm in voltage, suggesting left ventricular hypertrophy (LVH). However, the mean frontal plane QRS axis is markedly leftward, approaching −60°, invalidating the usefulness of limb-lead voltage criteria in the diagnosis of LVH (see Case 16). This patient has right bundle branch block (RBBB) and left anterior fascicular block (LAFB); unlike Case 17, anterolateral q waves are not present.

The T waves are inverted in leads I, II, aVL, and V1-6. It must be remembered that in BBB, the T wave direction is expected to be opposite to the terminal QRS vector (the characteristic secondary T wave changes). If this pattern is not present, another process is occurring. In RBBB, the terminal portion of the QRS complex is upright in lead V1 and inverted in lead V6. Consequently, inverted T waves in lead

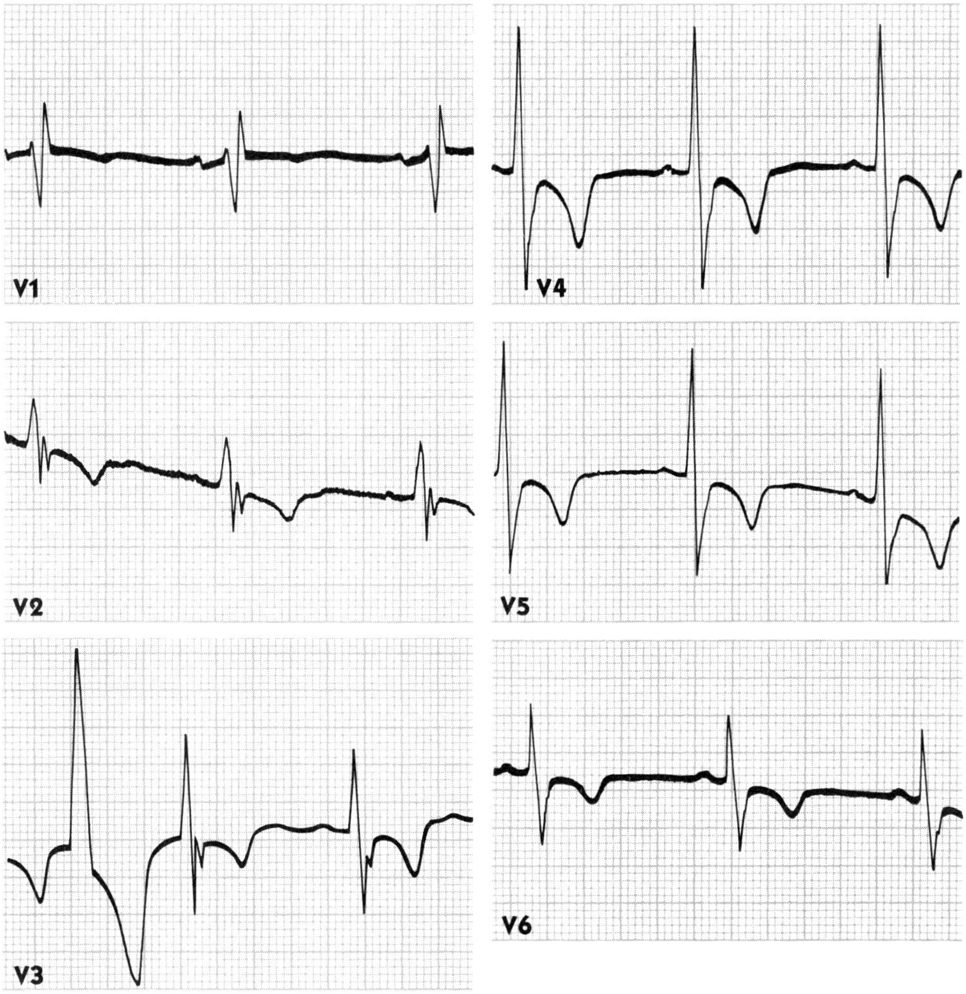

V1 are not worrisome. But the deep T wave inversions present in all the precordial leads here strongly suggest myocardial ischemia or infarction.

Serial ECGs and enzyme determinations documented myocardial infarction in this patient.

CASE 19

Right Bundle Branch Block and Left Posterior Fascicular Block With Anterior Wall Myocardial Infarction

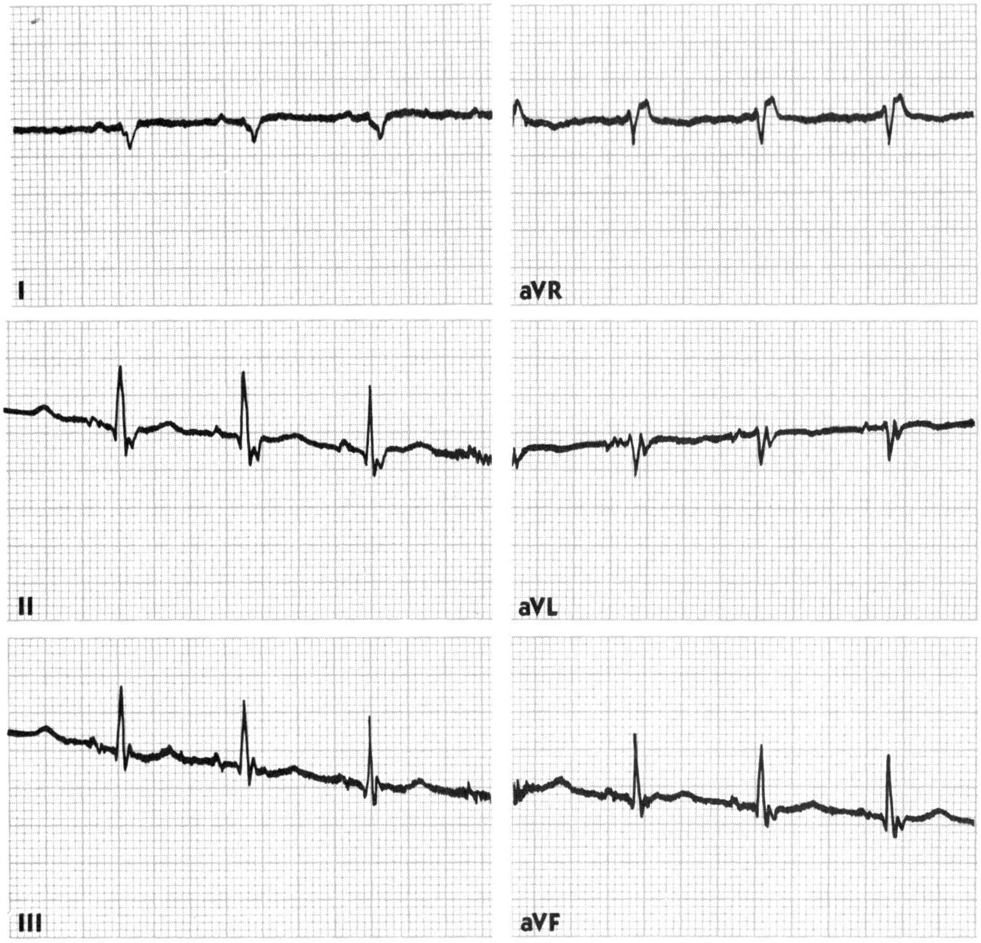

This ECG was recorded from a 68-year-old man with congestive heart failure that had developed after a myocardial infarction (MI) several months earlier. It shows an abnormally rightward mean frontal plane QRS axis of about +120° and a prolonged QRS duration of 0.12 second. The QRS complexes have an rS pattern in leads I and aVL and a qR pattern in leads II, III, and aVF. Broad, deep Q waves are present across the precordial leads. There are delayed terminal R waves in lead V1 and broad terminal S waves laterally. The T waves are upright inferiorly, inverted anteriorly, and flattened laterally.

This patient has right bundle branch block (RBBB). However, the right axis deviation (RAD) is not explained by that diagnosis, but is consistent with lateral wall MI or left posterior fascicular block (LPFB). In LPFB, initial depolarization of the left ventricle occurs anteriorly, superiorly, and leftward via the anterior fascicle of the left bundle branch. This is followed by propagation of the wave front inferiorly and rightward through the remainder of the ventricle, resulting in RAD. The initial anterosuperior vector generates a small, nonpathological q wave in the inferior leads II, III, and aVF, and a small r wave in leads I and aVL. Pure LPFB is unusual, but its association with RBBB is common.

The deep, wide Q waves across the precordial leads reflect the patient's recent anterior wall MI. LPFB can mimic anterior wall MI, with *small* q waves in the anterior precordial leads (V1-3), when

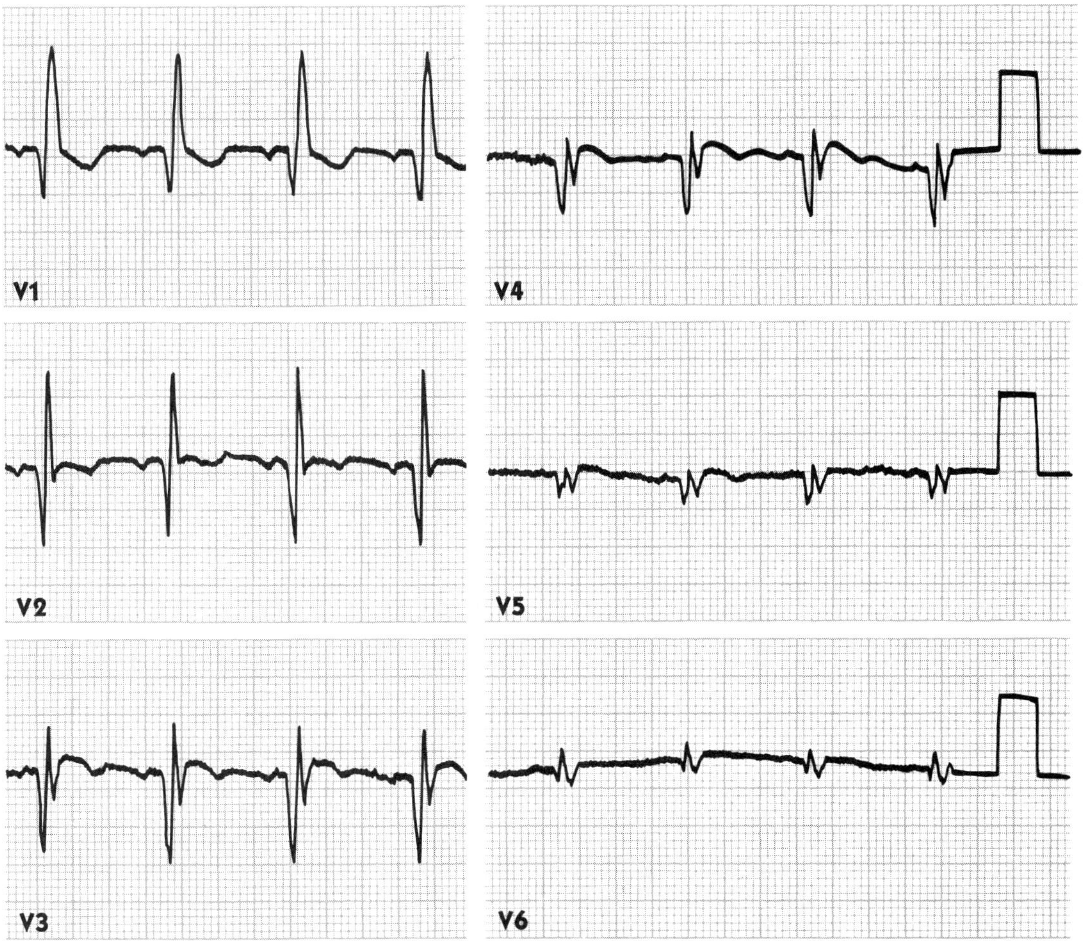

the initial QRS vector occurs somewhat below (and thus away from) the anterior surface leads. This can result from slightly high placement of the leads on the chest wall or from inferior displacement of the heart in the chest cavity, as occurs in obstructive pulmonary disease. However, the Q waves in this ECG are up to 11 mm deep, more than 0.04 second wide, and appear in all the precordial leads. Thus they are the Q waves of infarction, rather than a pseudoinfarction pattern caused by the fascicular block.

CASE 20

Inferolateral Wall Myocardial Infarction Mimicking Left Posterior Fascicular Block

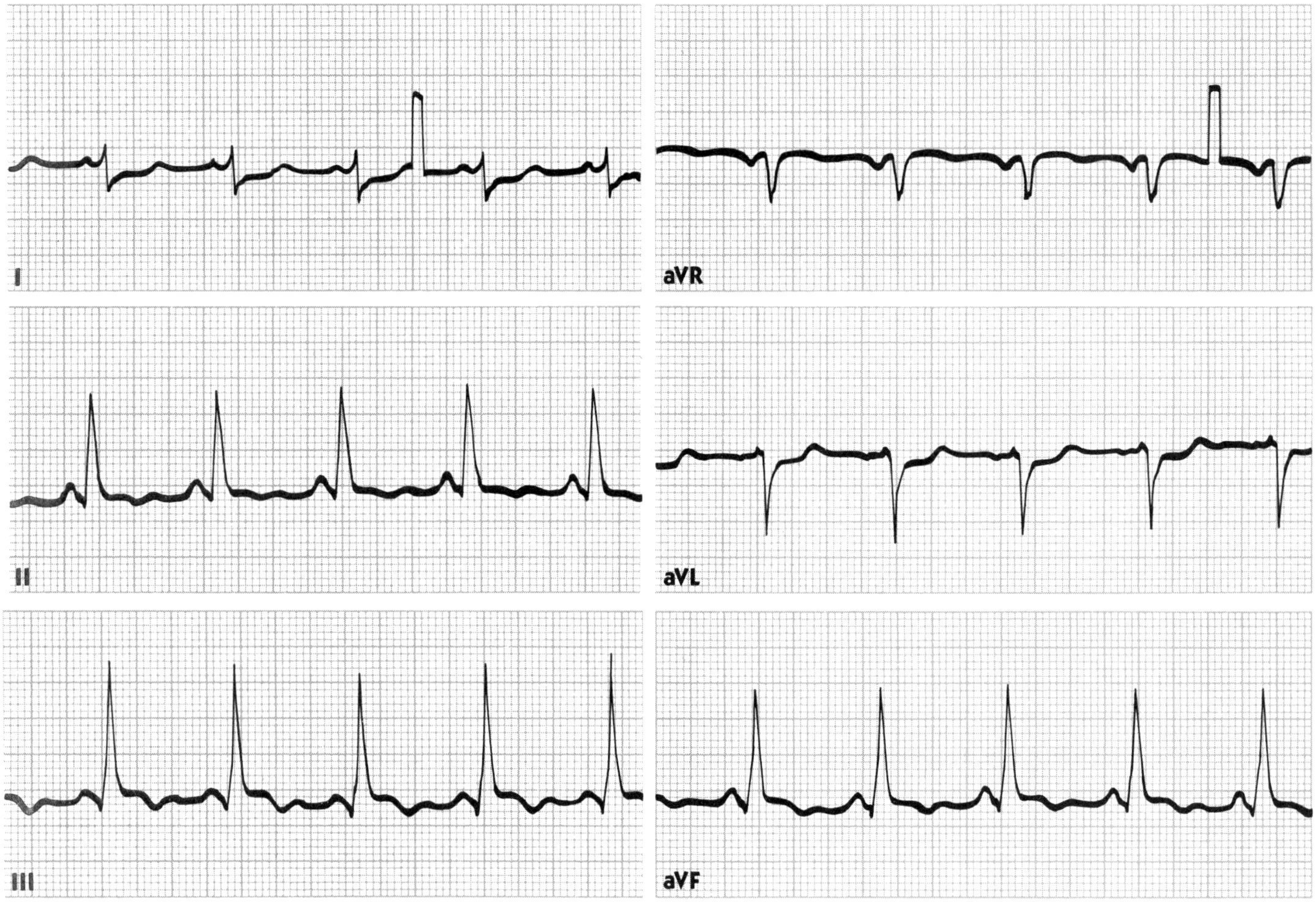

This 64-year-old woman complained of severe, prolonged, substernal chest pain. Her ECG shows a mean frontal plane QRS axis deviated to the right at + 100°, a prolonged QRS duration (0.12 second) indicating intraventricular conduction delay (see Case 21), and a prolonged QT interval (0.44 second). The P wave is biphasic in lead V1, but does not meet the criteria (≥ 0.12 second long, with the terminal negative portion at least 0.04 second long and 1 mm deep) for left atrial abnormality (see Case 9). Small q waves are present in leads II, III, and aVF. The ST segment is depressed in leads I, aVL, and V5-6 and elevated 1 mm in leads III, aVF, and V1-3. The T waves are inverted in leads II, III, aVF, and V5-6.

The small q waves and ST segment elevation inferiorly and the right axis deviation (suggesting loss of high lateral forces) are compatible with acute transmural inferolateral wall myocardial infarction (see Case 26). Although the differential diagnosis of this pattern includes left posterior fascicular block (LPFB), several observations militate against this possibility: First, the history of severe, prolonged chest pain raises the clinical suspicion of acute ischemia. Second, the inferior ST segment elevation suggests acute myocardial infarction (MI), but is not expected in LPFB. Third, the ST segment depression in the lateral leads suggests ischemia and/or infarction. Fourth, fascicular block is not expected to measura-

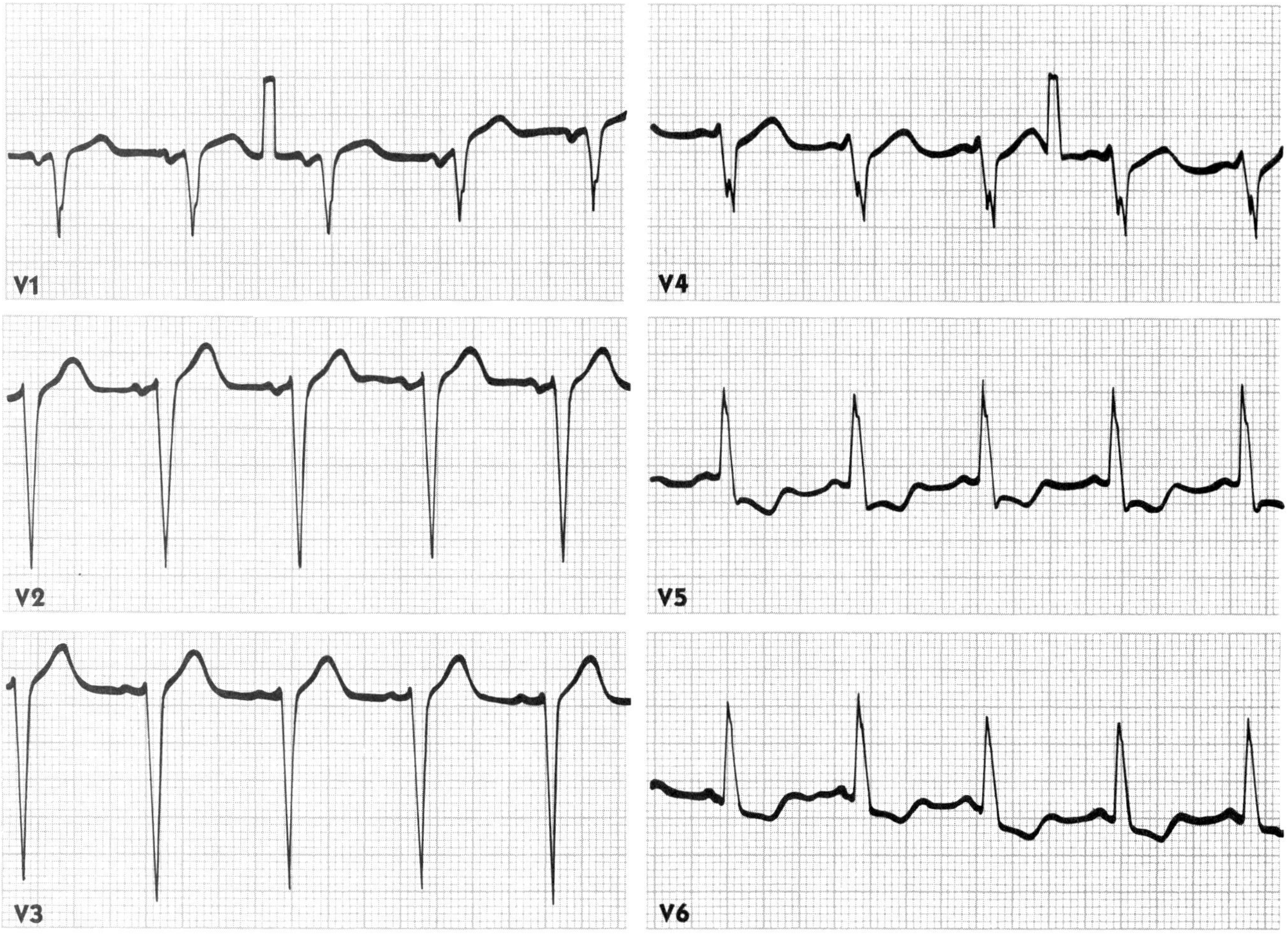

bly increase the QRS duration. Finally, QT interval prolongation unexplained by a medication history is frequently seen in acute ischemia and infarction, but not in fascicular block.

Serial ECGs and enzyme determinations documented acute inferolateral wall MI in this patient.

CASE 21

Intraventricular Conduction Delay, Unspecified Type

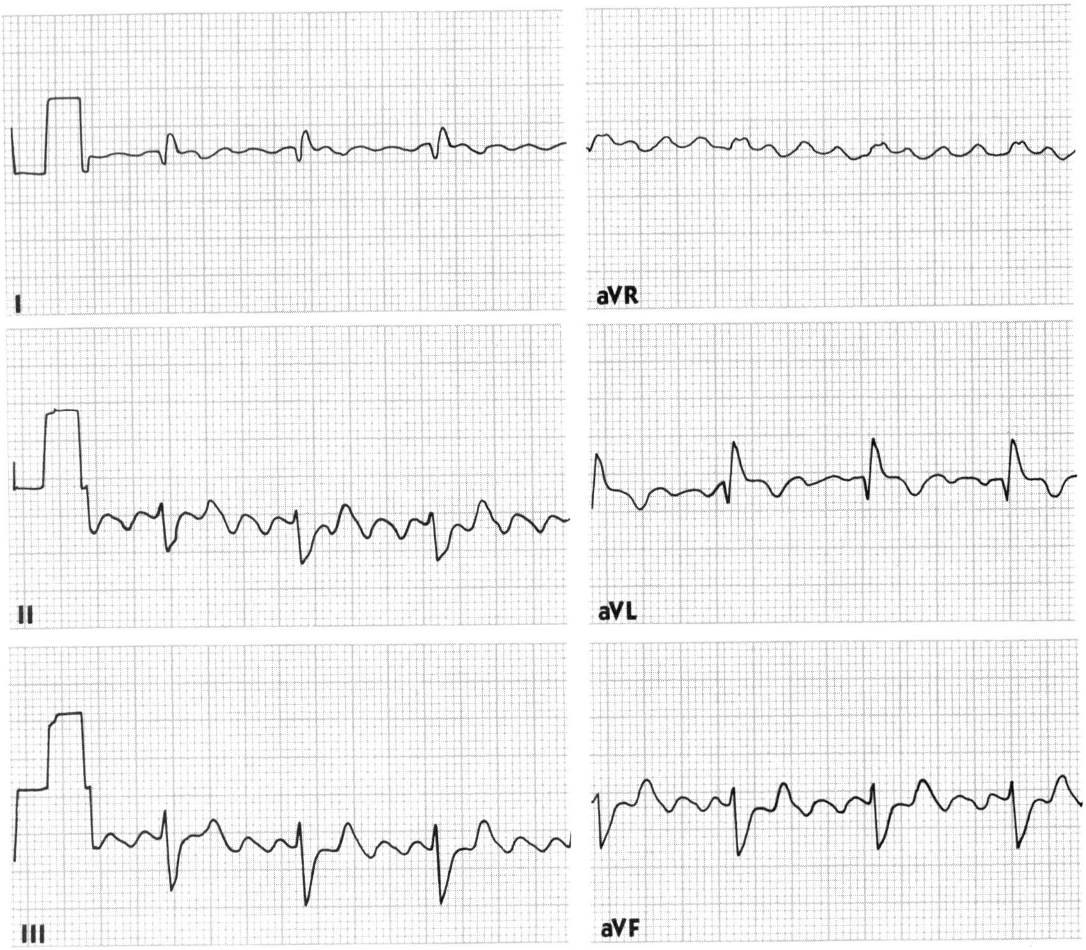

This 63-year-old man had an extensive anterior wall myocardial infarction (MI) seven years prior to this ECG, followed by an aneurysmectomy for congestive heart failure two years later. This record was made upon his admission for therapy of persistent congestive heart failure.

The ECG shows atrial flutter with a 4:1 AV conduction ratio and a ventricular rate of about 76 per minute. The QRS complexes are widened to 0.13 second, and the mean frontal plane QRS axis is shifted leftward to about − 75°. There are qR complexes in leads I and aVL and small r waves in the anterior and inferior leads. The morphology of the ST segment and T wave is difficult to assess because of superimposed atrial flutter waves.

This patient has a prolonged QRS duration suggesting intraventricular conduction delay, but the pattern does not precisely fit either left or right bundle branch block (BBB). Although the deep S wave in lead V1 suggests LBBB, there are no broad, notched monophasic R waves in lead V6. Moreover, although the deep, broad terminal S wave in lead V6 suggests RBBB, an rSR′ configuration is not present in lead V1. This pattern is therefore best termed intraventricular conduction delay of undetermined or unspecified type.

Left axis deviation plus a pattern of initial r waves in leads II, III, and aVF and initial q waves in leads I and aVL meet the criteria for left anterior fascicular block. But LAFB alone does not cause mea-

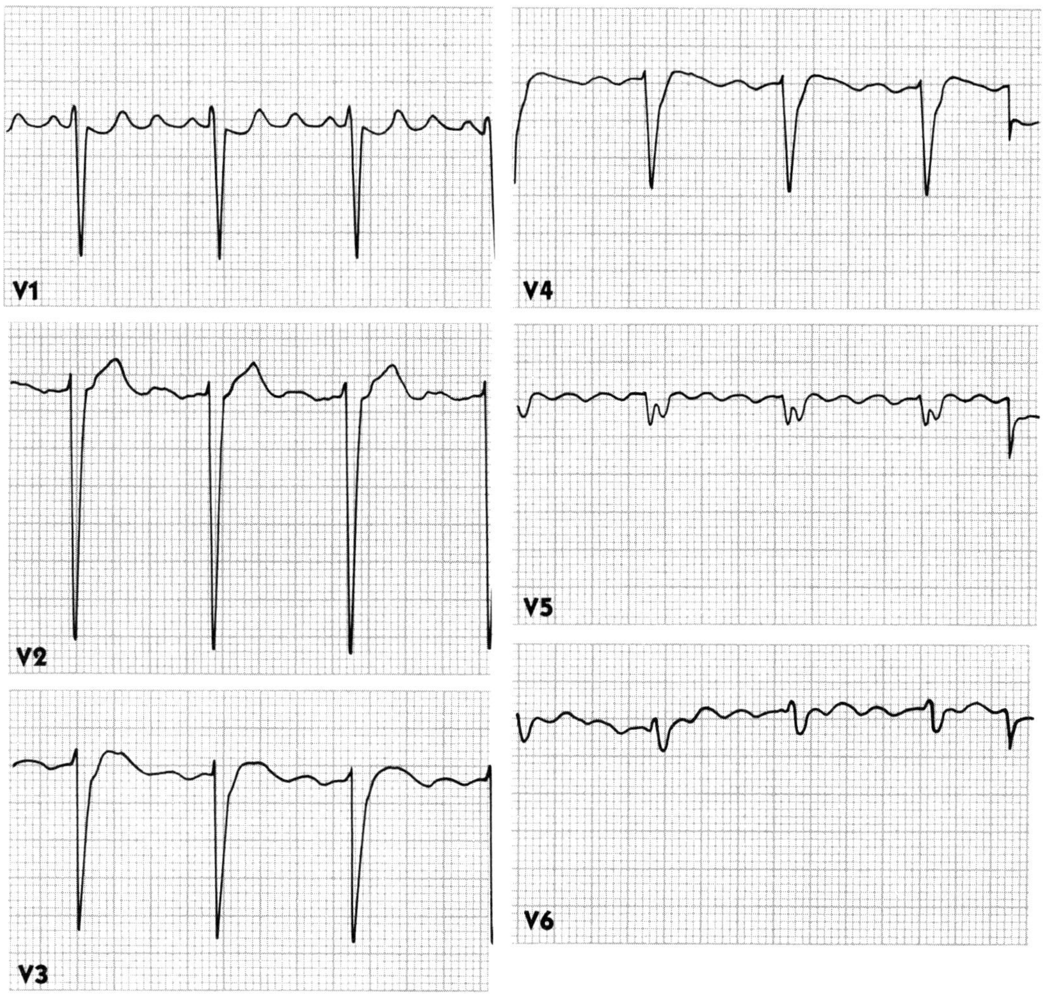

surable prolongation of the QRS duration. In addition, the lateral q waves are too broad to result solely from LAFB and probably reflect past anterolateral wall MI. The lack of R wave progression across the precordial leads reflects loss of anterior ventricular free wall due to either MI or aneurysmectomy in the past.

CASE 22

Permanent Cardiac Pacemaker—Right Ventricular Location—Mimicking Left Bundle Branch Block

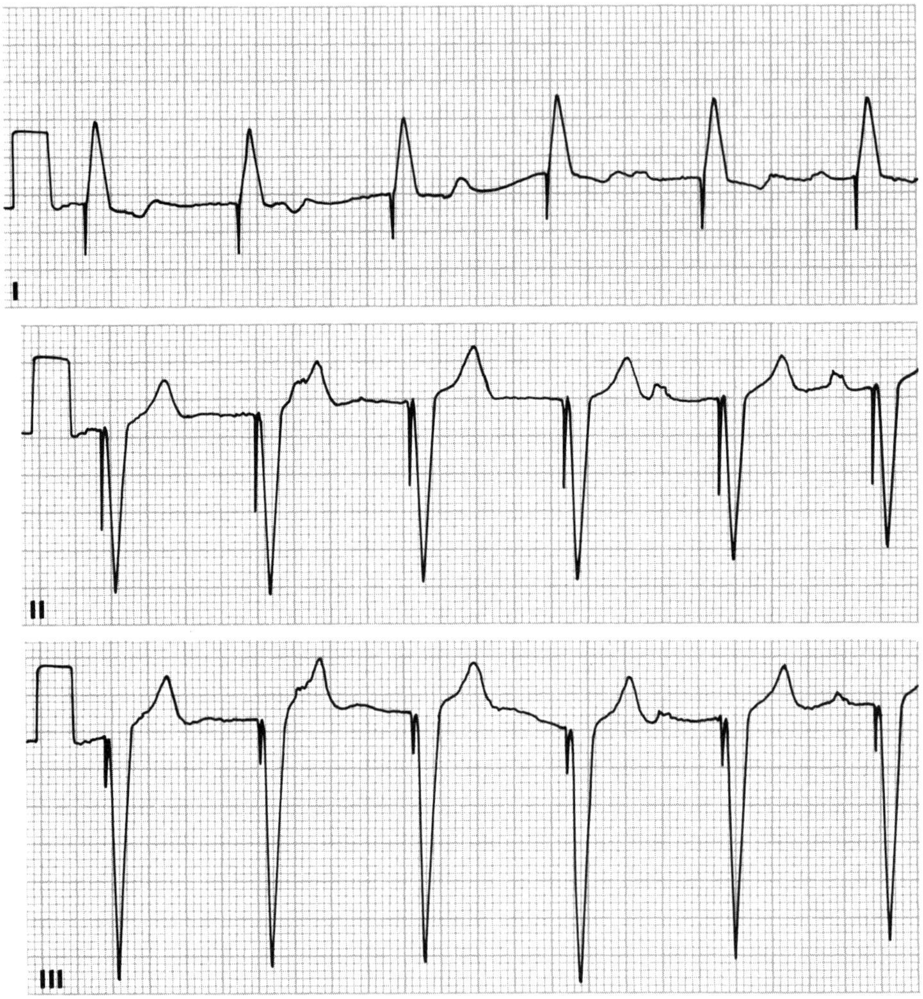

This 87-year-old woman's permanent pacing system was implanted due to complete heart block with syncope. Her ECG shows the normal pacing function of a demand ventricular pacemaker. The P waves occur independently of the paced rhythm. The paced complexes are 0.16 second wide. There are monophasic R waves in leads I, aVR, and aVL and QS complexes in leads II, III, and aVF. The markedly superior mean frontal plane QRS axis of paced complexes indicates that depolarization of the apical area of the heart is occurring before depolarization of the base. The precordial leads show a left bundle branch block (LBBB) pattern (see Case 13), with a QS configuration in lead V1 and a broad R wave in lead V6.

From which chamber is the heart being paced? This is the simplest rule to use: A pacemaker wire in or on the right ventricle creates an LBBB pattern, since the right ventricle is depolarized first; and one in or on the left ventricle creates a right bundle branch block (RBBB) pattern, since the left ventricle is depolarized first (see Case 23). This patient's ECG shows an LBBB pattern; thus, her permanent pacing lead is in the right ventricle.

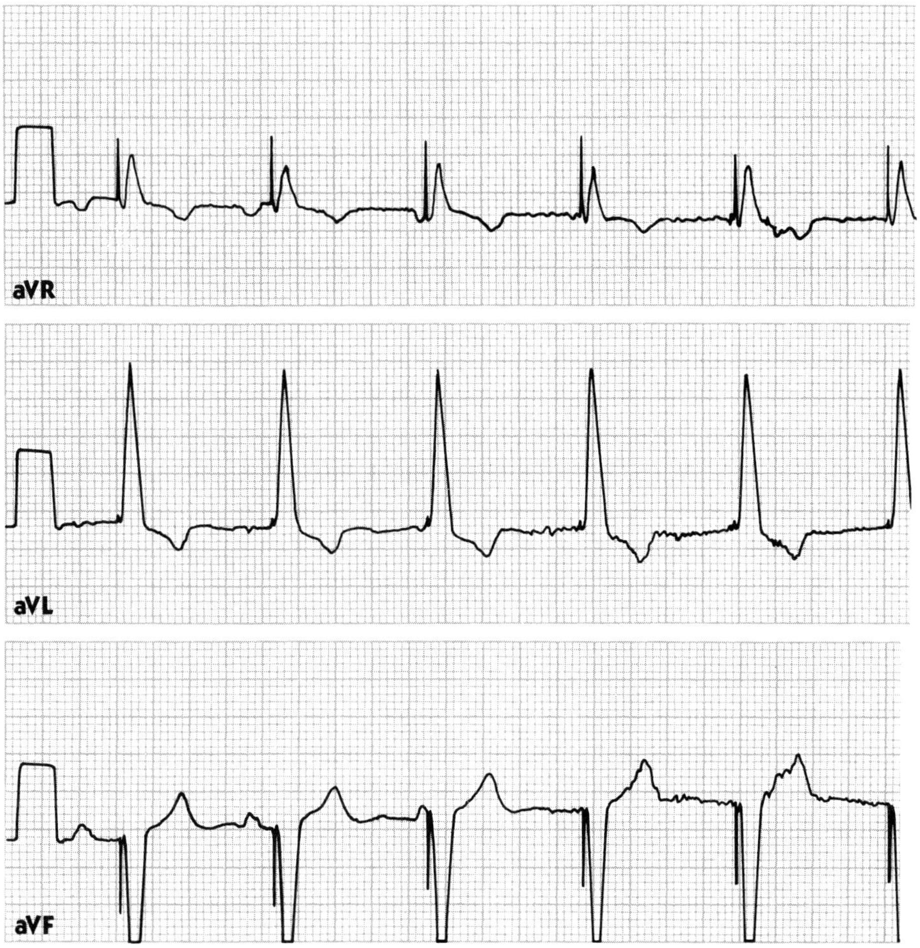

continued

When a pacemaker wire in (or on) the right ventricle initiates ventricular activation, the depolarization wave front begins in the right ventricle and spreads through the interventricular septum to the left. Left ventricular depolarization is delayed and prolonged, since the left ventricle's conduction system (the left bundle branch) is effectively bypassed. Because of the proximate location of a transvenously placed pacing wire to the right bundle branch and right ventricular myocardium, depolarization of the right ventricle proceeds in normal or near-normal fashion. This may not be true if the pacing wire is placed on right ventricular epicardium. The surface ECG's reflection of the conduction delay in left ventricular myocardium results in an LBBB pattern.

In BBB caused by organic heart disease involving abnormal ventricular depolarization and repolarization, ventricular hypertrophy and myocardial infarction cannot be diagnosed with certainty from the ECG. This is also true in cases of pacemaker-generated BBB patterns. These diagnoses must be assessed by other means.

CASE 22 *(continued)*

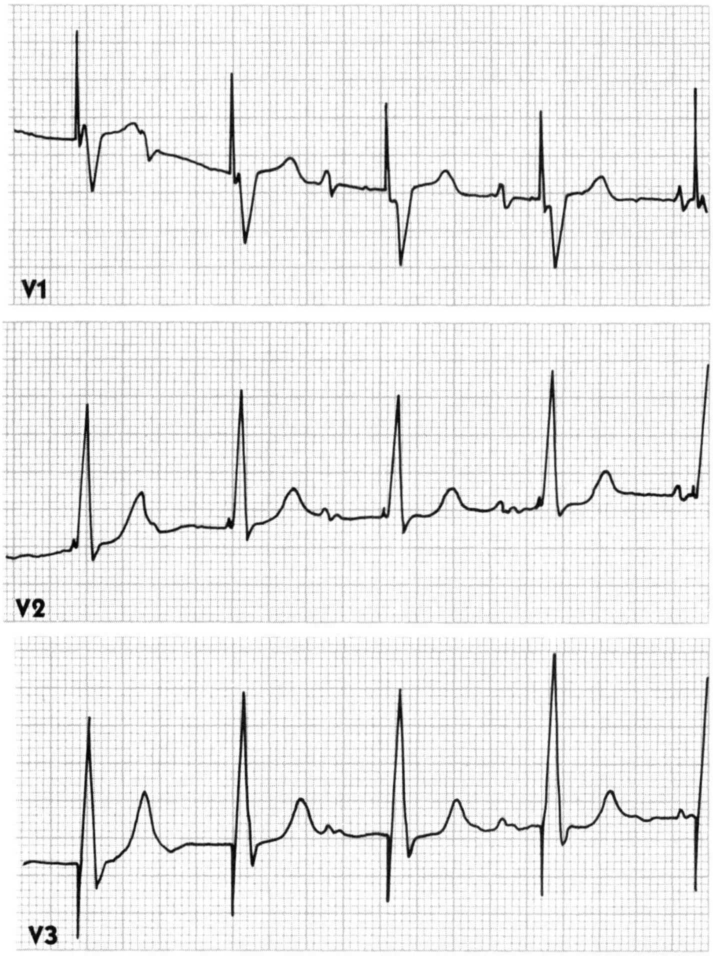

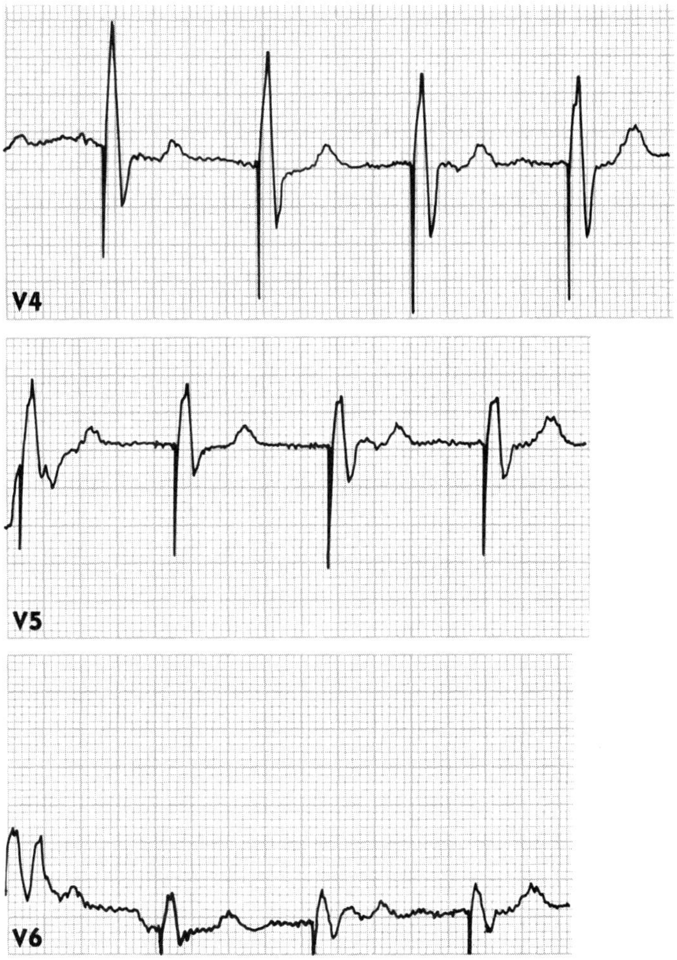
V4
V5
V6

CASE 23

Permanent Cardiac Pacemaker—Left Ventricular Epicardial Location—Mimicking Right Bundle Branch Block

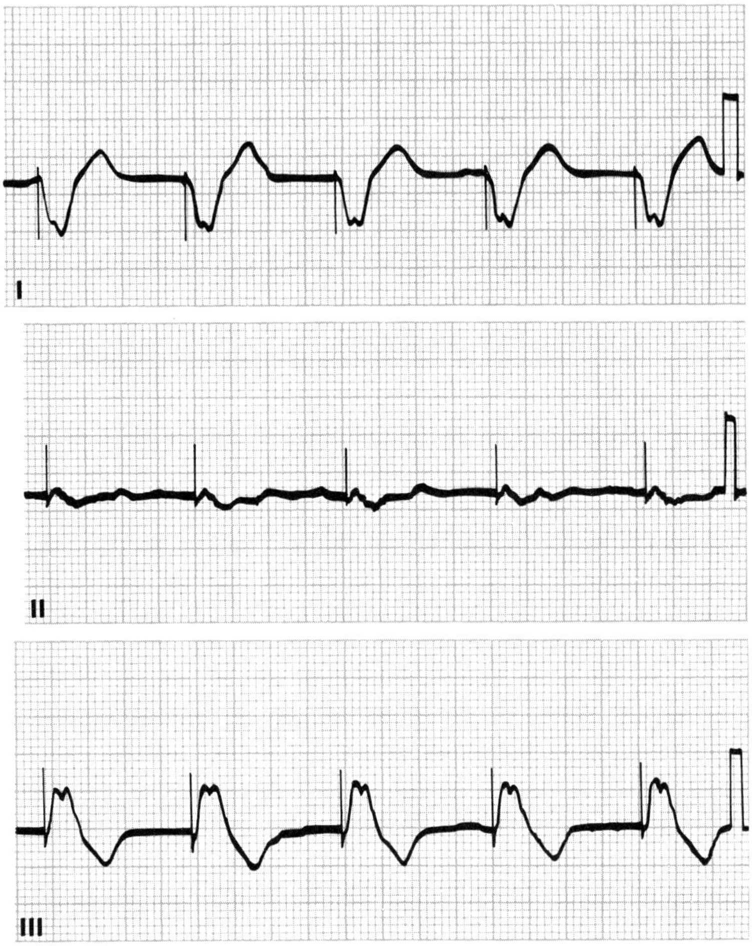

This 67-year-old woman had a permanent cardiac pacemaker placed on the epicardial surface of the left ventricle at the time of thoracotomy. Her ECG shows predominantly paced rhythm, although there are occasional fusion complexes (the narrow QRS complexes). P waves can be seen without relationship to the paced beats. The paced QRS duration is prolonged to 0.20 second and the QT interval to 0.42 second. The mean frontal plane QRS axis of the paced complexes is +150°. There are RR′ complexes in lead V1 and essentially QS configurations laterally (the initial positive deflection in these leads represents the decay curve artifact of the pacing stimulus). The T wave vectors are opposite to the terminal QRS vectors, representing secondary changes caused by altered ventricular depolarization.

As would be expected with a pacemaker lead located on the left ventricular epicardial surface, this ECG shows a right bundle branch block (RBBB) pattern of intraventricular conduction. If the pacemaker lead is placed on the anterolateral free wall of the left ventricle (LV apical lead placement is not used due to thinness of the tissue), depolarization begins in the left ventricle and sweeps medially (rightward) via intramuscular spread through the left ventricular free wall and interventricular septum to the right ventricle. Thus, right ventricular depolar-

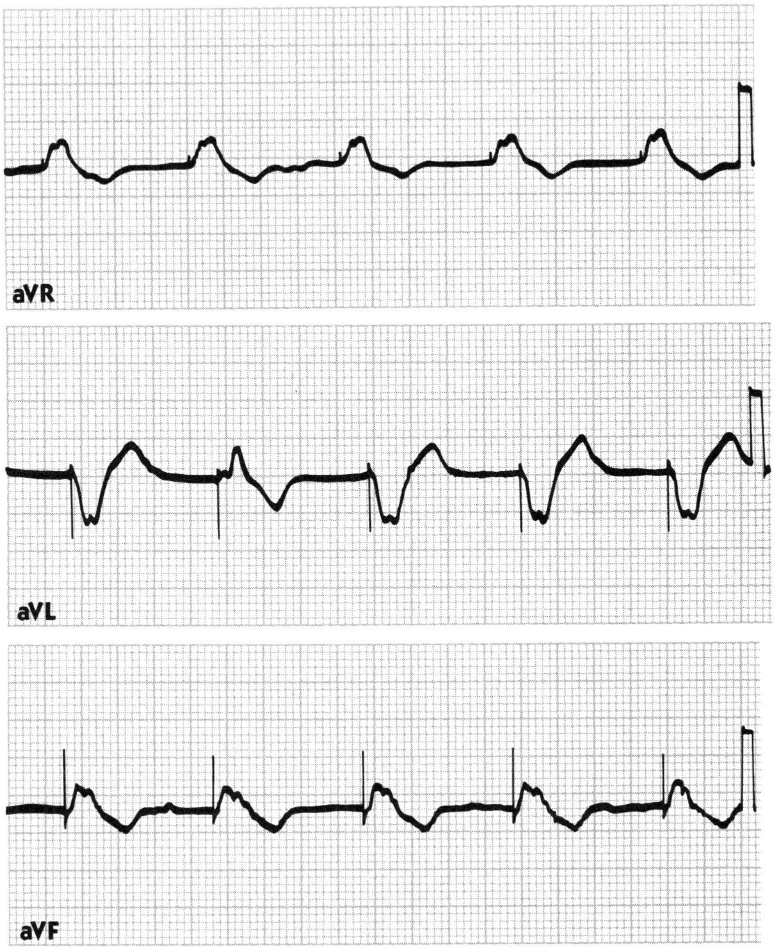

continued

ization is delayed, and an RBBB pattern is generated. Although right axis deviation does not occur in non-paced RBBB without an underlying reason—such as right ventricular hypertrophy or left posterior fascicular block (see Cases 12 and 19)—its occurrence in pacemaker-caused RBBB patterns may be understood, since both initial and net QRS vectors are directed rightward.

Because depolarization of both left and right ventricles is abnormal, it is not possible to diagnose right ventricular hypertrophy, left posterior fascicular block, or lateral wall myocardial infarction from the ECG alone in patients with pacemaker-generated RBBB patterns.

CASE 23 *(continued)*

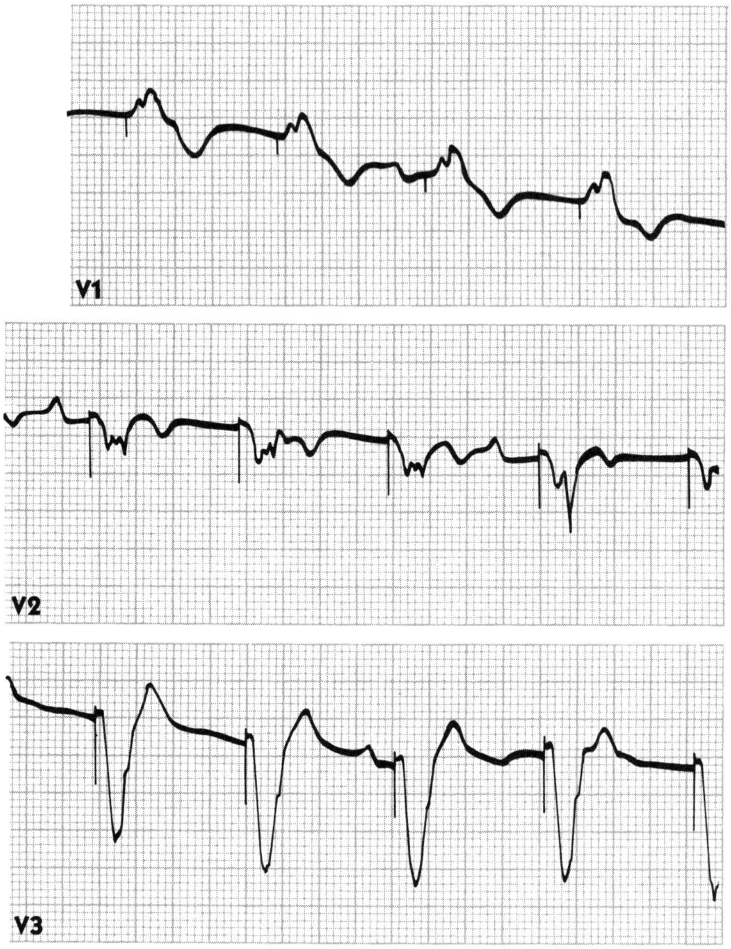

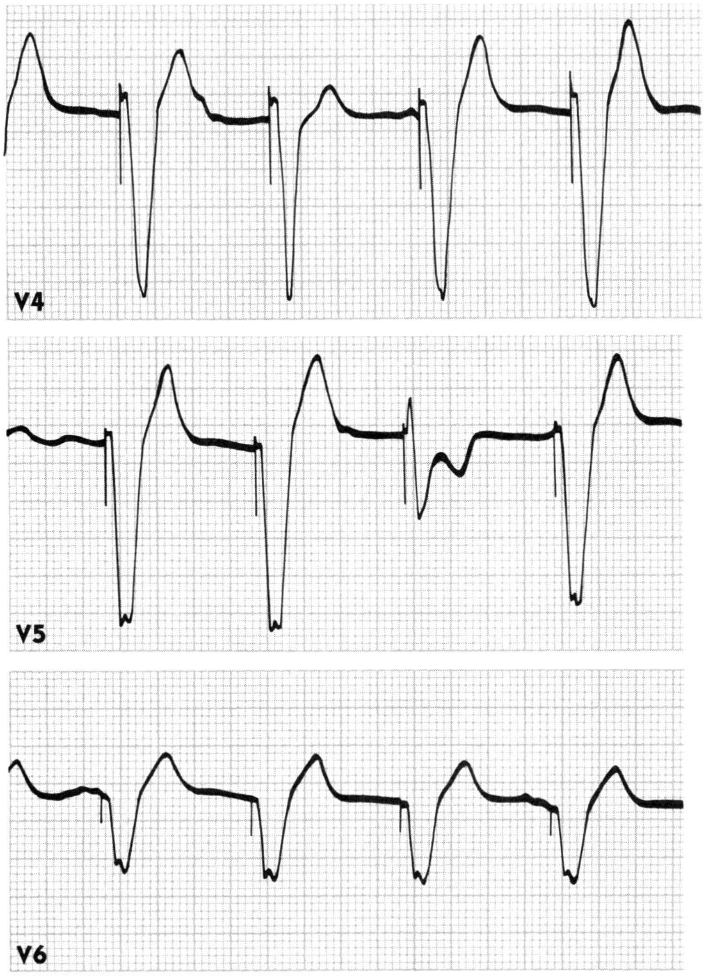
V4
V5
V6

SECTION IV

Myocardial Infarction and Ischemia

CASE 24A

Anterior Wall Myocardial Infarction

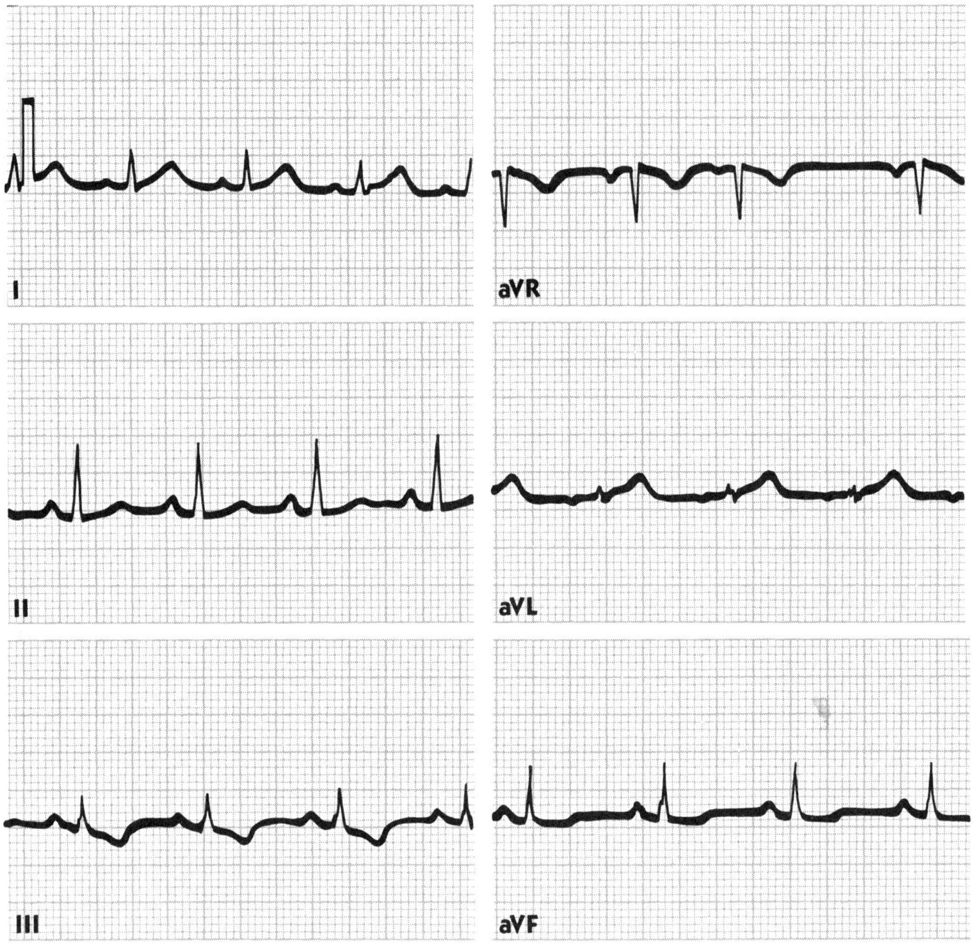

This 31-year-old man with hypercholesterolemia was admitted with severe substernal chest discomfort of several hours' duration. His ECG shows sinus rhythm, normal intervals, and a normal mean frontal plane QRS axis. The QRS complexes are unremarkable. Considerable ST segment elevation and abnormally tall (over 5 mm) T waves are present in the anterior precordial leads V1-5. The ST segment is elevated 1 mm in leads aVL and V6 and depressed slightly in lead aVF. The T wave is inverted in leads III and aVF.

These ECG abnormalities represent acute myocardial infarction (MI) or transmural ischemia (usually due to coronary artery spasm). During the early stages of MI, tall, peaked ("hyperacute") T wave abnormalities occur, rapidly followed by ST segment elevation resulting from a current of injury generated by damaged myocardium. As cell death occurs, myocardial electrical activity ceases and the classic Q waves of transmural MI develop in the involved areas.

The genesis of Q waves can be elucidated by this theoretical image: In a symmetrically and simultaneously depolarizing cylinder, all vectors point outward, perpendicular to the cylinder's surface. If any portion of the cylinder is removed, the forces on the opposite side will be unopposed and the net dipole will move in that direction. For example, in anterior wall MI, the loss of anterior myocardial tissue leaves posterior forces unopposed; thus the net dipole is directed posteriorly, away from the anterior leads. This causes loss of R waves anteriorly and inscription of Q waves. Further evolution of the MI produces eventual resolution of the ST elevation accompanied by developing T wave inversion.

The above Q wave process is similar in anterior, inferior, and lateral wall MI; however, posterior wall MI results in "reciprocal" changes (prominent R

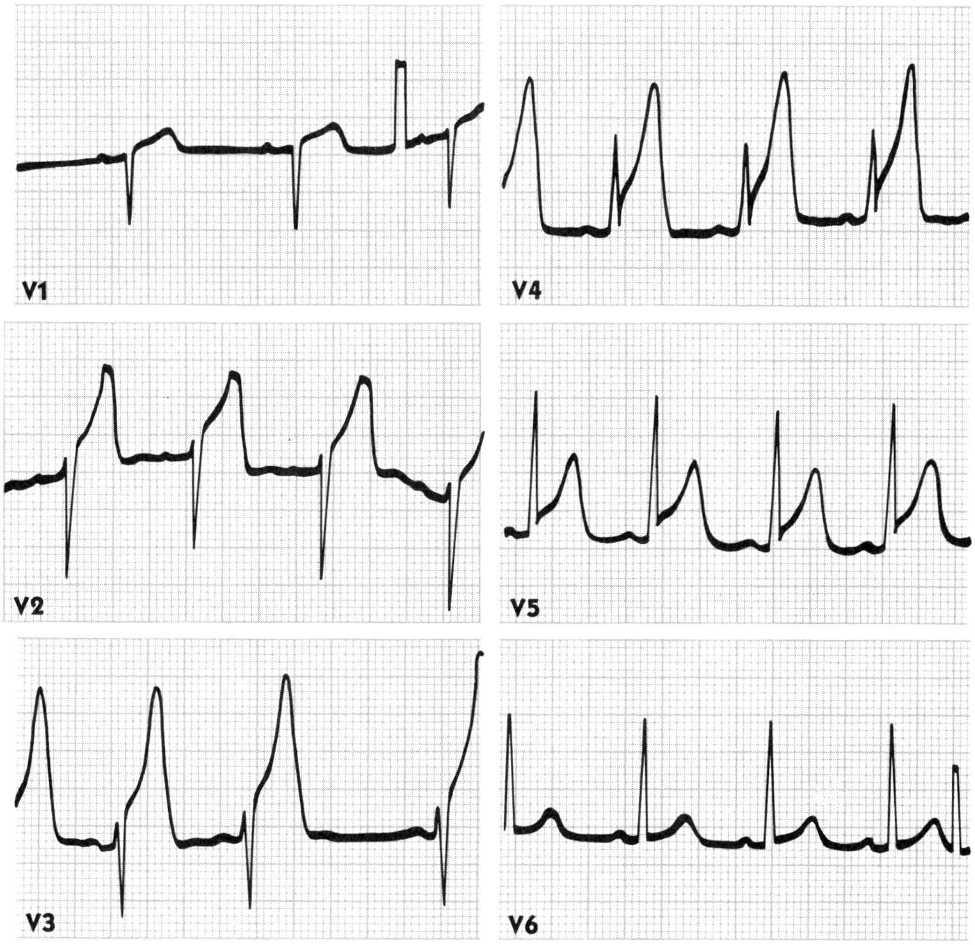

waves) in the anterior precordial leads, since the routine 12-lead ECG does not "see" the posterior wall (see Case 28). Posterior leads V7-10 may be used to assess posterior wall forces.

In this ECG, the acuteness of the MI can be ascertained from the marked ST segment elevation with hyperacute T waves. Neither Q waves nor T wave inversion, which generally appear hours to days after the acute event, are present in the anterior leads at this time.

ST segment elevation can be seen in normal individuals with early repolarization (see Case 61), as well as in patients with several different types of cardiac conditions, notably pericarditis (see Cases 40 and 42). The following specific ST segment abnormalities suggest MI: upward convexity; elevation exceeding 5 mm; obscuration of the terminal portion of the QRS complex by the elevated ST segment; prolongation of the QT interval; simultaneous ST segment elevation and inverted or hyperacute T waves; confinement of the abnormalities to a specific area of coronary artery perfusion; and reciprocal changes in opposing leads.

The differential diagnosis of reciprocal ST changes (ST segment depression and elevation appearing in opposite leads) includes a second area of ischemia or infarction. The diagnosis cannot be made from the ECG alone; an independent test, such as myocardial scintigraphy, is also necessary.

CASE 24B

Evolution of Anterior Wall MI

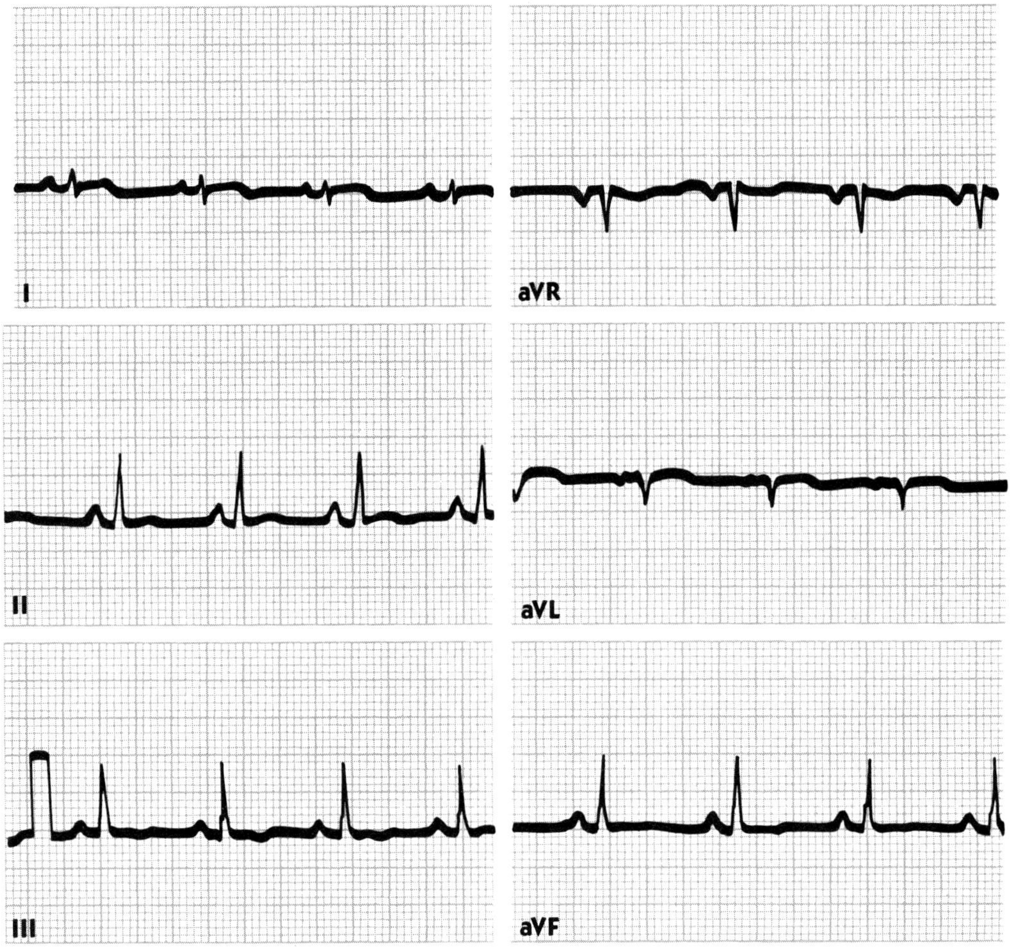

This ECG was recorded from the patient in Case 24A, one day later. The mean frontal plane QRS axis is now about +90°, due to loss of lateral forces. The QT interval (0.36 second) is slightly prolonged for the heart rate. ST segment elevation is still present in leads V1-5, but T wave inversions have replaced the hyperacute T waves in those leads. In leads III and aVF, the T wave inversion has partially resolved. There is loss of R wave amplitude in the anterior precordial leads, but Q waves have not yet developed.

The development of Q waves on the surface ECG is not mandatory for the diagnosis of transmural MI. Depending on the amount of myocardium lost and the magnitude of unopposed posterior forces, the initial anterior vector can be either diminished (with resultant poor R wave progression across the precordial leads) or completely absent (with resultant QS complexes).

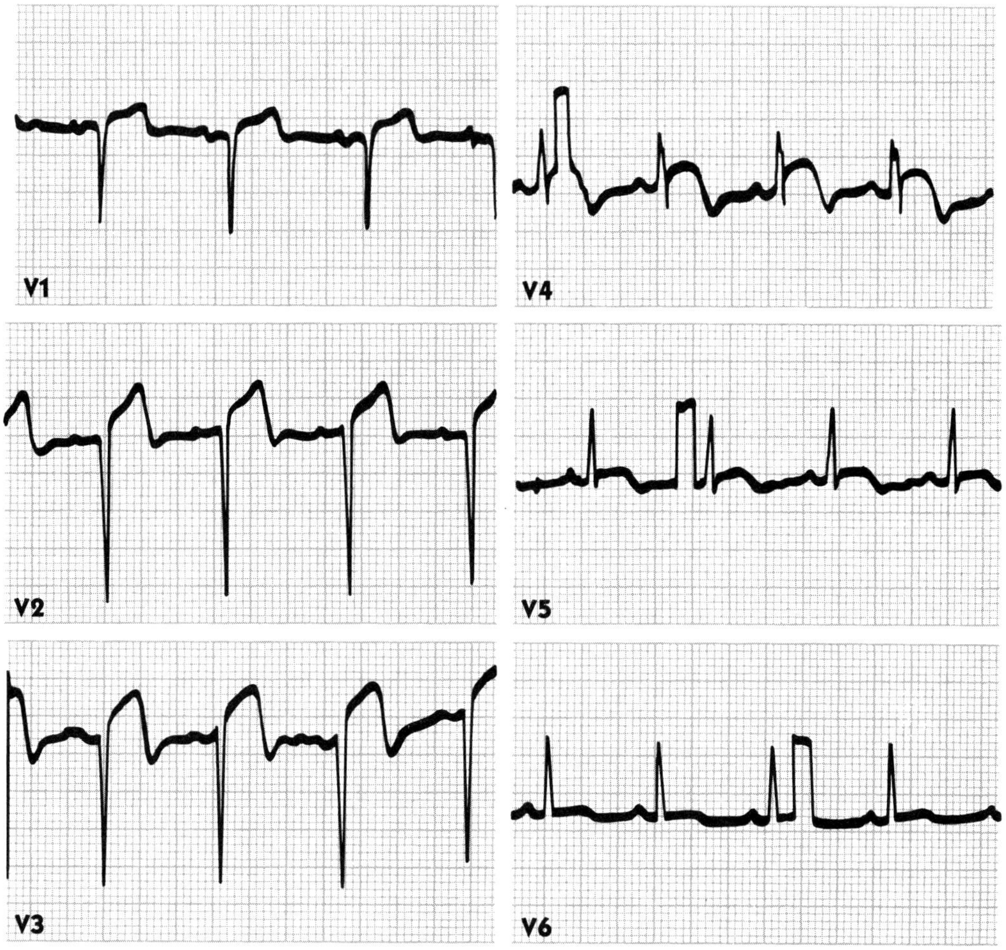

Poor R wave progression can appear in a number of other situations, including overly high placement of the precordial leads, left ventricular hypertrophy, and chronic obstructive pulmonary disease with hyperinflation of the chest (see Table 2 in the Appendix). Thus, this finding alone is not diagnostic or even suggestive of anterior wall MI unless serial ECG changes or accompanying ST-T abnormalities compatible with MI are present.

CASE 24C

Continued Evolution of Anterior Wall MI

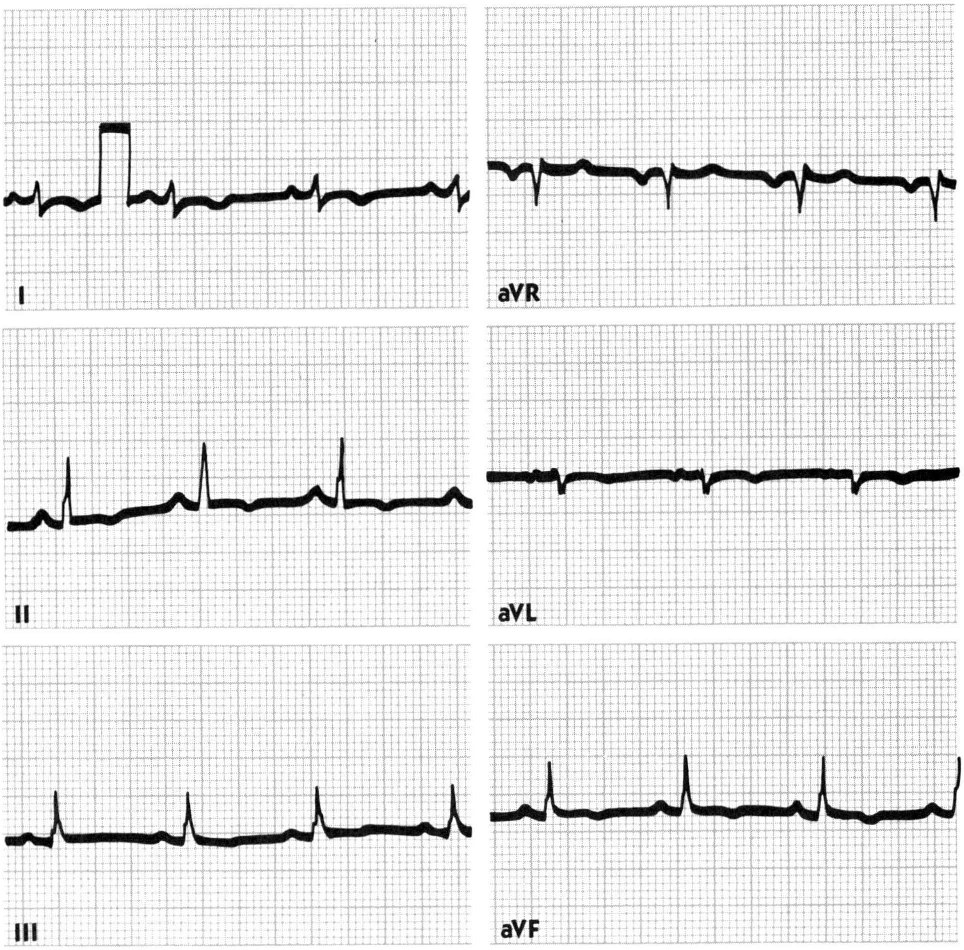

This ECG was recorded from the same patient two weeks later. ST segment elevation is still present in leads V1-2 but is now resolved in V3-5. The T waves are deeply inverted across the precordial leads V2-6. A QS complex has developed in lead V1, with small r waves in leads V2-3 and marked R wave loss in V4. Minimal changes in the inferior leads persist.

Evolution of the anterior MI has been characterized by (1) the acute stage, with marked ST segment elevation and hyperacute T waves; (2) the intermediate stage, with continuing ST segment elevation but of lesser degree, T wave inversion, and loss of R wave amplitude; and (3) the later stage, with deepening T wave inversion and development of Q waves.

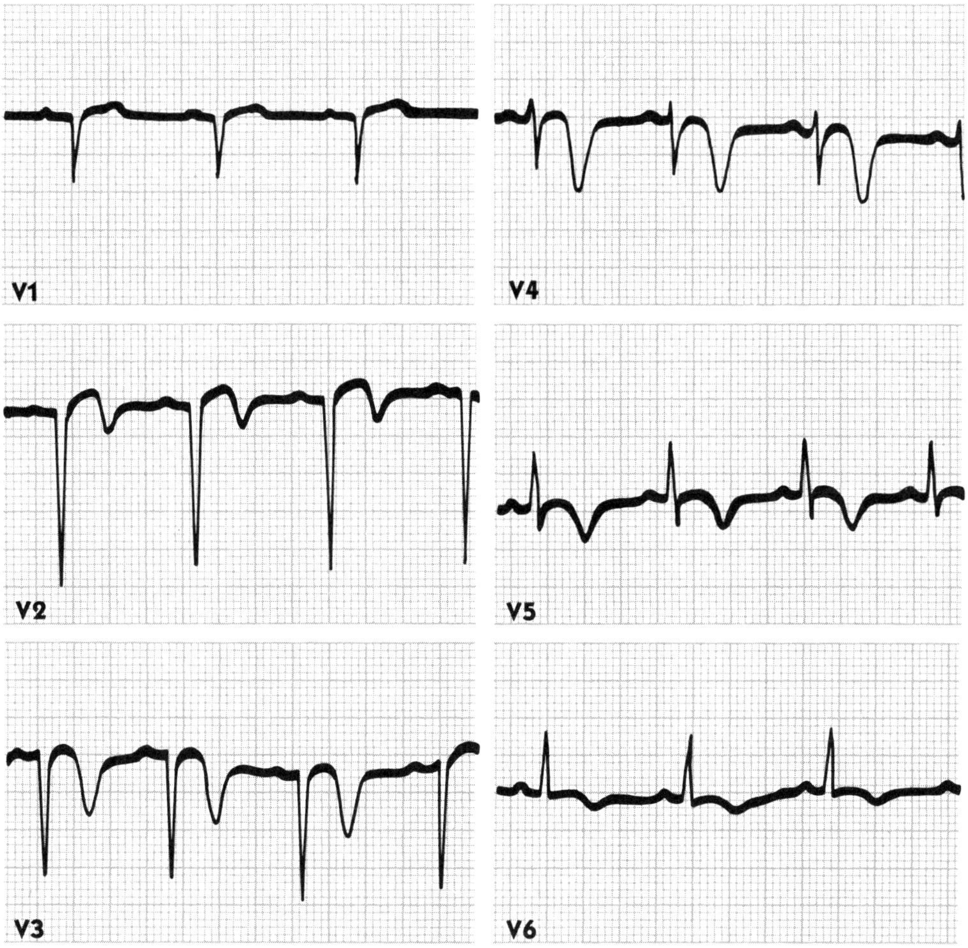
V1
V4
V2
V5
V3
V6

CASE 24D

Remote Anterior Wall MI

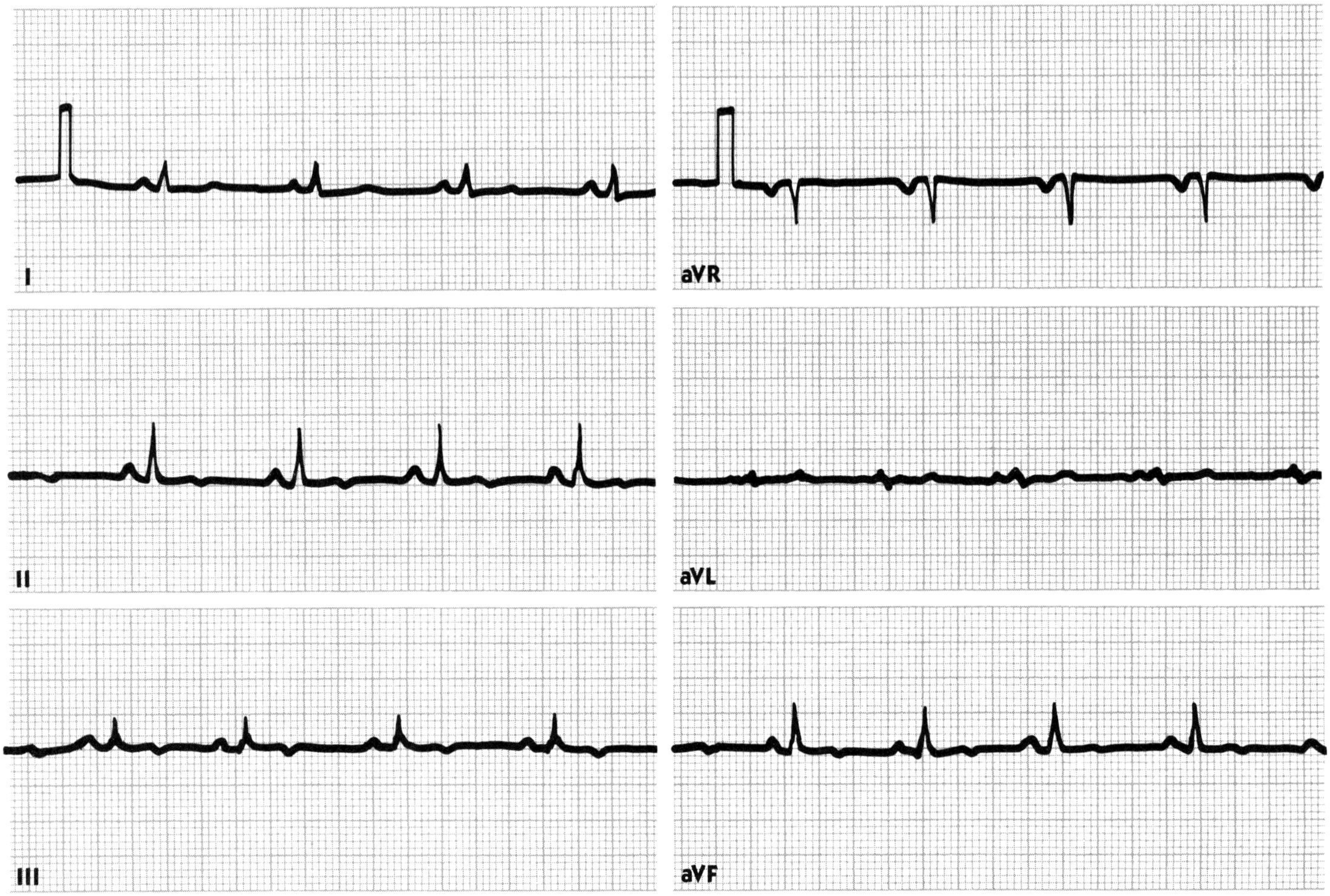

The final ECG in this series was recorded five years later. The ST segment elevation has resolved virtually completely, and the deep T wave inversion is no longer present. Anterior and lateral wall forces have been regained (note the mean frontal plane QRS axis of +60° and the absence of QS complexes, except in lead V1). T wave abnormalities persist, but are no longer specific for past MI (unless the evolutionary history is known). In fact, if this ECG were the sole available tracing from this patient, anterior wall MI would not be diagnosable.

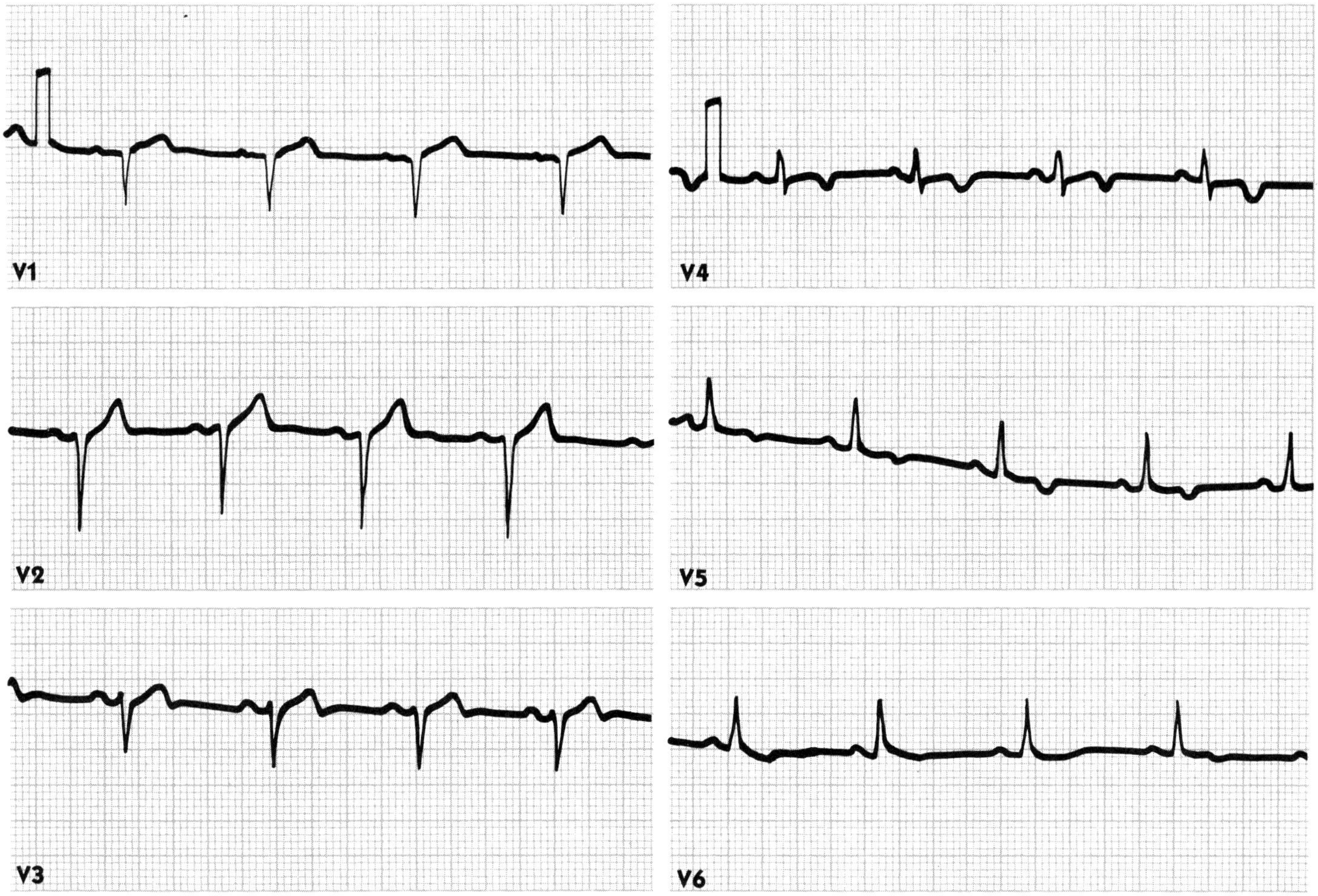
V1
V2
V3
V4
V5
V6

CASE 25

Remote Anterolateral Wall Myocardial Infarction With Left Atrial Abnormality

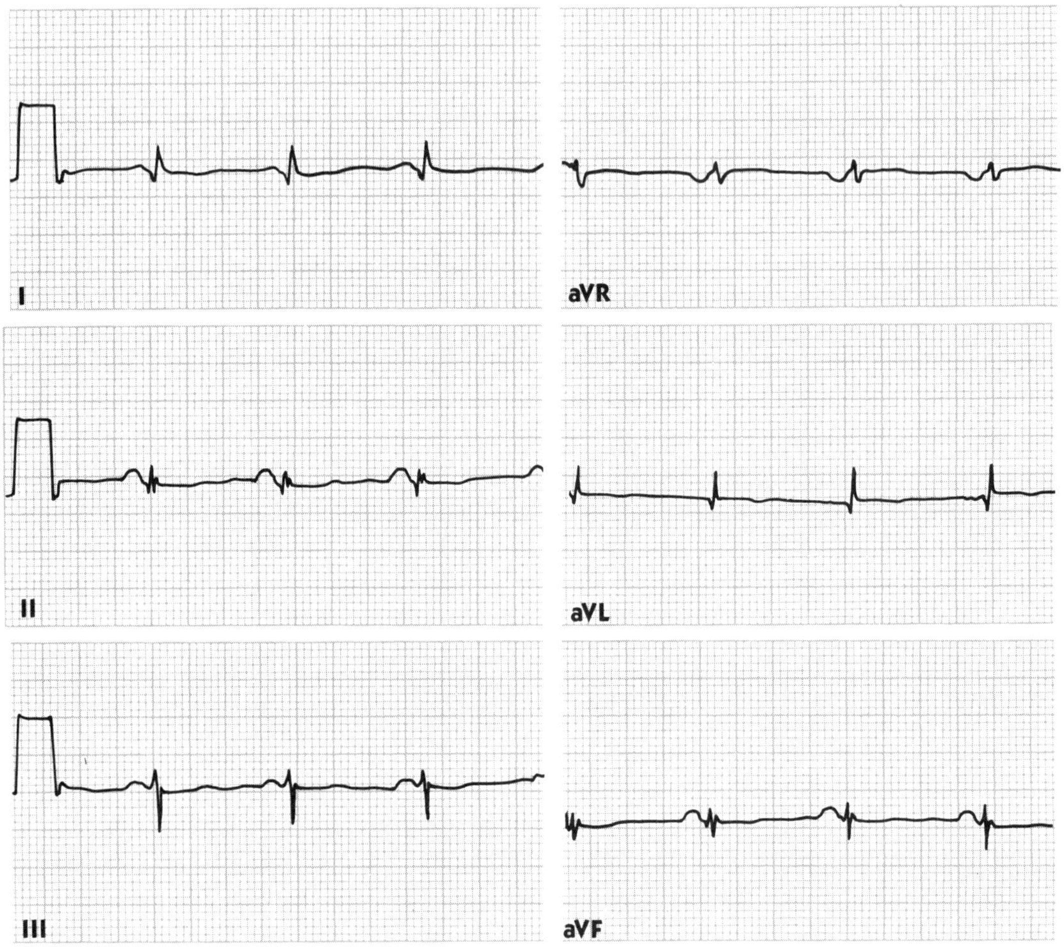

This 38-year-old man has congestive heart failure and a history of a myocardial infarction (MI) two years previously. The ECG shows normal intervals and a mean frontal plane QRS axis of 0°. In lead II, the P wave is 0.12 second wide; in lead V1, it has a deep and wide terminal negative component, compatible with left atrial abnormality (LAA) (see Case 9). There are significant Q waves in leads I, II, aVL, V5, and V6 and QS complexes in leads V1-4. The T waves are flattened inferiorly and laterally.

Deep Q waves in the lateral and anterior leads without acute ST segment changes suggest past anterolateral MI. However, any process causing destruction of myocardium, such as cardiomyopathy, can result in similar ECG findings. With loss of anterior and lateral myocardium, the depolarization forces from the right and inferoposterior portions

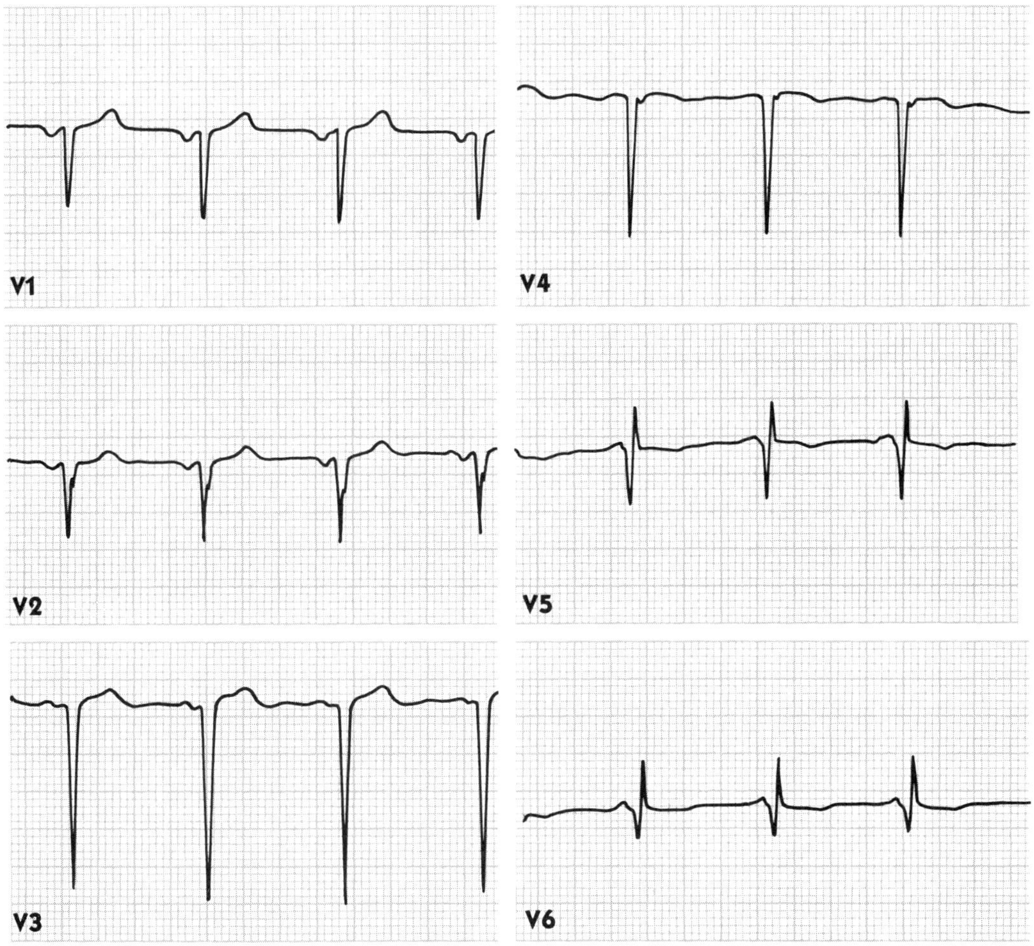

of the heart are unopposed. Consequently, the surface ECG "sees" the initial dipole directed posteriorly and slightly rightward, and deep initial Q waves are inscribed anteriorly and laterally. The terminal lateral forces reflected in the anterolateral terminal R waves are generated by the remainder of the left lateral ventricular free wall.

This patient has severe congestive heart failure as a result of his past MI; thus, his LAA pattern is more likely related to an intra-atrial conduction delay caused by left atrial dilatation than by left atrial hypertrophy. Treatment of left ventricular failure will often result in normalization of the LAA pattern.

CASE 26A

Inferior Wall Myocardial Infarction

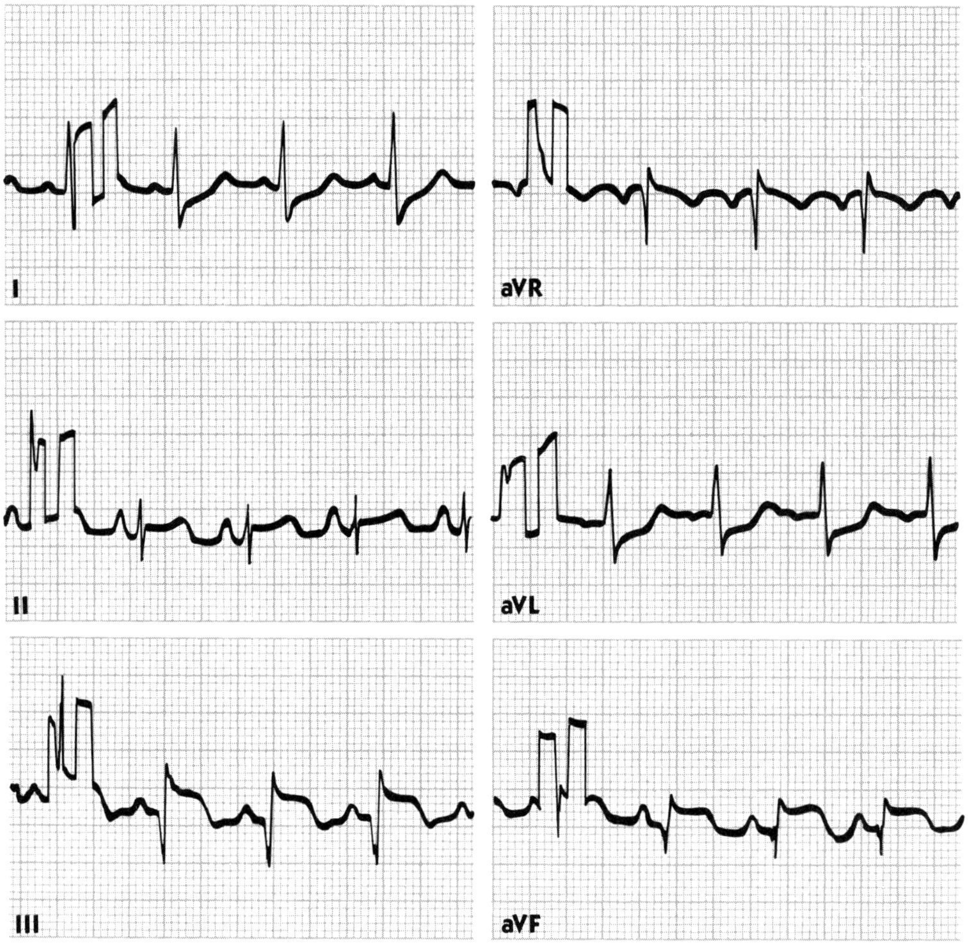

This 36-year-old woman developed severe substernal chest pain and was brought to the Emergency Room, where she suffered a cardiac arrest. Her post-resuscitation ECG, shown here, reveals sinus tachycardia, a mean frontal plane QRS axis of −20°, and a slightly prolonged QT interval of 0.36 second. There are deep Q waves in leads III and aVF. The ST segment is elevated 1-3 mm in leads II, III, and aVF; the 1-mm ST elevation in lead V1 has upward convexity. Slowly upsloping ST segment depression is present in leads I, aVL, and V3-4.

This patient has transmural inferior wall myocardial infarction (MI), with Q waves and ST segment elevation in the inferior leads. The Q waves reflect loss of myocardium inferiorly, and the ST segment changes reflect the injury current. Because hyperacute T waves are not present and Q waves have already evolved, the MI is probably minutes to hours old and most likely accounted for, rather than occurred during, the cardiac arrest.

The anterior and lateral ST segment depression could represent anterolateral wall ischemia occurring concomitantly with the MI or changes reciprocal to the inferior wall MI. Reciprocal ST depression, the inverse of acute ST elevation, appears in leads opposite to the MI. If the vector of the injury current is directed inferiorly, for instance, the inferior leads will show ST segment elevation. The injury current will thus be directed away from the anterior and/or high lateral leads, and these will show ST segment depression. In anterior MI, the injury current is directed anteriorly, inscribing ST segment elevation in the anterior leads, while the inferior leads record reciprocal ST segment depression.

Thus it is somewhat disconcerting to see ST segment elevation in lead V1 in this ECG, when ST

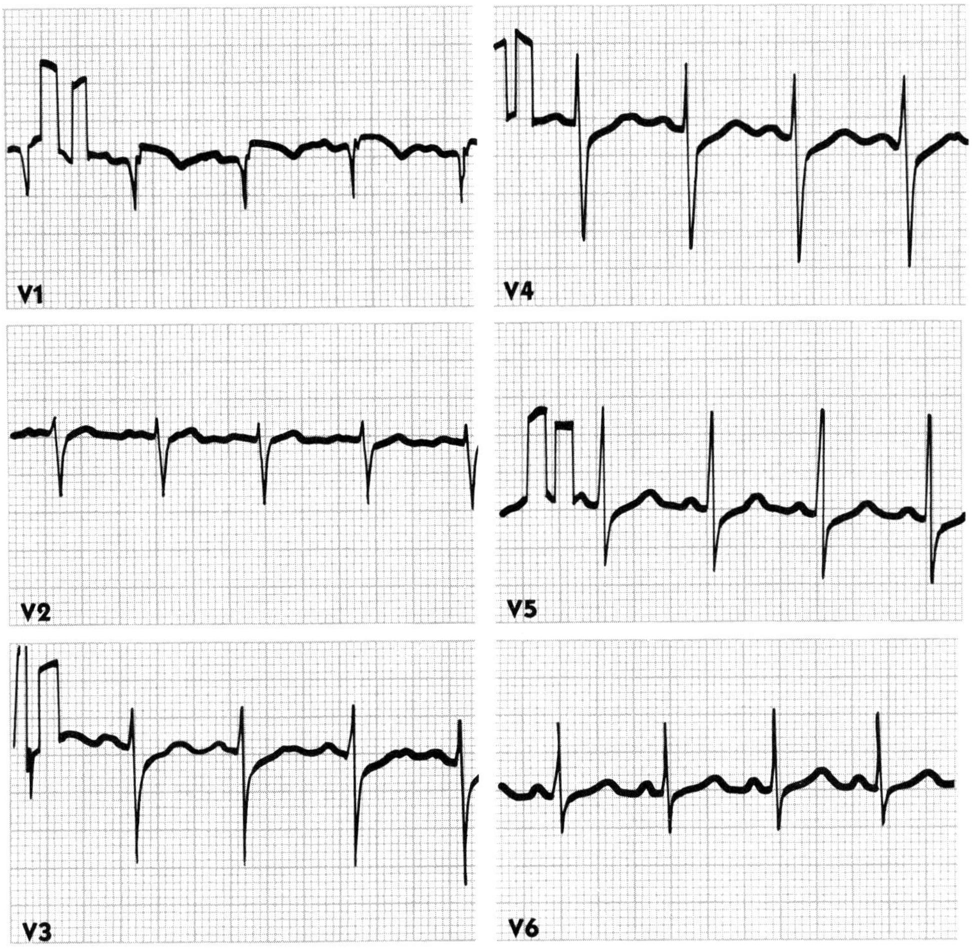

depression or a normal ST segment might be anticipated. This unexpected finding in lead V1 should raise the question of right ventricular MI (which could be confirmed with leads V3R and V4R) or septal MI.

CASE 26B

Evolution of Inferior Wall MI

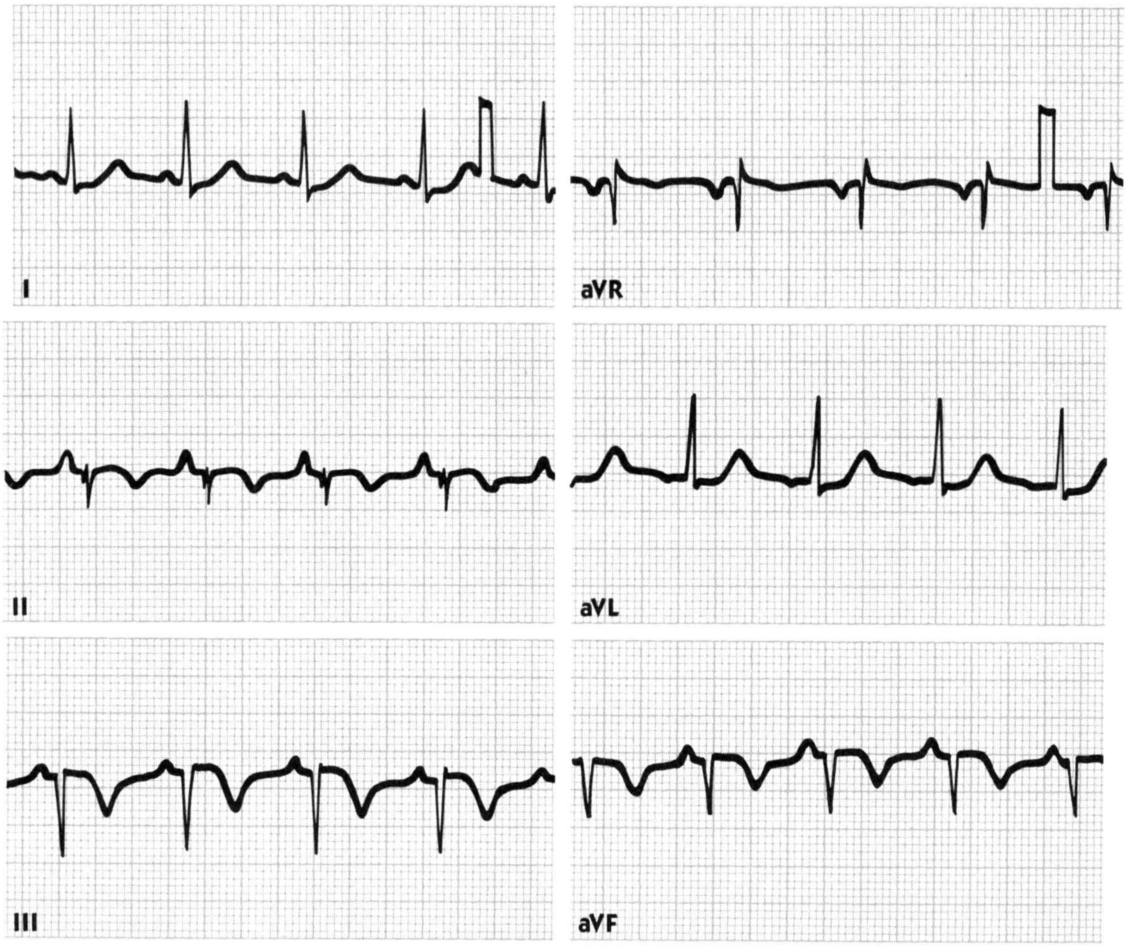

Two days later, this patient's ECG shows a leftward shift of the mean frontal plane QRS axis to −45°. Q waves now appear in leads II, III, and aVF, with associated T wave inversion and only minimal ST segment elevation. The lateral ST abnormalities have nearly resolved. These two ECGs illustrate the evolution of a transmural inferior wall MI.

With loss of inferior myocardium, the net dipole has shifted toward the remaining myocardium—anterior, superior, and lateral. The QRS vector is thus directed superiorly and leftward, causing abnormal left axis deviation. It is important to recognize that in transmural inferior wall MI, superior axis deviation is *not* due to conduction system disease involving the anterior fascicle of the left bundle branch (see Case 16). It actually results from loss of inferior forces due to the MI.

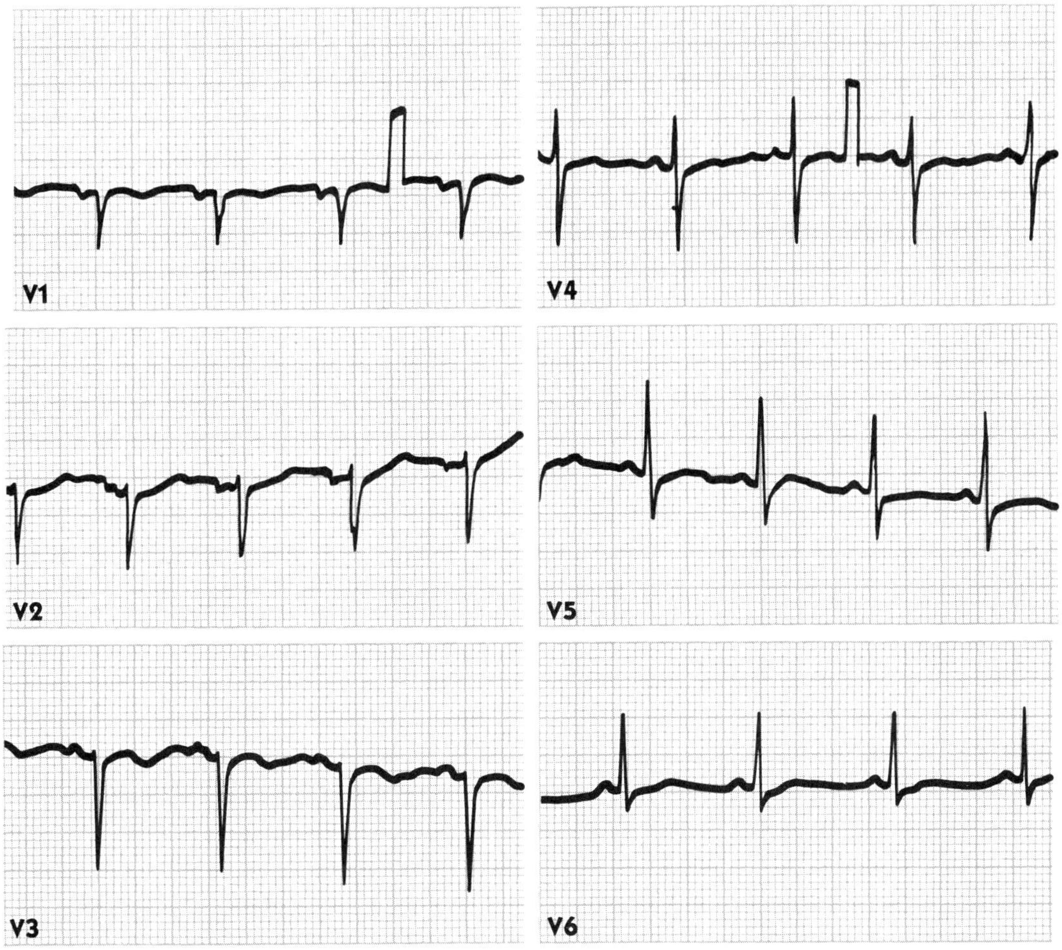
V1
V4
V2
V5
V3
V6

CASE 27

Inferior Wall Myocardial Infarction With Profound Anterolateral ST Segment Depression

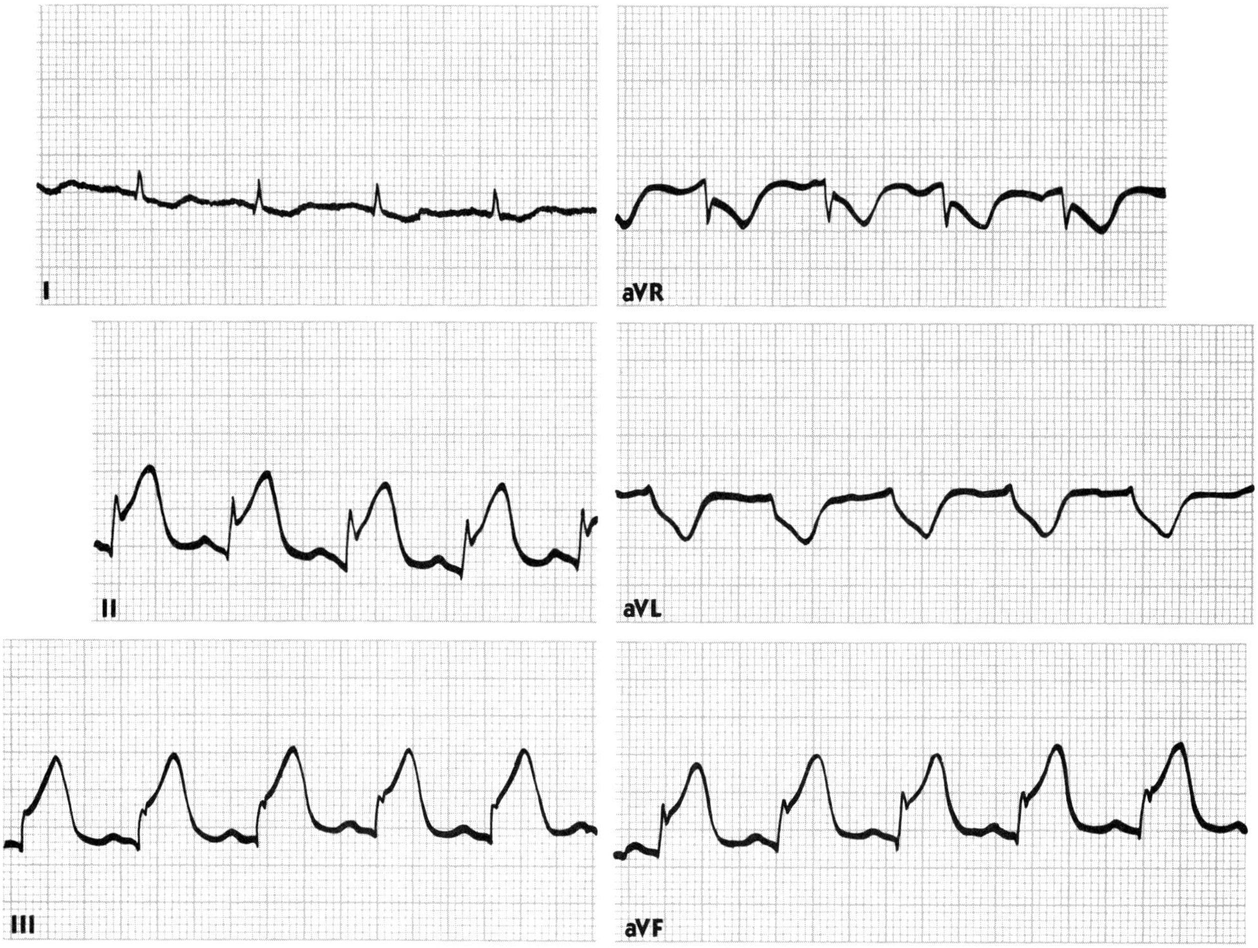

This 80-year-old man had 1½ hours of severe substernal chest pain, accompanied by diaphoresis, nausea, and palpitations. His ECG shows normal intervals and a normal mean frontal plane QRS axis. There are small q waves, considerable ST segment elevation, and tall T waves in leads II, III, and aVF. The ST elevation is so marked that the QRS complexes are partially obscured. All other leads show marked ST segment depression, with terminal upright T waves.

The ST segment elevation and tall T waves are compatible with acute transmural inferior wall myocardial infarction (MI) or coronary artery spasm (see Case 31). Despite the diffuse and marked ST segment depression in all but the inferior leads, reciprocal ST

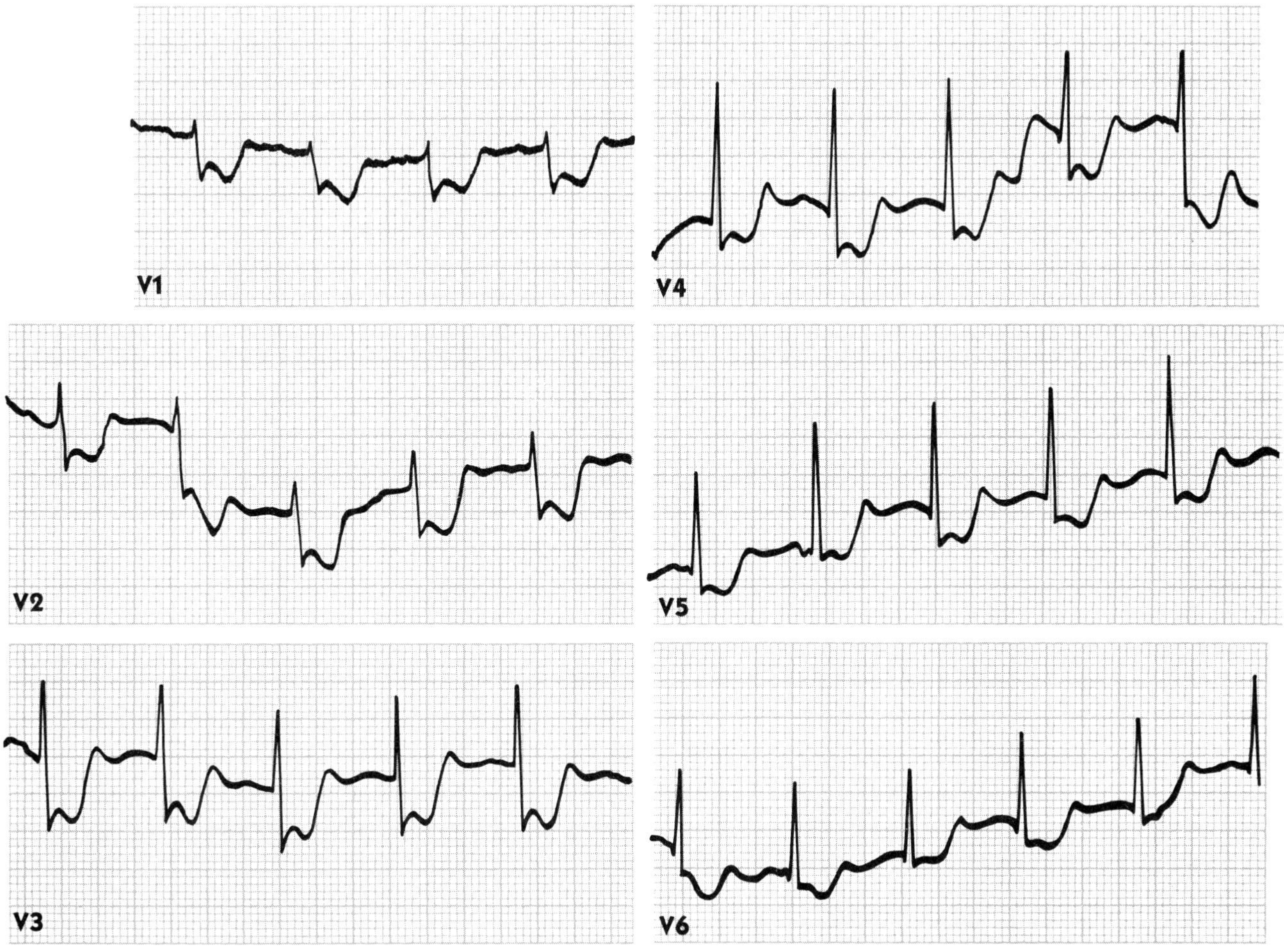

changes and diffuse ischemia cannot be differentiated with certainty from the ECG alone. While reciprocal ST changes generally involve ECG leads opposite to the MI, they are sometimes diffuse. Thus the differential diagnosis cannot be determined without independent clinical evidence.

CASE 28

Inferior and Posterior Wall Myocardial Infarction

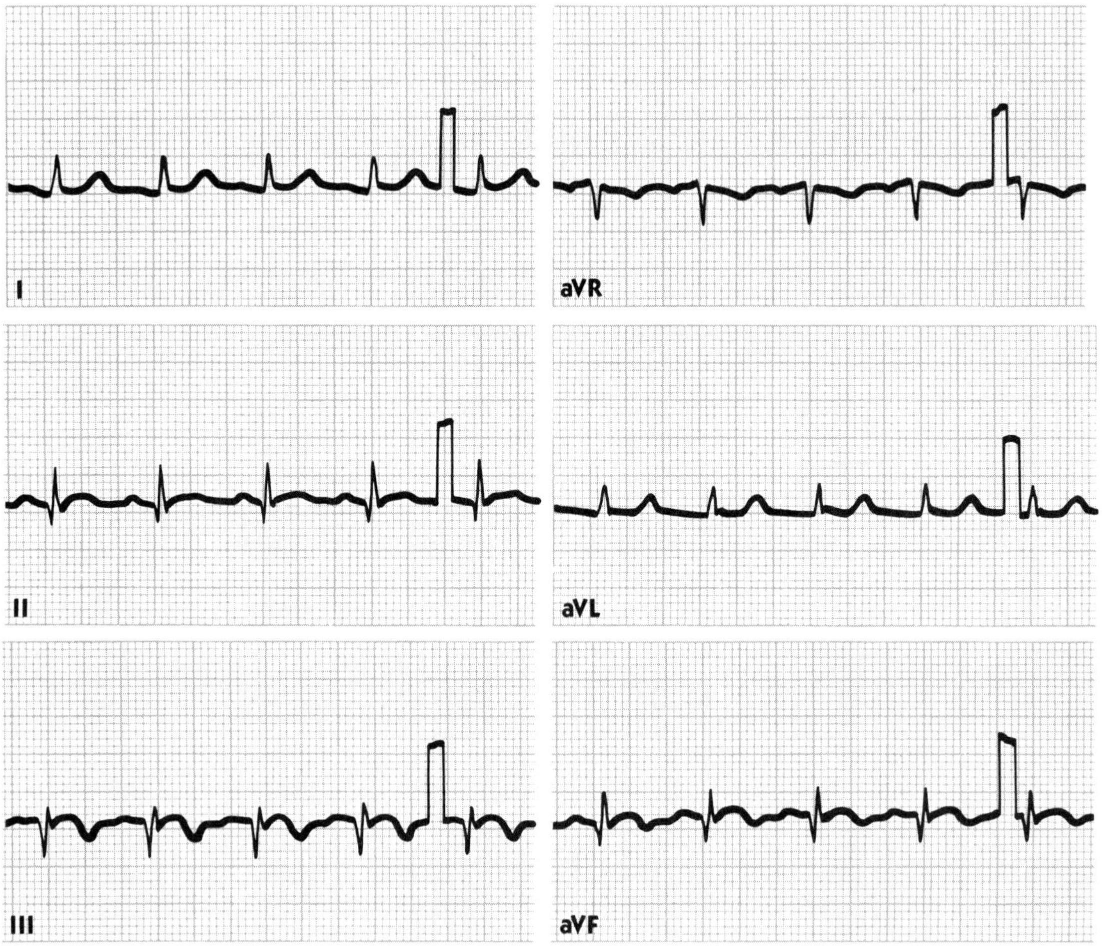

This patient presented to the Emergency Room with severe, prolonged chest pain. His ECG shows sinus rhythm and normal PR, QRS, and QT intervals. There are deep Q waves in leads II, III, and aVF, with associated ST segment elevation of upward convexity and T wave inversion. Tall R waves are seen in leads V1-2, with 3 mm of ST elevation and tall, peaked T waves in V2. Lead I shows slight ST segment elevation.

This patient has an acute inferior wall myocardial infarction (MI), with Q waves and ST elevation inferiorly. The dominant R wave in lead V1 and the pure R wave in lead V2 suggest concomitant posterior wall MI. This is not infrequently seen in conjunction with inferior and/or lateral wall MI, since all these areas lie in ventricular myocardium subserved by either the right or the left circumflex coronary artery.

Anterior R wave inscription in posterior MI is the inverse of Q wave inscription. Using the model of the depolarizing cylinder (see Case 24A), when posterior forces are lost, anterior forces are left unopposed, resulting in tall R waves in the anterior leads. Since the anterior precordial leads "see" the reciprocal changes of the posterior MI, ST segment depression (the reciprocal of ST elevation) would be expected. The isolated ST elevation in lead V2 is difficult to explain, but could represent septal MI or posterior wall myocardial ischemia seen reciprocally. The ST elevation in lead I probably represents lateral involvement in the infarction.

The differential diagnosis of prominent anterior R waves includes right ventricular hypertrophy (RVH) and Wolff-Parkinson-White conduction, type A (see

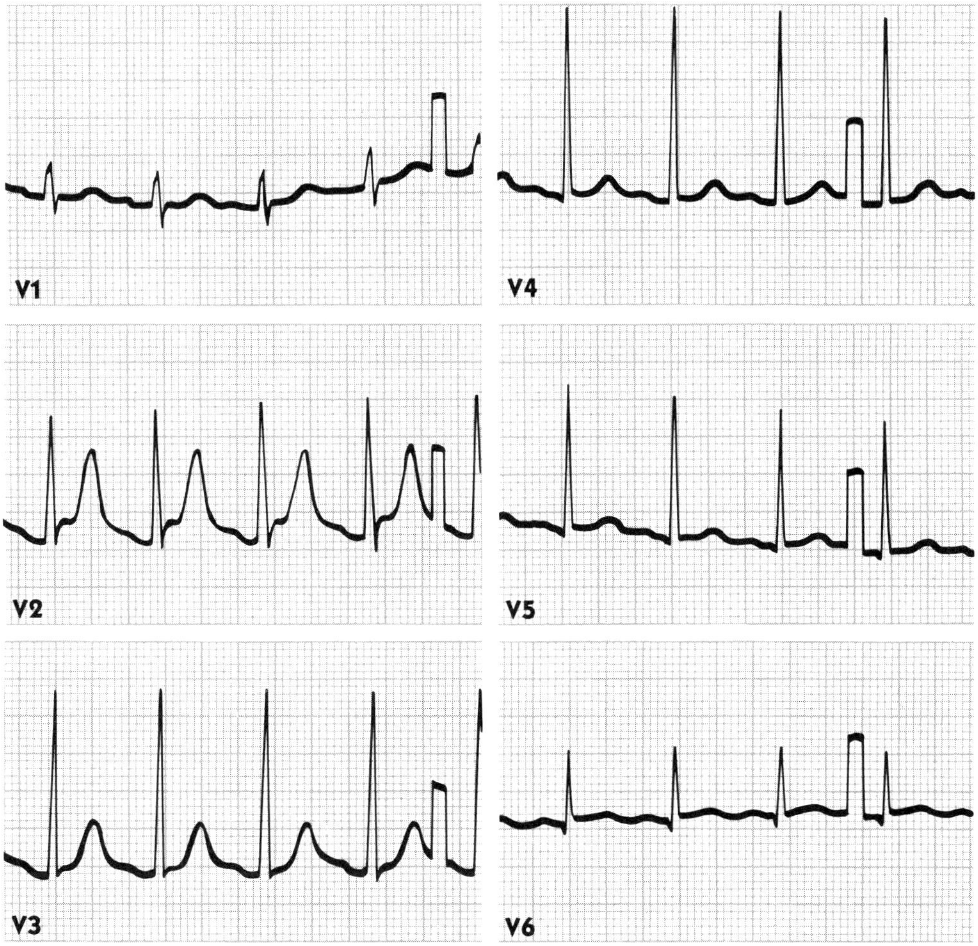

Cases 5, 6, and 34). The latter can usually be distinguished by the presence of a short PR interval and delta waves. The distinction from RVH can be more difficult; however, RVH is unlikely in the absence of rightward axis shift (see Table 3 in the Appendix). Other conditions that can produce prominent anterior forces (see Table 4) include normal variants, asymmetric septal hypertrophy (see Case 4), and certain forms of muscular dystrophy.

CASE 29

Acute Nontransmural Anterior Wall Myocardial Infarction

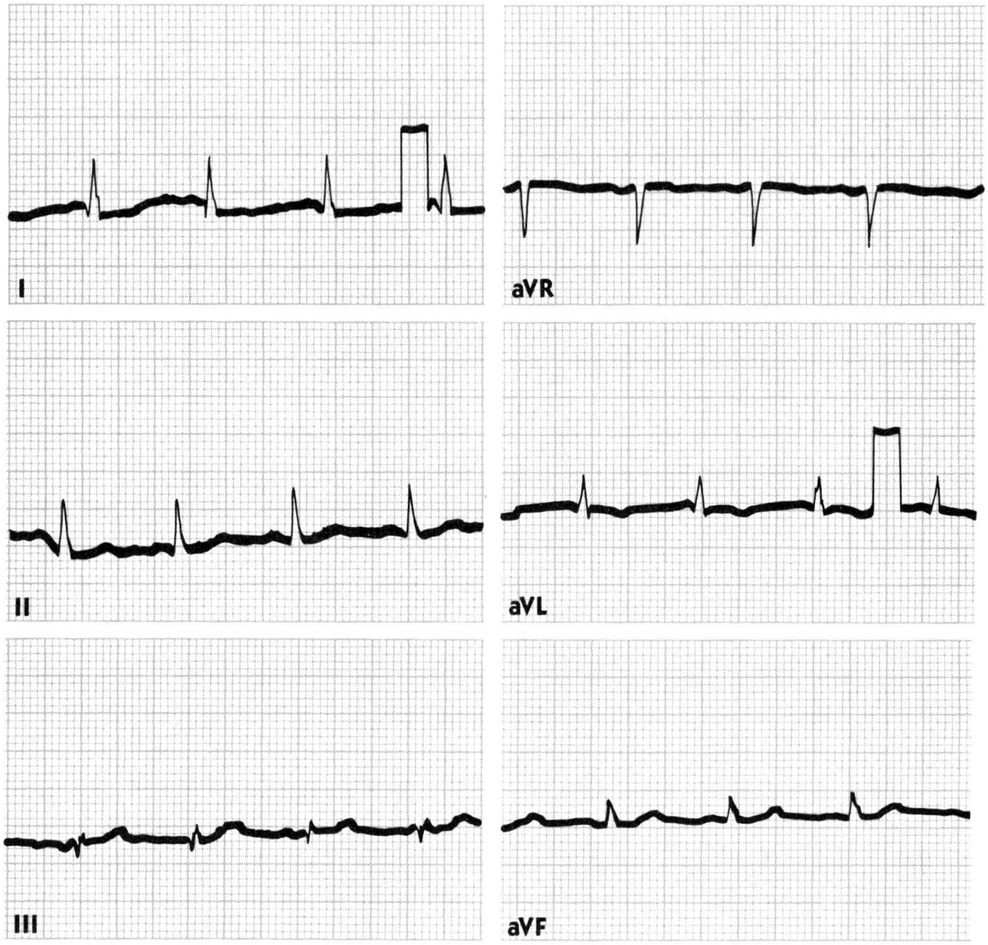

When this 64-year-old man was admitted with substernal chest pain, his ECG was normal. The ECG shown here, recorded on the following day, has a mean frontal plane QRS axis of +30° and normal PR and QRS intervals. The QT interval is 0.36 second, prolonged for the rate ($QT_C = 0.45$). The P waves are normal, and no pathological Q waves are present. However, the T waves are inverted in leads aVL and V1-4 and flat in lateral leads I and V5-6. There is J point depression of 1 mm in leads V3-4.

New symmetrical T wave inversions in a setting suggesting myocardial infarction (MI) are compatible with the diagnosis of nontransmural MI. During ventricular systole, blood flow is decreased to the subendocardial layers of the heart due to pressures generated in the left ventricle; thus, the subendocardium receives most of its blood supply during diastole. Further compromise in subendocardial blood flow can lead to ischemia and necrosis of the subendocardium.

Early work suggested that the subendocardium contributes little to the surface ECG; subendocardial MI was expected to subtract little from the QRS configuration and to produce no pathological Q waves. From the 1950s until recently, MIs without associated changes in QRS configuration were routinely labeled "subendocardial" or "nontransmural." However, newer data indicate that QRS changes are, in fact, present in many pathologically documented *non*transmural MIs. Conversely, a sizable proportion of pathologically documented transmural MIs have *no* associated QRS changes. Thus, the surface ECG cannot reliably distinguish between nontransmural and transmural MI; as an ECG finding, the distinction is misleading.

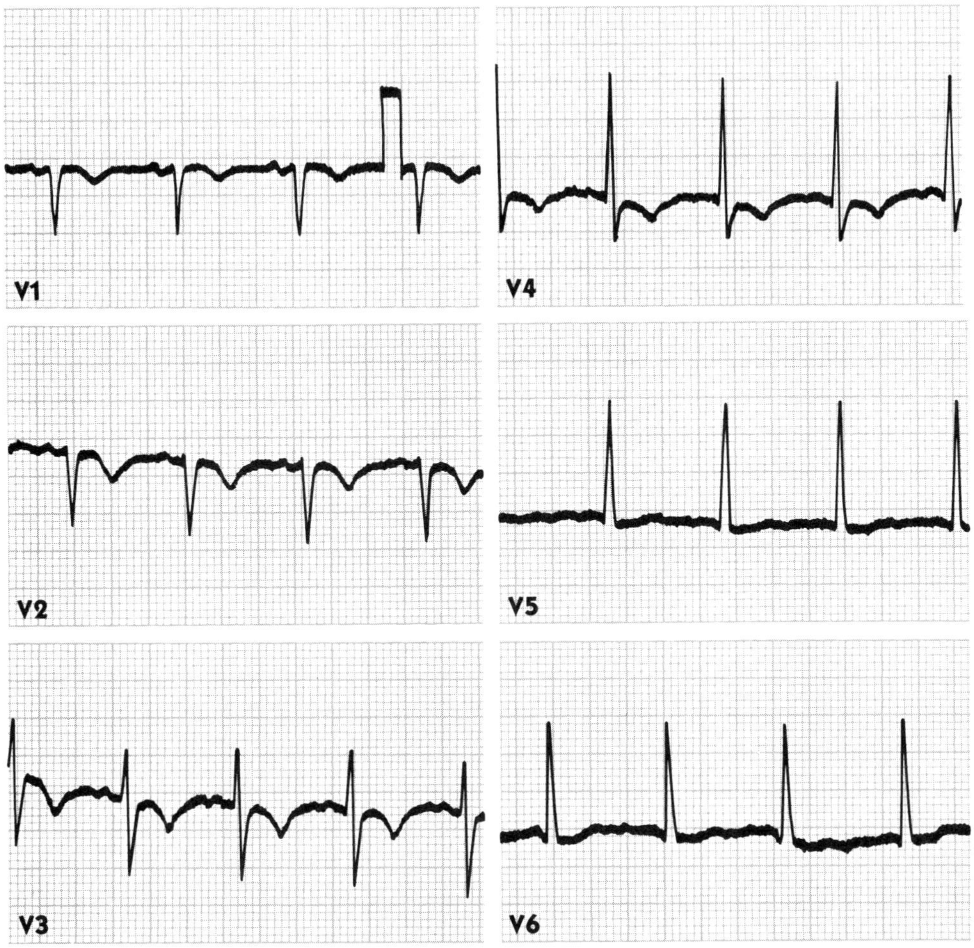

For the ECG diagnosis of nontransmural MI, four points must be kept in mind: (1) The T wave inversions must be new. Old MI can leave inverted T waves in the involved areas as its sole residuum (see Case 24D). (2) The T wave inversions must persist over time. Subendocardial ischemia without MI can lead to symmetrical T wave inversions during the ischemic episode, but these changes are reversible with resolution of the ischemia. (3) Other recognized causes of T wave abnormalities—such as hypertrophy, bundle branch block, pericarditis, and early repolarization—must be excluded (see Table 5 in the Appendix). (4) The clinical setting must always receive prime consideration. In this case, the initial ECG was normal, but the history of substernal chest pain prompted hospital admission. MI was subsequently documented by serial ECGs and enzyme studies.

CASE 30—A and B

Nontransmural Myocardial Ischemia

CASE 30A

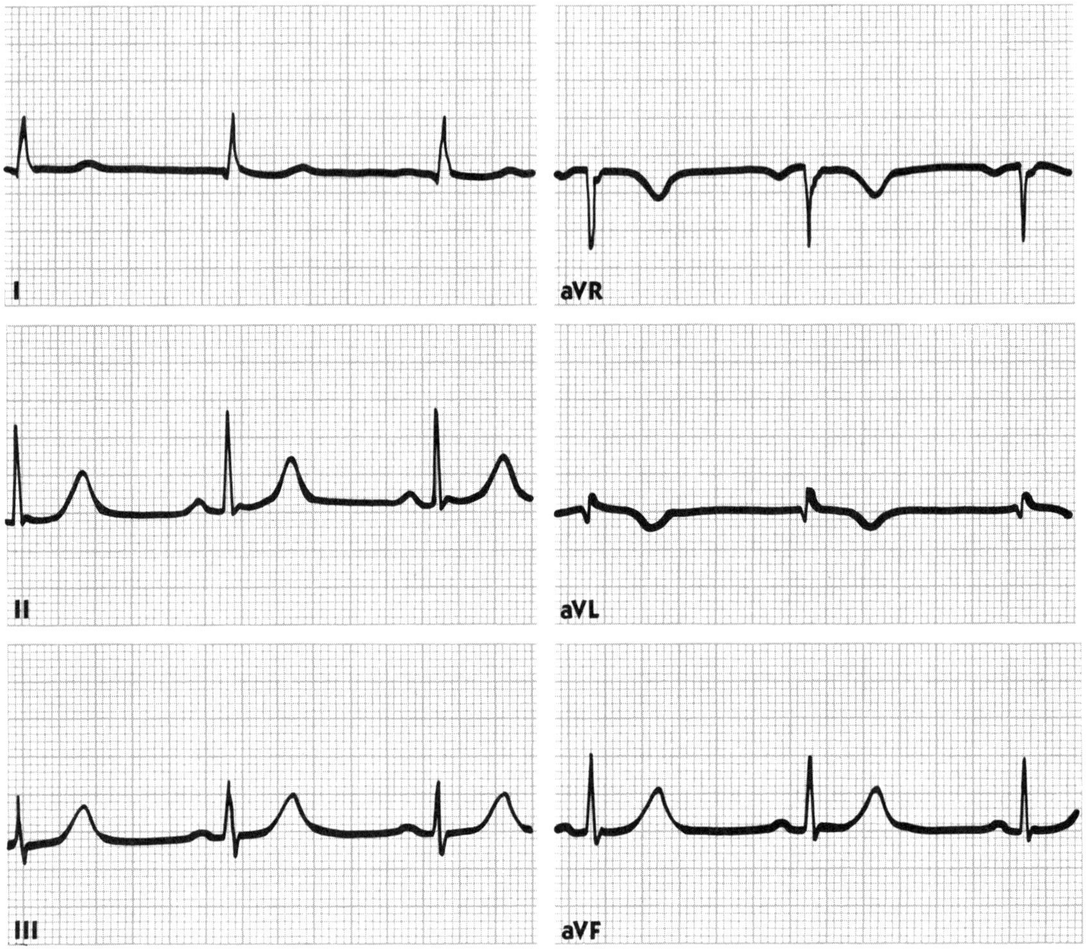

This case involves a patient with exertional angina of recent onset undergoing exercise testing to document coronary artery disease. His resting ECG (A) shows sinus rhythm, normal intervals, and a mean frontal plane QRS axis of +60°. A qR pattern with T wave inversion appears in lead aVL; isolated q waves confined to this lead probably reflect the transition zone of the QRS axis. In the patient's exercise ECG (B), recorded during chest pain, the QRS axis has shifted to −10°. Downsloping ST segment depression is present in leads II, III, aVF, and V3-6. There is mild ST segment elevation in lead aVL.

These two sets of tracings illustrate several ECG features of nontransmural myocardial ischemia. ST segment depression, either downsloping or horizontal, is suggestive of ischemia in the appropriate clinical setting. The ST depression may be isolated or accompanied by T wave inversion or peaking. (These T wave changes may also occur without ST depression; sometimes they are the sole manifestation of ischemia.) If the baseline ECG displays ST-T abnormalities, acute ischemia can "normalize" them, probably by vectorial cancellation (see Cases 14 and 32). The QT interval may be prolonged. Ischemia can occasionally cause transient alterations in intraventricular conduction, producing a shift of the mean frontal plane QRS axis (as in this case), as well as fascicular block and bundle branch block patterns. Transient loss of R wave amplitude is also sometimes seen.

Unfortunately, none of these ECG findings is specific for myocardial ischemia. However, these findings can strongly suggest ischemia if: (1) the clinical

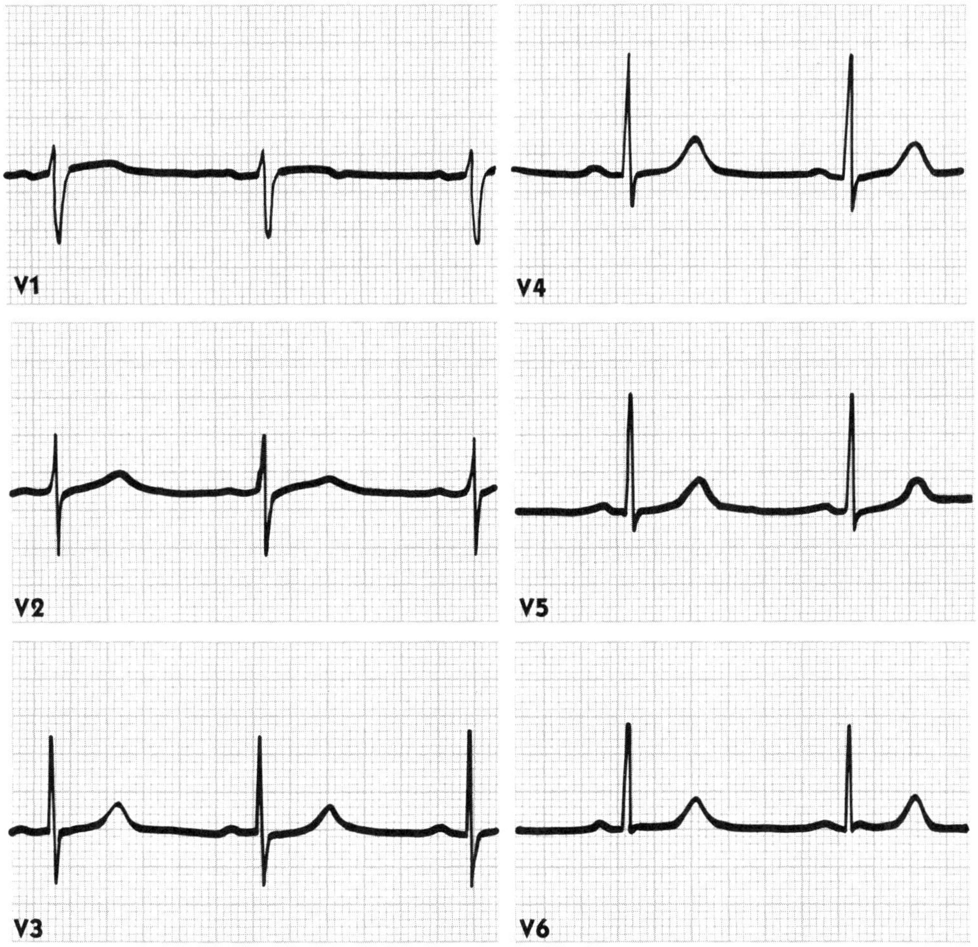

continued

setting is appropriate; (2) the abnormalities return to baseline after the acute event; and (3) the ST-T abnormalities cannot be explained by other possible causes of similar changes (see Table 5 in the Appendix).

CASE 30B

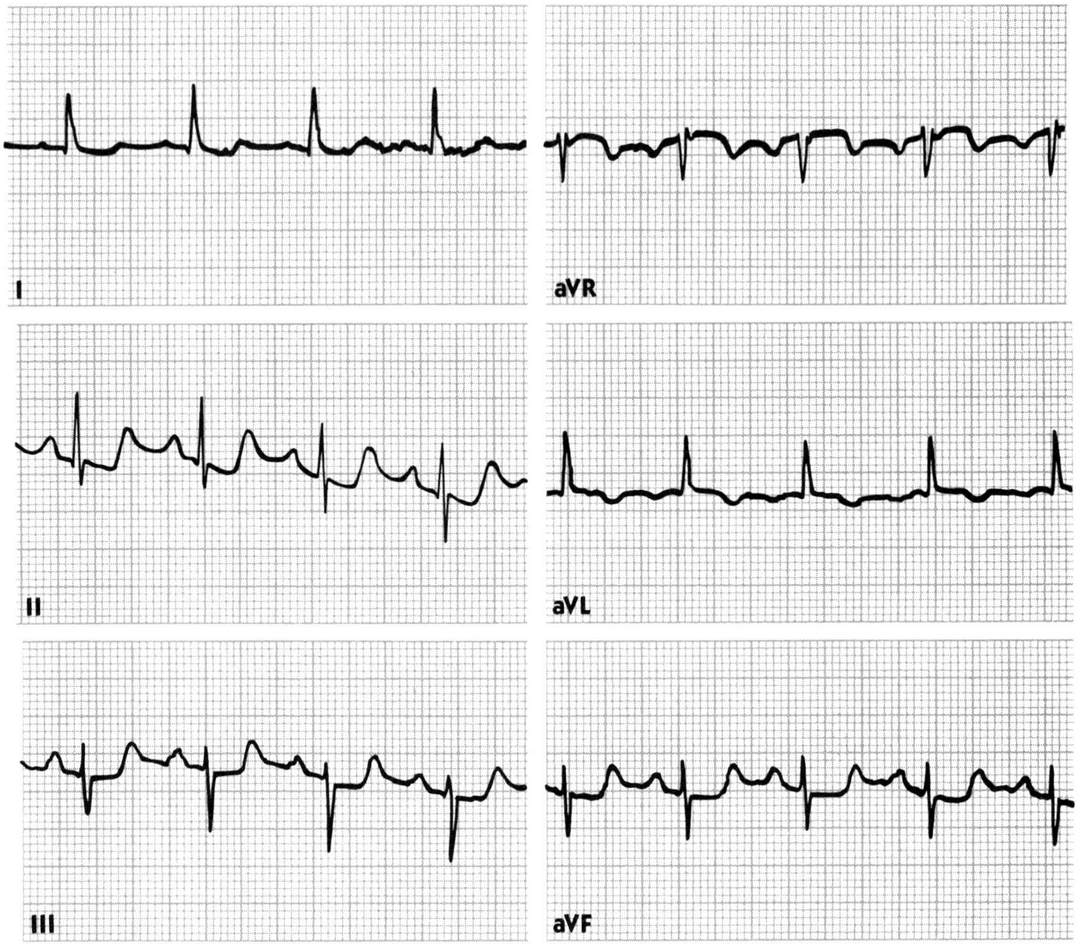

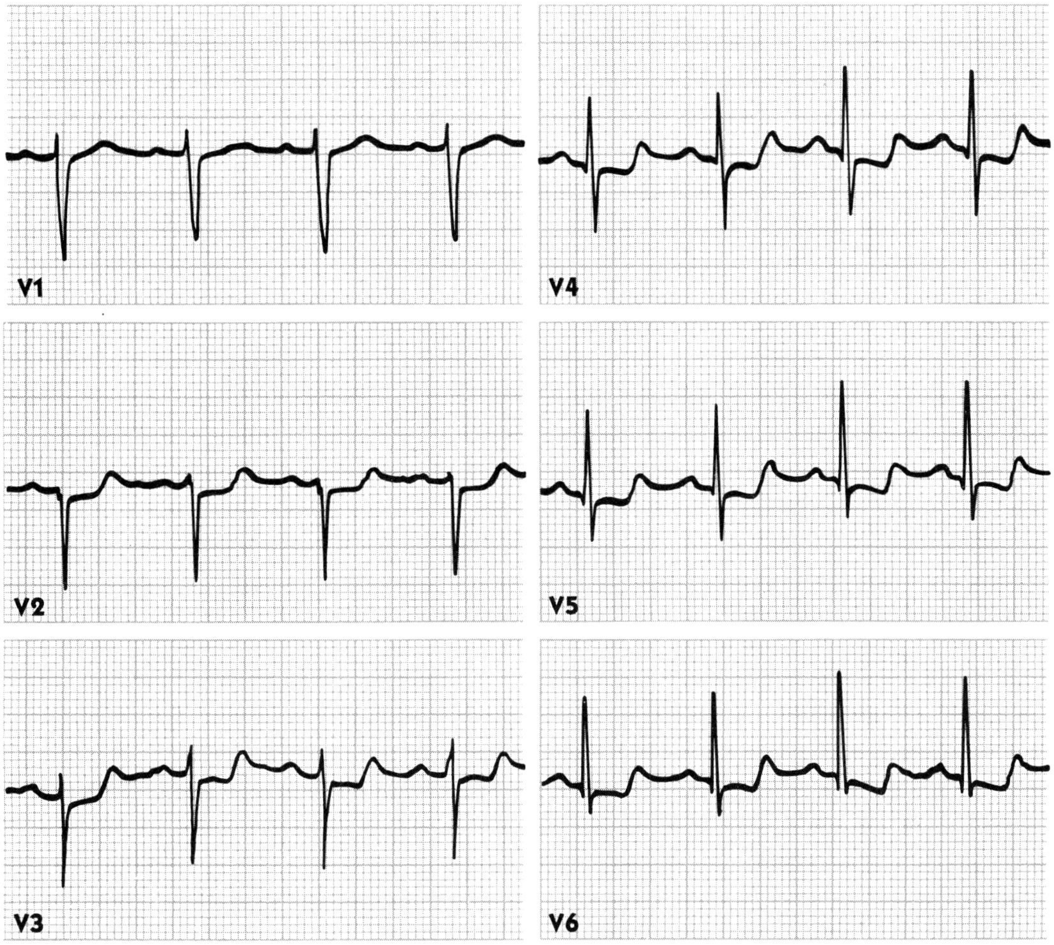
V1
V4
V2
V5
V3
V6

CASE 31—A and B

Transmural Myocardial Ischemia Due to Coronary Artery Spasm

CASE 31A

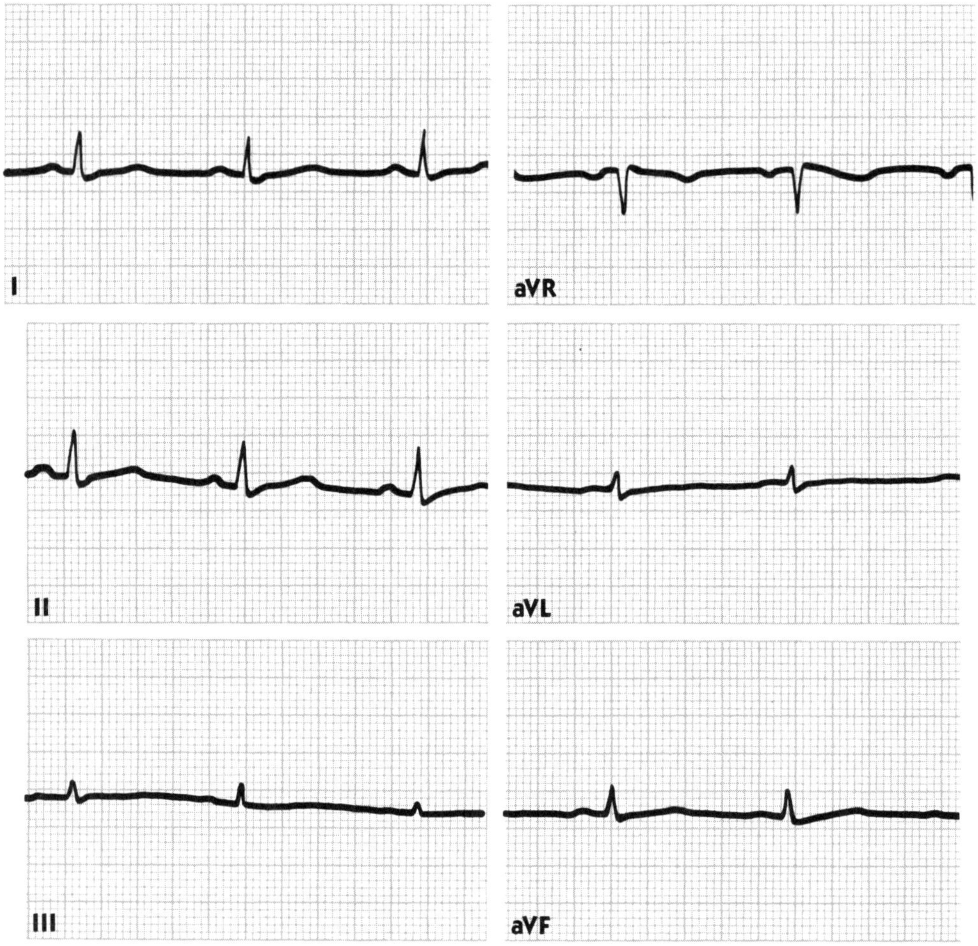

This 42-year-old man had angina at rest as well as during exertion. His admission ECG (A) is normal. Shortly after admission he developed severe chest pain at rest, and the second ECG (B) was recorded. It shows sinus rhythm, normal intervals, and a mean frontal plane QRS axis of +30°. The P wave and QRS morphology is normal, but the S wave amplitude in leads V2-3 has decreased since the admission ECG (A). Most noteworthy are the considerable ST segment elevation and increased T wave amplitude in the anterior precordial leads V1-4 and the similar, but less prominent, elevations in leads I, aVL, and V5. Leads III and aVF show ST segment depression with upright T waves, consistent with reciprocal changes or inferior wall myocardial ischemia. With resolution of the chest pain 20 minutes later, the ECG returned to baseline. Acute myocardial infarction (MI) was ruled out by serial enzyme determinations. Subsequent coronary angiography revealed single-vessel coronary artery disease, with a high-grade obstruction of the left anterior descending coronary artery.

This patient's history and ECG findings are classic for vasospastic (Prinzmetal's) angina. This condition is characterized by coronary artery spasm in a normal or stenotic vessel, causing a profound reduction in blood flow and transmural ischemia in the area of the vessel's distribution. Injury currents produced by the transmural ischemia generate ST segment ele-

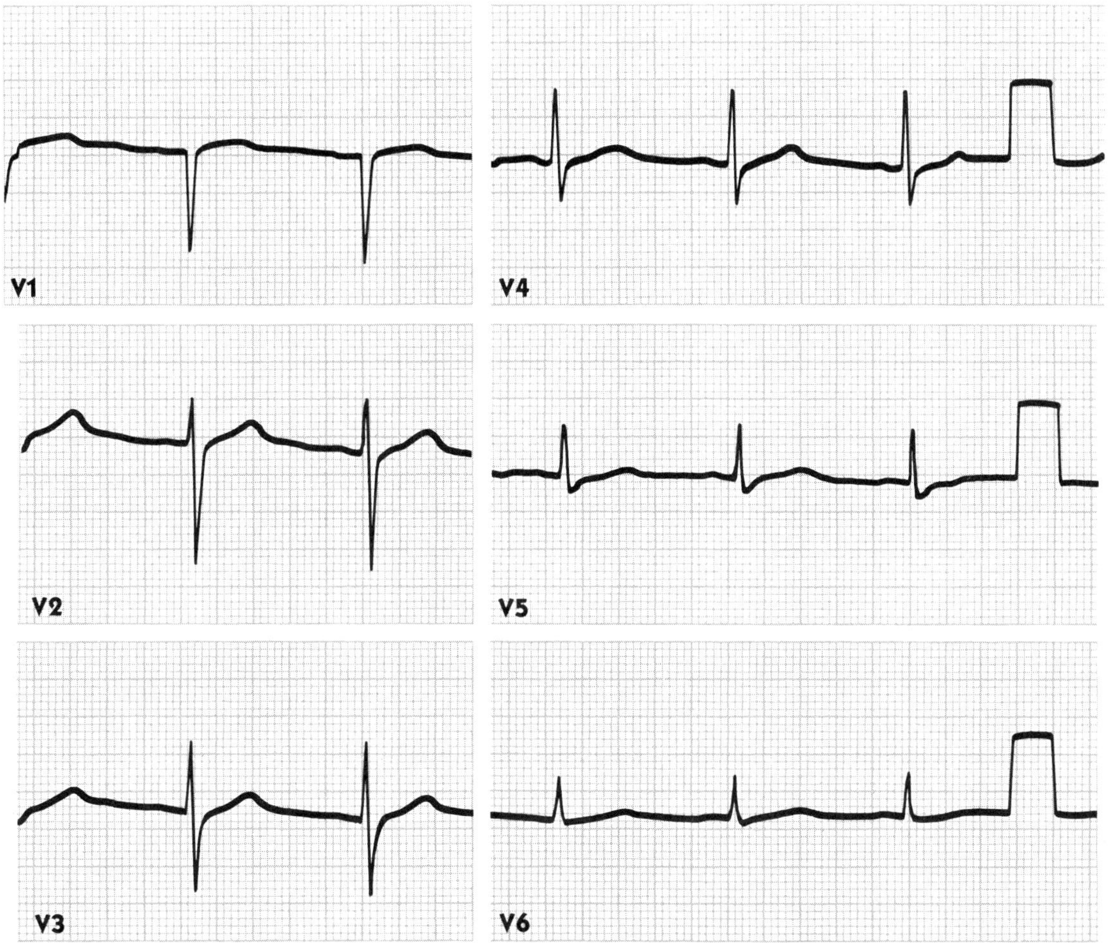

continued

vation and hyperacute T wave changes on the surface ECG. In this case, the patient undoubtedly developed spasm in the left anterior descending artery at the site of stenosis, creating anterior wall myocardial ischemia reflected by the marked ST-T abnormalities. The ST elevation in coronary artery spasm is classically (but not always) marked, confluent with the terminal portion of the QRS complex, associated with markedly increased T wave amplitude and increased R wave (or decreased S wave) amplitude, and localized to specific leads reflecting the area supplied by the vessel in spasm. ST depression is frequently seen in distant leads, where it could be reciprocal or secondary to ischemia. Ventricular arrhythmias and various degrees of AV block may also be associated with episodes of coronary artery spasm.

Of major diagnostic importance is the *reversibility* of all these changes with resolution of the ischemia. Except for this feature, an episode of coronary artery spasm cannot be distinguished from acute MI on the ECG. In acute MI, the ECG changes persist and evolve (see Cases 24 and 26).

CASE 31B

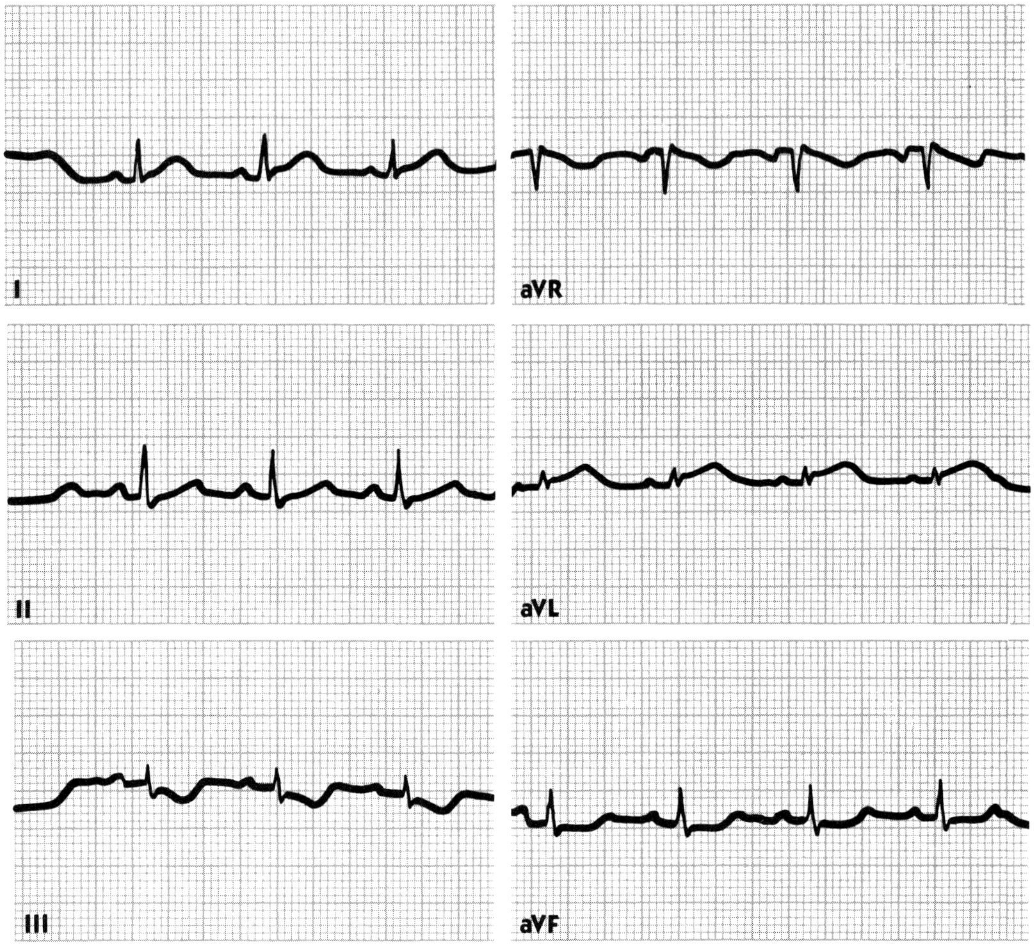

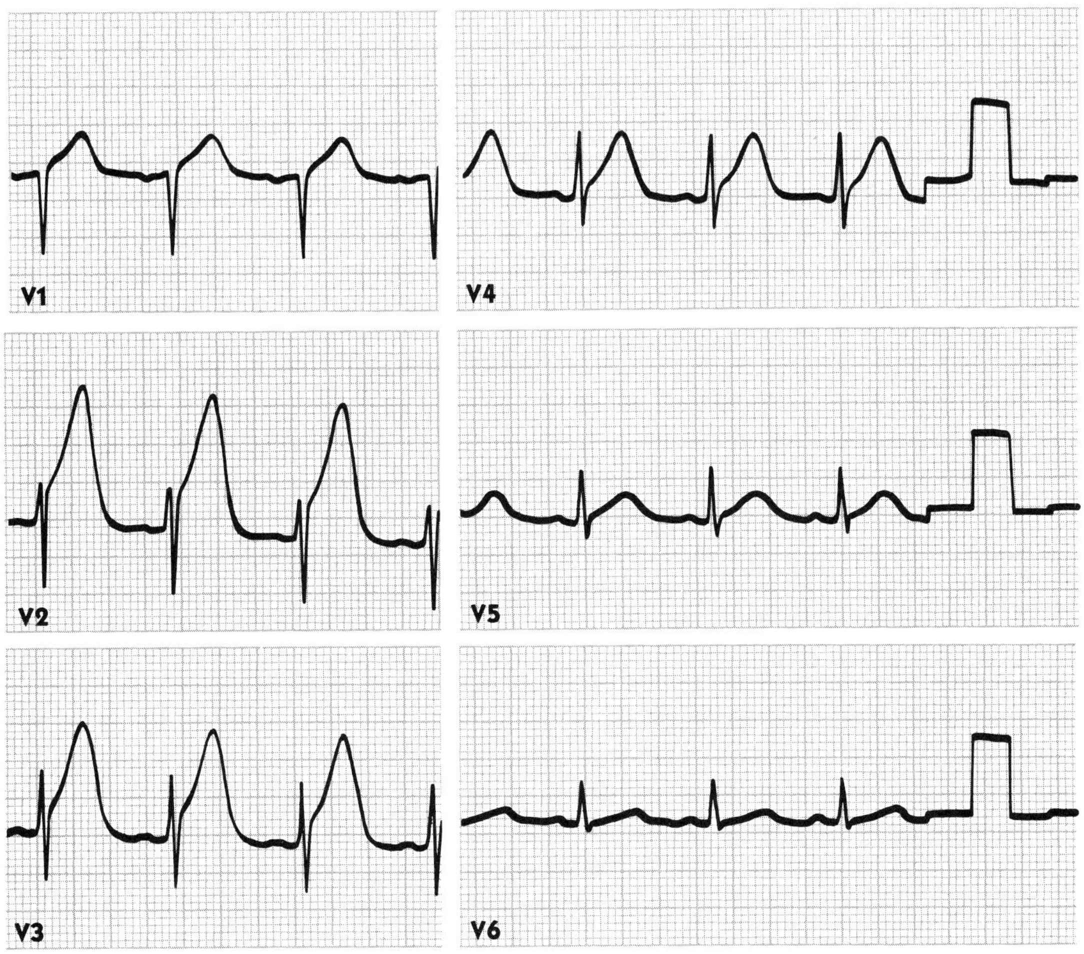
V1
V4
V2
V5
V3
V6

CASE 32—A and B

Coronary Artery Spasm Mimicking Posterior Wall Myocardial Infarction

CASE 32A Pain-free

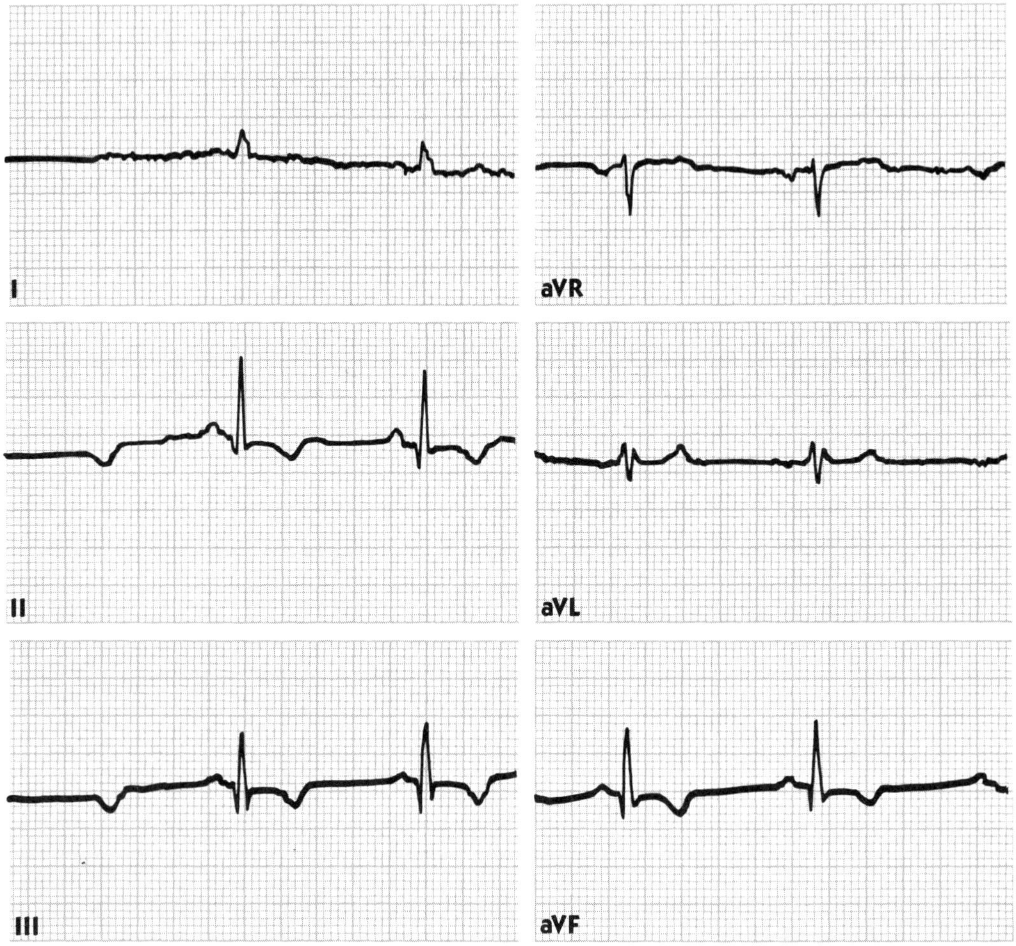

The first ECG (A) was recorded from a patient with previous inferior wall myocardial infarction (MI), unstable angina, and severe three-vessel coronary artery disease documented angiographically. The rhythm is sinus, the intervals are normal, and the mean frontal plane QRS axis is +60°. There are deep Q waves in leads II, III, and aVF and T wave inversion in these leads and in V5-6. These abnormalities were known to be unchanged from previous ECGs and therefore are compatible with remote MI involving the inferior wall.

The second ECG (B) was recorded during an episode of severe chest pain. Slight but definite ST segment elevation, taller R waves, and newly *upright* T waves appear in leads II, III, and aVF. There is ST segment depression in leads V1-4. Tall R waves are now present in lead V1, and the QRS duration is slightly longer (0.10 second) than in the previous ECG (0.08 second). When the chest pain resolved, these ECG abnormalities also resolved, and a third ECG (not shown) was unchanged from the first (A). MI was ruled out by serial enzyme determinations.

This patient's ECG during pain shows evidence of transmural myocardial ischemia inferoposteriorly (although the ST elevation is not as marked as in Case 31). The anterior ST depression most likely represents posterior ST elevation seen reciprocally rather than anterior ischemia. Transmural ischemia may cause an

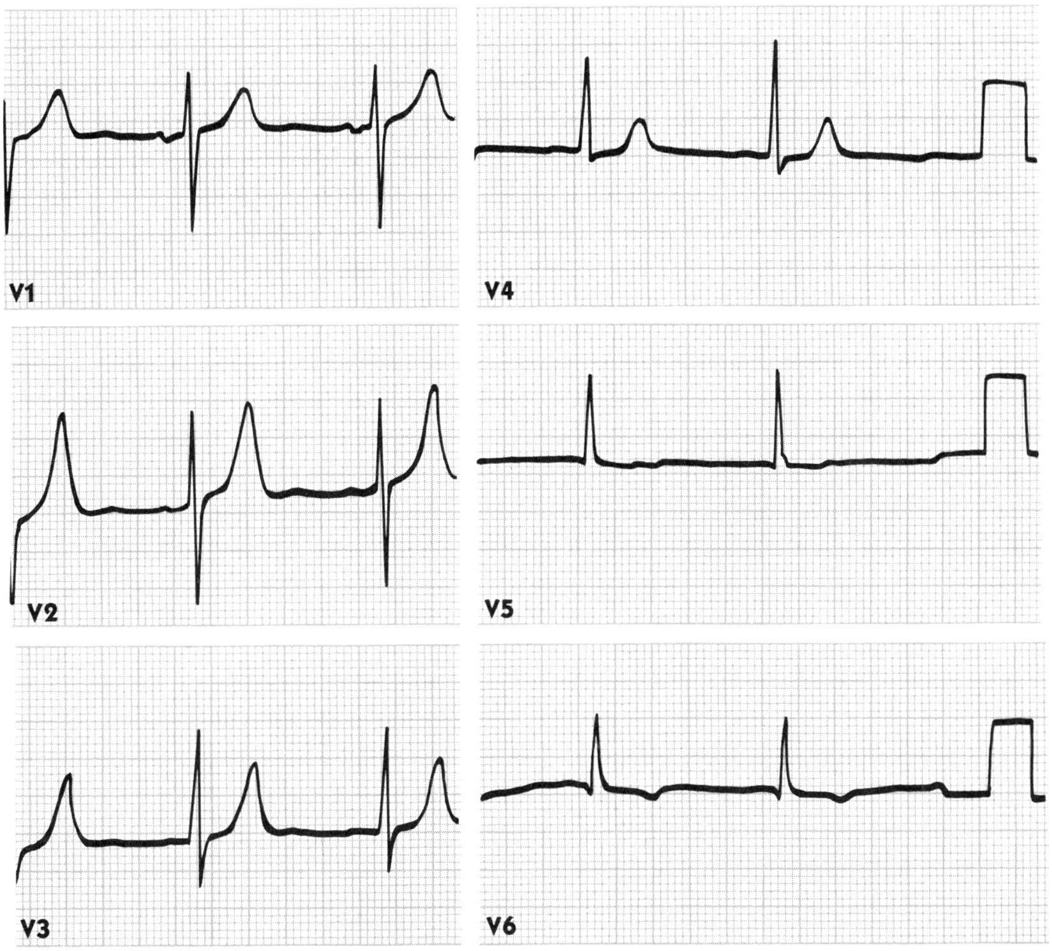

continued

increase in R wave amplitude in affected leads. Although the precise mechanism is uncertain, it may involve Brody effect or local conduction delay. In this case, there is increased R wave amplitude in lead V1 recorded during pain suggesting posterior wall transmural ischemia with transient loss of posterior forces. The slight increase in QRS duration suggests the possibility of ischemia-induced conduction delay. The transience of the ECG findings implicates coronary artery spasm in the distribution of the right or left circumflex coronary artery.

Of special note is the nearly normal appearance, during the ischemic episode, of the inferior T waves that were inverted in the baseline ECG. This phenomenon is termed "pseudonormalization." It can result from any process that alters T wave morphology, but in the appropriate setting it suggests myocardial ischemia or infarction.

CASE 32B During pain

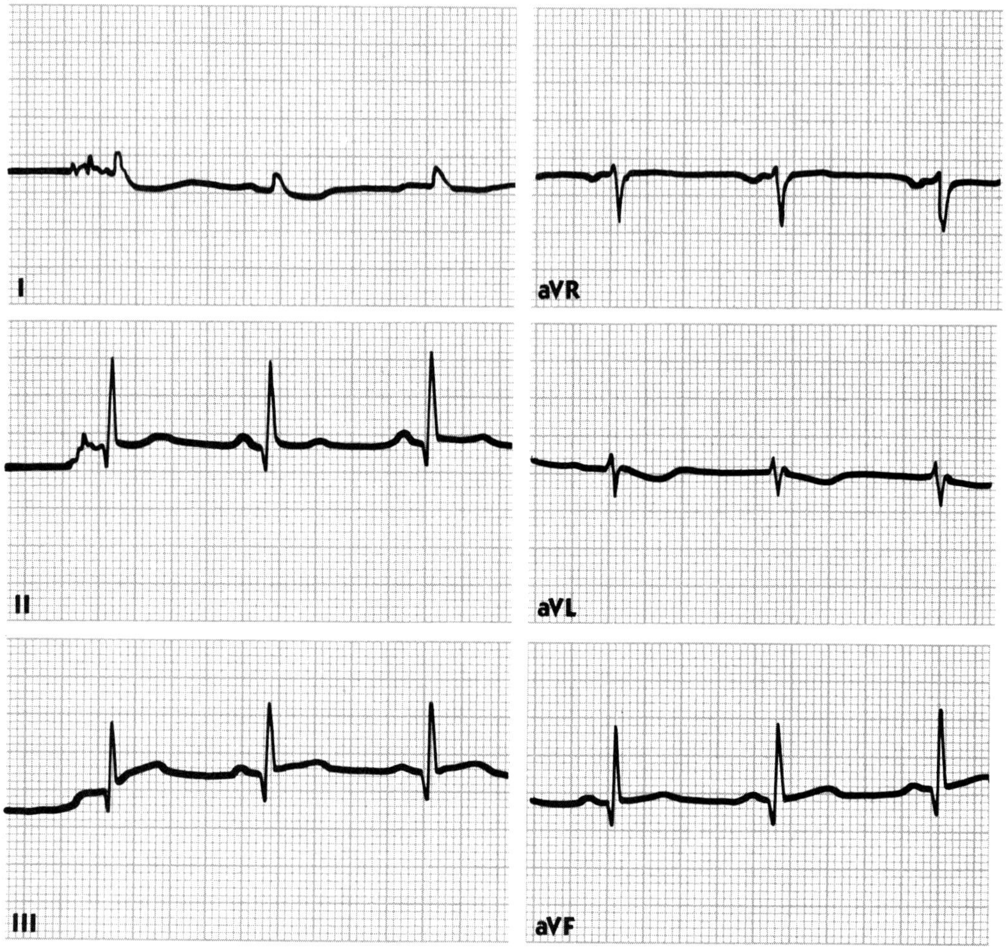

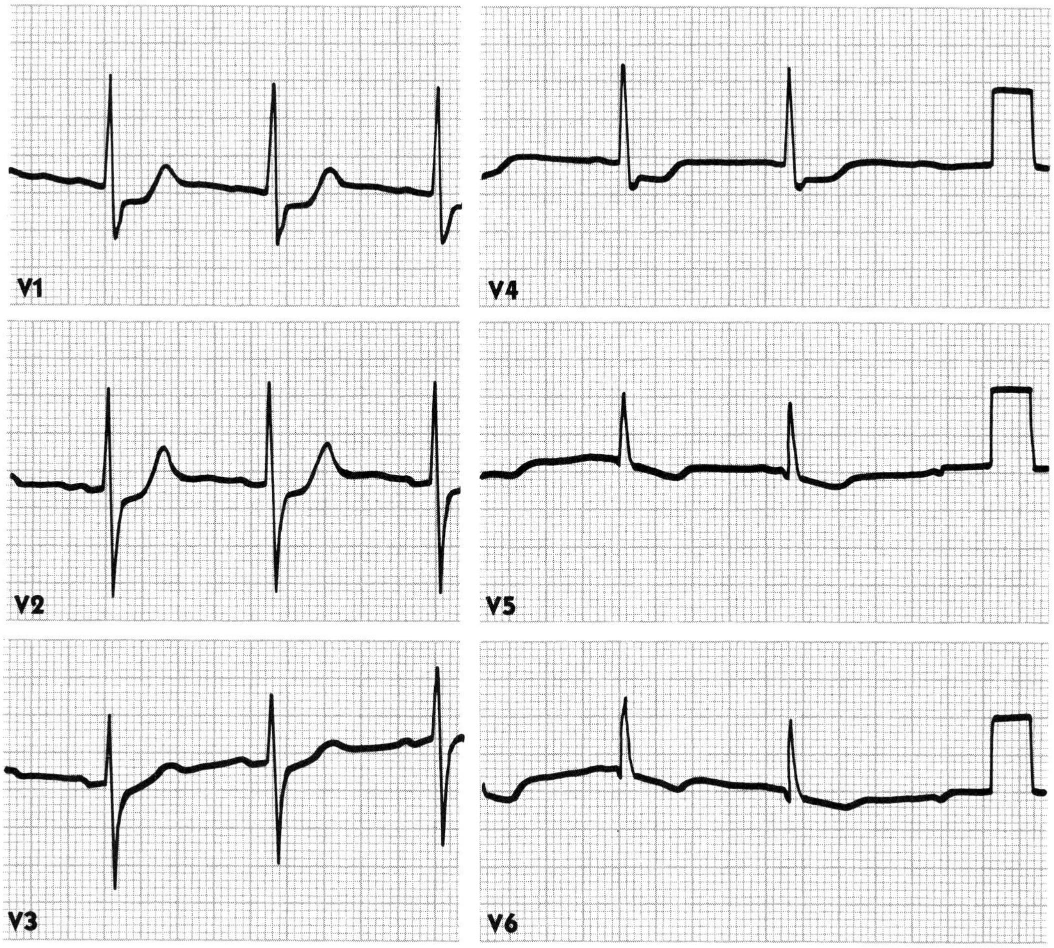
V1
V2
V3
V4
V5
V6

CASE 33

Myocardial Contusion

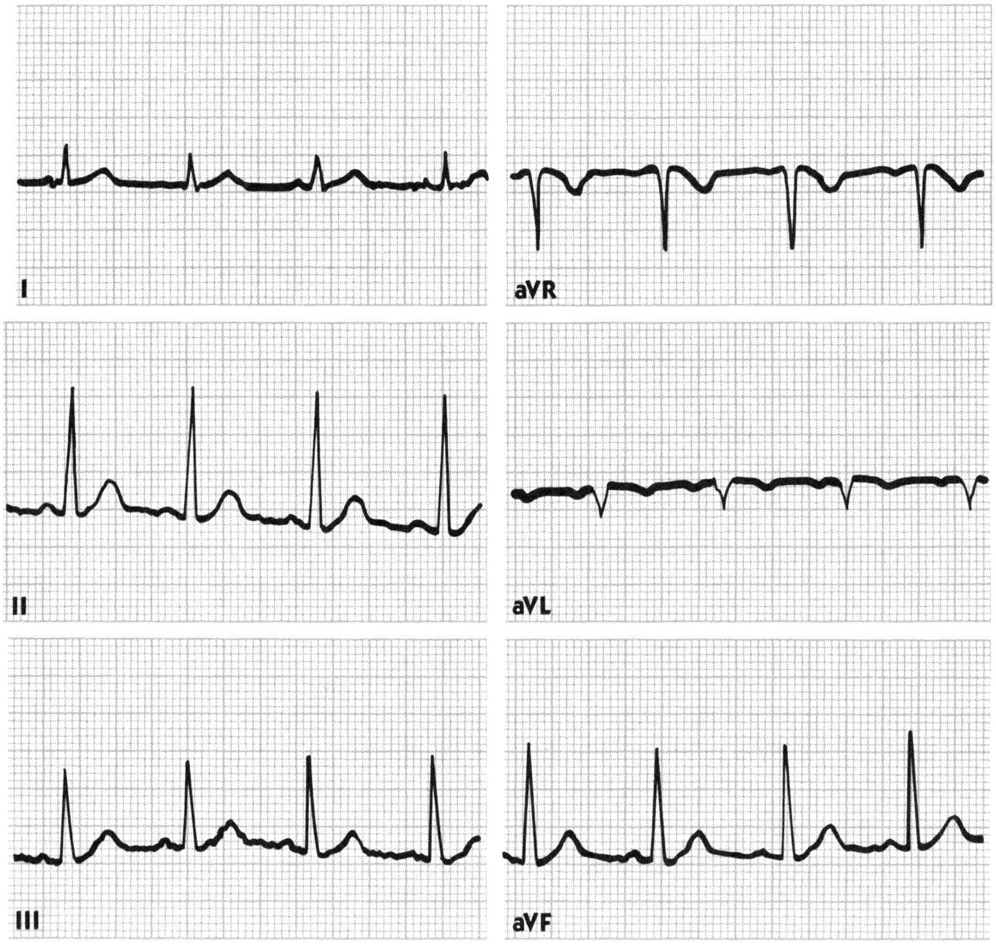

This ECG was recorded from a 25-year-old man with a steering wheel injury of the chest from an automobile accident. The ECG is normal except for marked J point and ST segment elevations in leads V1-4. In the anterior precordial leads, the downsloping portions of the ST segments obscure the terminal portions of the QRS complexes and merge with tall T waves, deforming their onsets. These abnormalities suggest injury currents and thus resemble those in acute anterior wall myocardial infarction (MI). However, MI due to coronary artery disease is unlikely in this young, healthy patient. Cardiac trauma can lead to coronary thrombosis with resulting myocardial damage. But much more common is cardiac contusion from blunt trauma to the chest involving the anterior myocardium. The surface ECG reflects myocardial injury regardless of the underlying mechanism(s). In cases like this one, depending on degree of myocardial cell damage, typical ST segment elevation and hyperacute T wave abnormalities can evolve into transmural MI patterns. T wave inversions alone may reflect a nontransmural MI (see Case 29). In myocardial contusion, the early risk is the same as in MI due to coronary disease, although the prognosis is generally benign.

The ST alterations in this ECG could represent early repolarization changes that occur as a normal variant in young persons. However, early repolarization changes usually do not obscure the QRS complex. In addition, the ST segment typically slopes gently upward in a concave pattern, rarely exceeds a few millimeters in amplitude, and may be accompanied by terminal T wave inversion in early repolarization (see Cases 61 and 62). None of these features

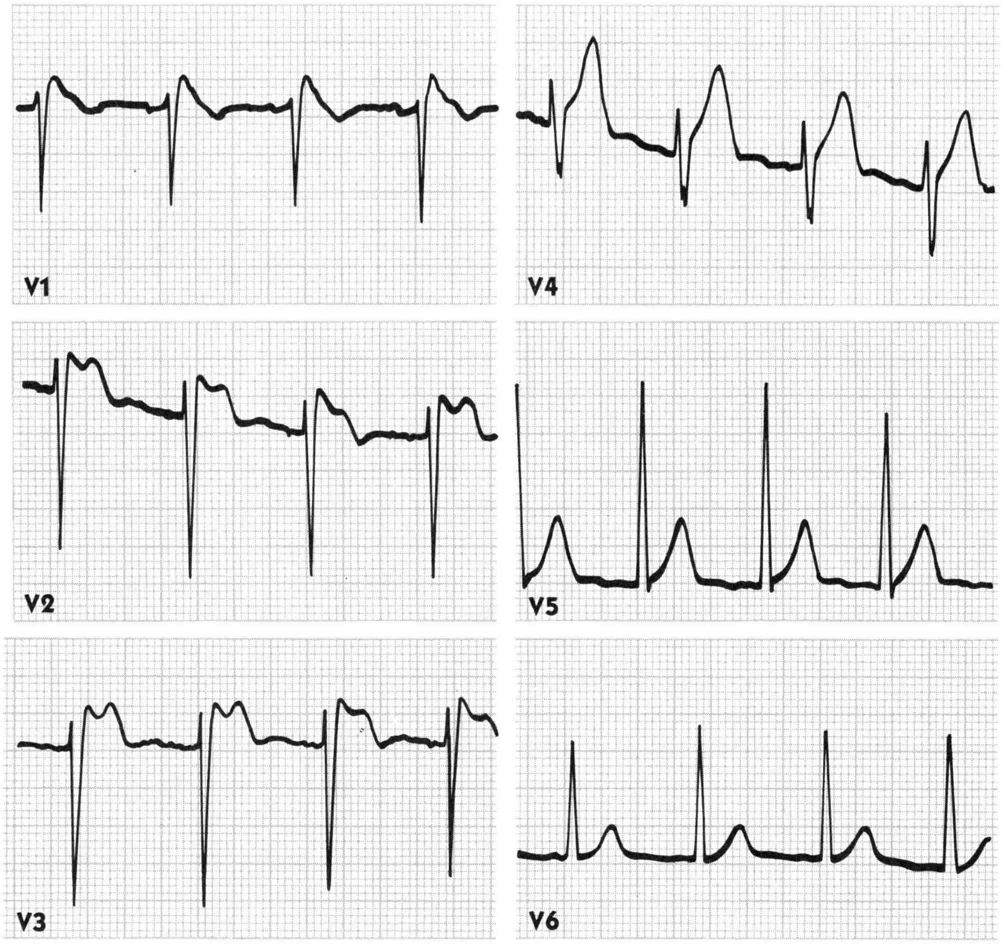

is present in this ECG. ST segment elevation can also result from epicardial inflammation and injury in pericarditis (see Cases 40 and 42). The distinction between traumatic pericarditis and myocardial contusion cannot be made on ECG grounds alone.

SECTION V

Accessory AV Conduction Syndromes

CASE 34

Wolff-Parkinson-White Conduction, Type A

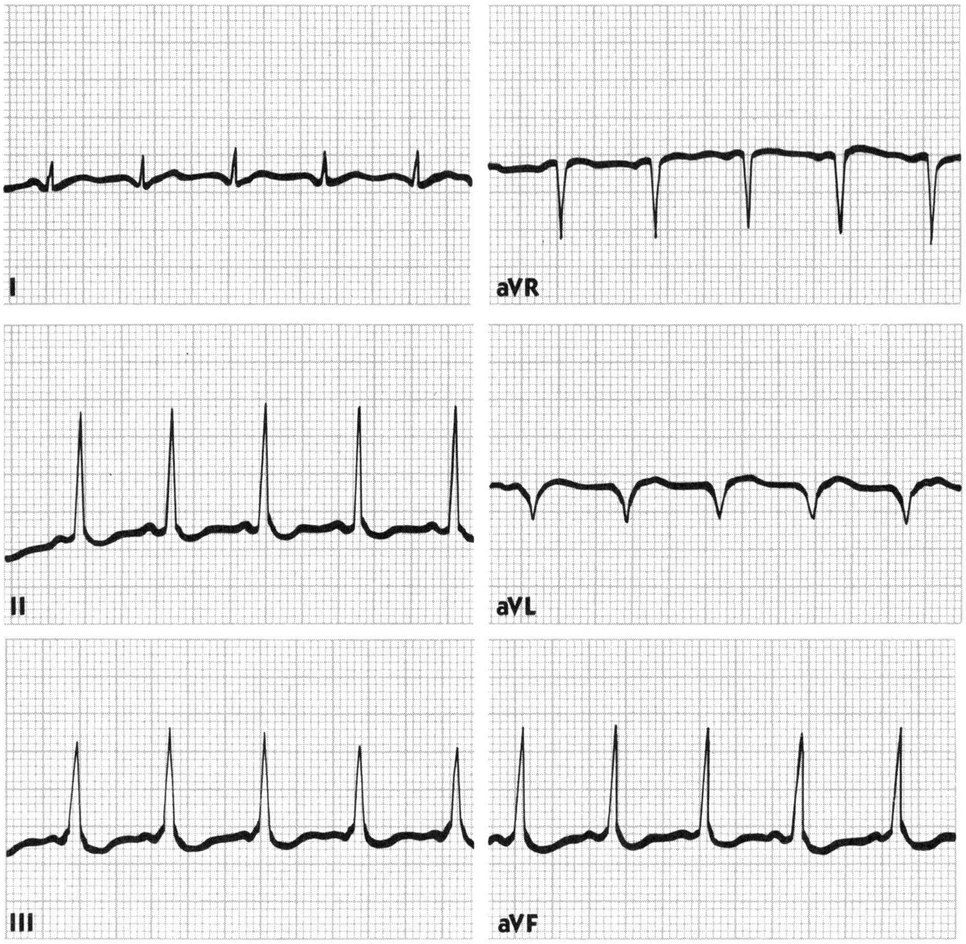

This ECG was recorded from a 25-year-old man who complained of episodic palpitations. The PR interval is short (0.11 second), the QRS duration is slightly prolonged (0.12 second), and the QT interval is normal. The mean frontal plane QRS axis is +80°. Some QRS complexes show an initial slur; this is best seen in leads III and V2-5. This initial slur is called a "delta" wave because of its resemblance to the Greek letter. A similar slurring, directed downward, appears in leads I and aVL. Nonspecific ST-T abnormalities are present and are probably related to the abnormality of ventricular depolarization described below.

The Wolff-Parkinson-White (WPW) syndrome is a form of ventricular pre-excitation (see Table 6 in the Appendix). The WPW syndrome is defined electrocardiographically by a short PR interval and a delta wave, and pathologically by accessory atrioventricular conduction pathways known as the bundles of Kent. Ventricular activation begins early in WPW conduction, since the AV node (where the greatest delay in atrioventricular conduction normally occurs) is bypassed. Intraventricular conduction can vary from normal to various degrees of pre-excitation; i.e., the ventricles may be depolarized: (1) entirely through the normal AV node-His-Purkinje system (see Fig. 2A in the Appendix); (2) entirely through the accessory pathway (see Fig. 2B); or (3) via both pathways (see Fig. 2C).

If an atrial impulse bypasses the AV node, the PR interval will be short, since impulses traverse the accessory pathway rapidly. However, if initial ventricular activation occurs via an accessory pathway inserting directly into ventricular muscle, it will proceed more slowly than it would if conducted via

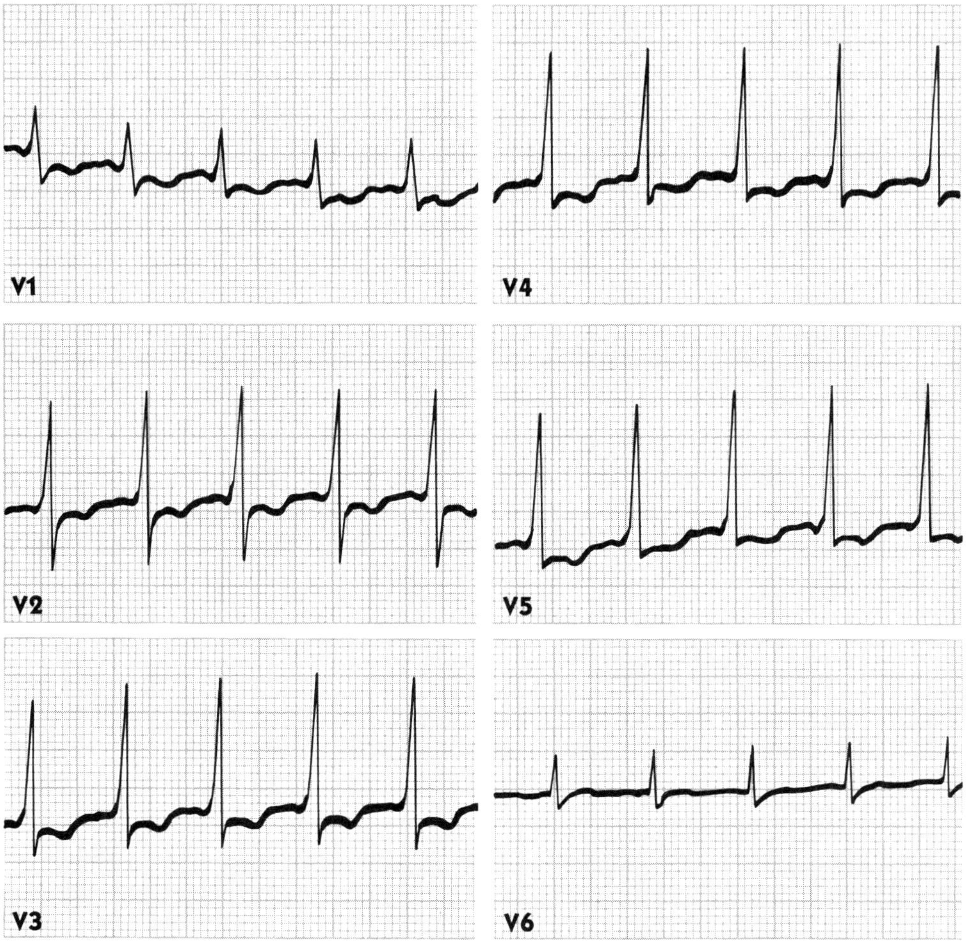

the His-Purkinje system, due to the slower intramuscular spread of the impulse. The delta wave on the ECG represents this early activation of ventricular muscle. The remainder of the QRS morphology represents later ventricular activation. If the ventricles are depolarized via both normal and accessory pathways, the QRS complex will be a fusion complex. If depolarization occurs entirely over the bypass tract, the QRS complex will be a "pure" WPW complex.

WPW conduction has been arbitrarily (and simplistically) separated into two types, A and B, depending on whether the delta wave is directed anteriorly or posteriorly. In type A WPW, the anteriorly directed delta waves describe initial slurred R waves in lead V1; in type B, the posteriorly directed delta waves describe slurred Q waves in V1. Variations in location of the accessory conduction pathway produce QRS patterns that are neither type A nor type B. The distinction actually carries little significance.

There are two reasons for recognizing WPW conduction. First, patients with this syndrome are prone to reciprocating supraventricular tachycardias, atrial flutter, and atrial fibrillation. Second, WPW conduction results in QRS morphology that is often misread as myocardial infarction (see Table 7 in the Appendix). In this case, the tall R waves in lead V1, the Q wave in lead I, and the QS complex in lead aVL might lead to the erroneous diagnosis of posterolateral MI or right ventricular hypertrophy. Measurement of the PR interval is helpful in determining the correct diagnosis.

CASE 35

Wolff-Parkinson-White Conduction, Type B

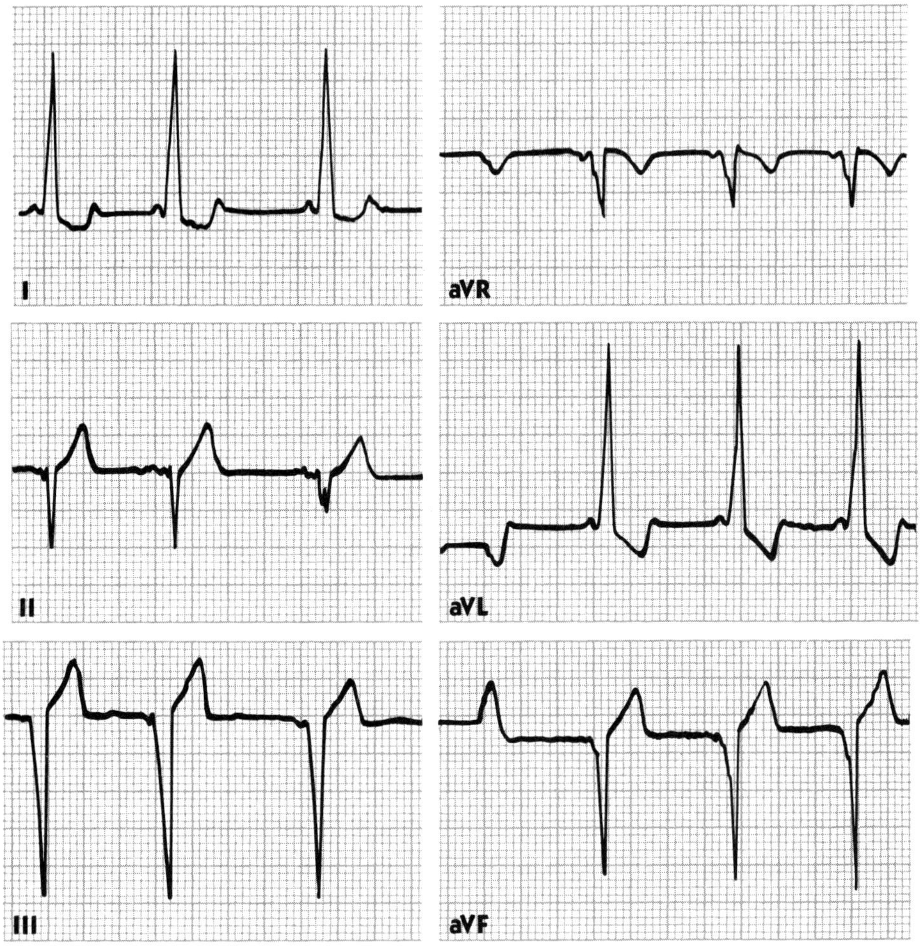

This ECG was recorded from a healthy 4-year-old child who had an episode of tachycardia with shortness of breath. It shows sinus rhythm with a short PR interval (0.08 second) and a slightly prolonged QRS duration (0.12 second). The mean frontal plane QRS axis is markedly superior at about $-70°$. Delta waves are best seen in leads I, aVL, and V4-6. There are QS complexes in leads II, III, aVF, V1-2, and V4R. The ST segments are depressed in leads I and aVL and elevated in leads II, III, aVF, V1-2, and V4R.

The short PR interval and the delta waves in the lateral leads indicate ventricular pre-excitation of the Wolff-Parkinson-White (WPW) type. The delta wave is directed posteriorly, superiorly, and laterally. Because of its posterior direction, it is inverted in lead V1 (type B WPW), causing a Q wave. Since the delta wave is also directed superolaterally, inverted delta

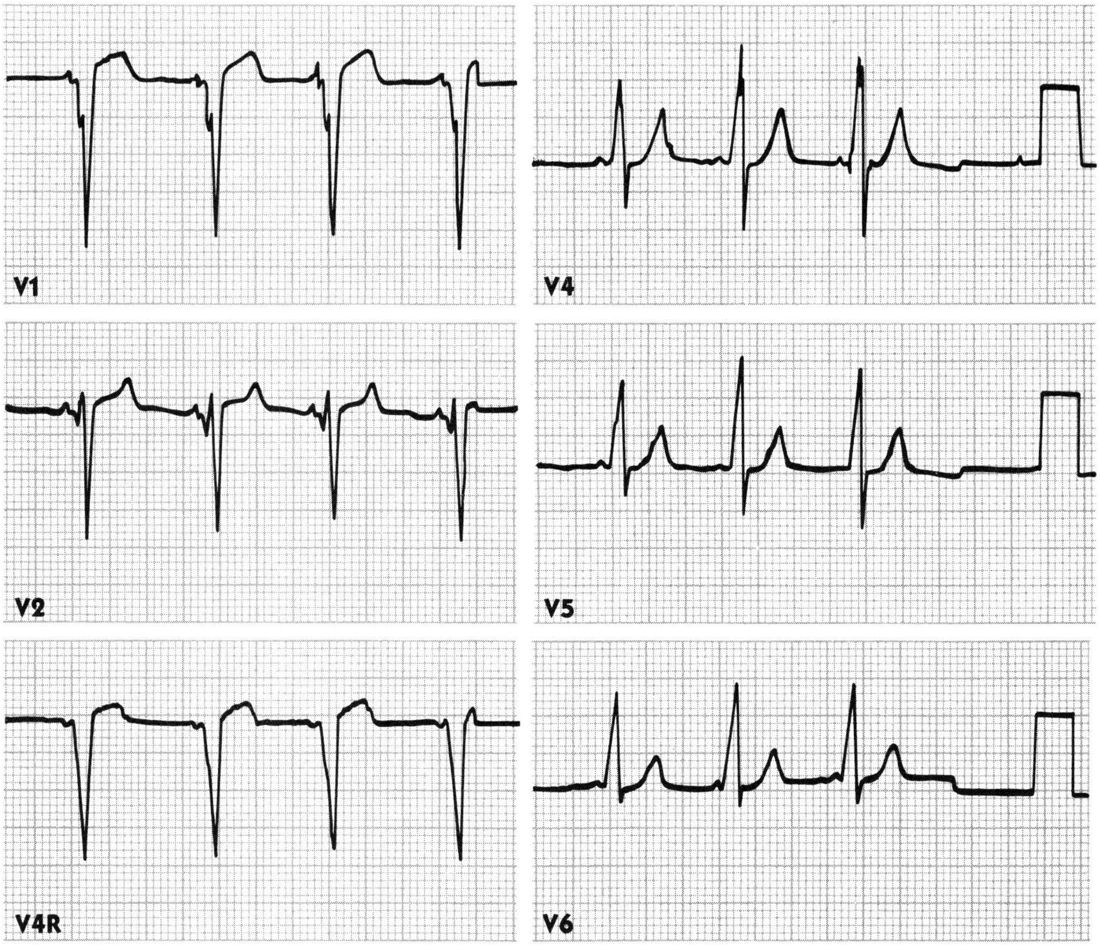

waves cause QS complexes in the inferior leads. WPW conduction represents ventricular depolarization via intramuscular spread, with variable contribution by the normal AV node-His-Purkinje system. Consequently, secondary ST-T abnormalities may occur in a direction opposite to the delta wave and in proportion to the degree of activation occurring via the accessory pathway. This explains the ST-T wave depression in the high lateral leads and the ST-T wave elevation in the anteroinferior leads in this ECG.

It is easy to see how these ECG findings could be mistaken for inferoseptal myocardial infarction. Indeed, the QS wave with ST segment elevation in lead V4R might suggest right ventricular infarction. Measurement of the PR interval, identification of the delta wave, and clinical correlation are all mandatory in arriving at the correct diagnosis.

CASE 36

Wolff-Parkinson-White Conduction Mimicking Inferoposterolateral Wall Myocardial Infarction

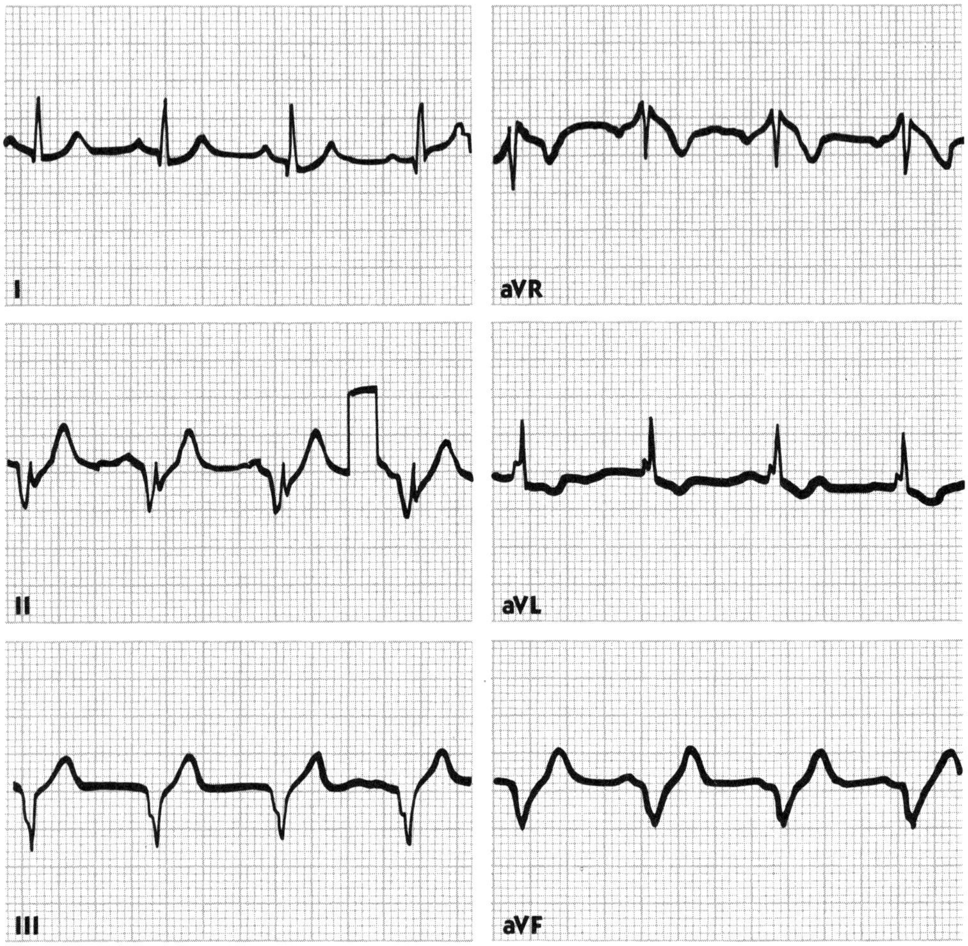

This 54-year-old man with hypertension was thought to have had a previous myocardial infarction (MI) on the basis of this routine ECG. The rhythm is sinus. The PR interval is at the lower limit of normal (0.12 second), and the QRS duration is mildly prolonged (0.11 second). The mean frontal plane QRS axis is directed abnormally superiorly. R waves appear in lead V1 and delta waves in leads aVL and V2-3. The R waves are markedly tall anteriorly (up to 40 mm). Inverted delta waves in leads II, III, aVF, and V5-6 cause QS and QR complexes and, thus, abnormal left axis deviation. There is ST segment depression anteriorly.

This patient has type A Wolff-Parkinson-White (WPW) conduction with an anteriorly directed delta wave—and not, as was thought, an inferoposterior and lateral wall MI. The prominent voltages anteriorly might be interpreted as right ventricular hypertrophy (RVH). But ventricular depolarization is abnormal; consequently, the diagnosis of RVH cannot be made. This case illustrates that WPW conduction is the "great imitator" of MI, ventricular hypertrophy, and abnormal axis deviation.

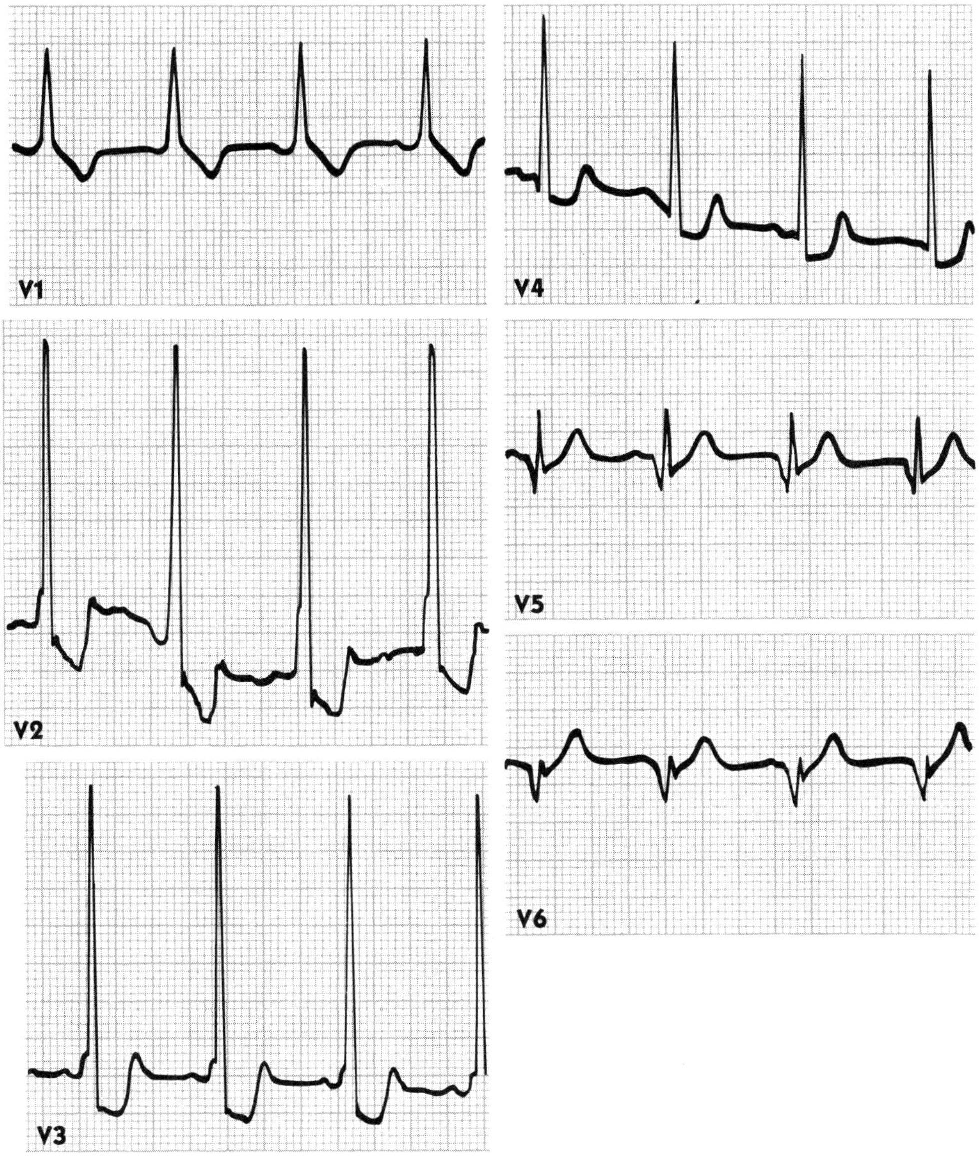
V1
V4
V2
V5
V3
V6

CASE 37

Wolff-Parkinson-White Conduction Mimicking Left Bundle Branch Block

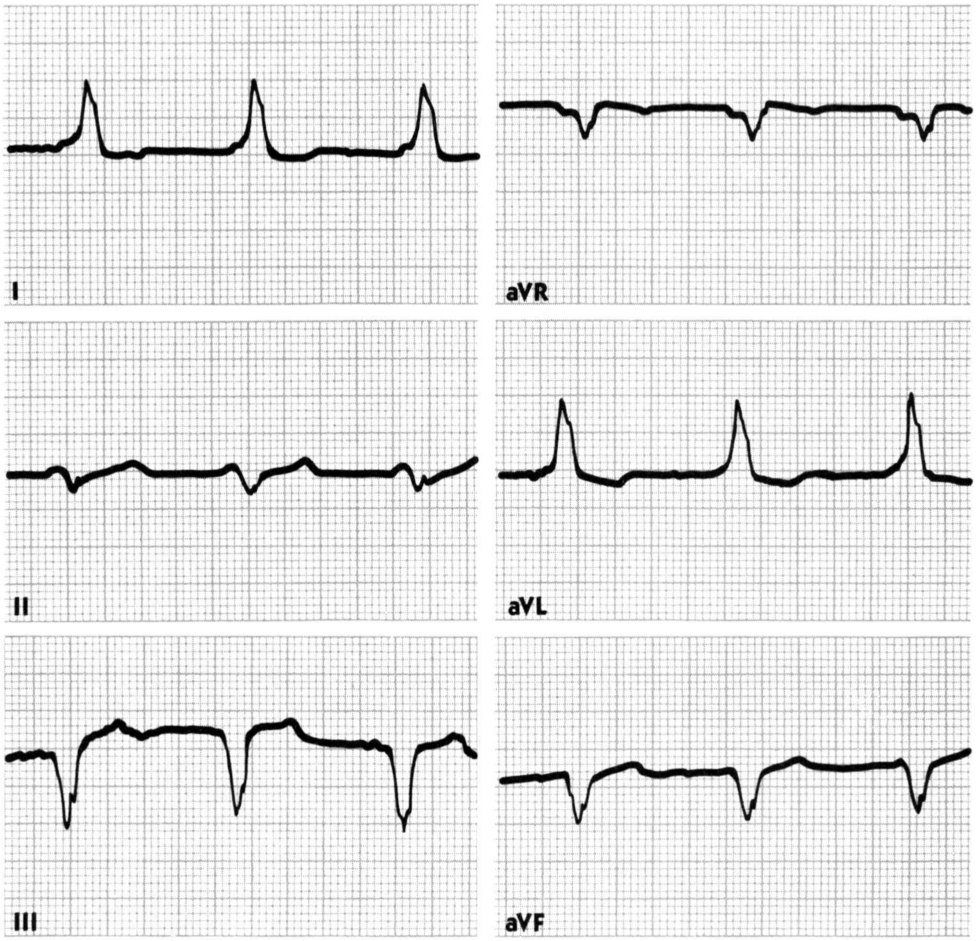

This ECG was recorded from a young man with symptomatic tachycardias. It shows sinus rhythm, although the P wave, just visible at the onset of the QRS complex, might be missed and the rhythm mistaken for junctional. The PR interval is 0.08 second, and the QRS duration is prolonged to 0.14 second. The mean frontal plane QRS axis is $-60°$.

The deep, broad QS complex in lead V1 and the monophasic R wave in lead V6 resemble the typical pattern of left bundle branch block (see Case 13). The QS complexes inferiorly could suggest old inferior wall myocardial infarction. However, this patient has Wolff-Parkinson-White (WPW) conduction, type B, with a delta wave that is directed posterosuperiorly. The diagnosis can be made by the very short PR interval. The markedly prolonged QRS duration indicates

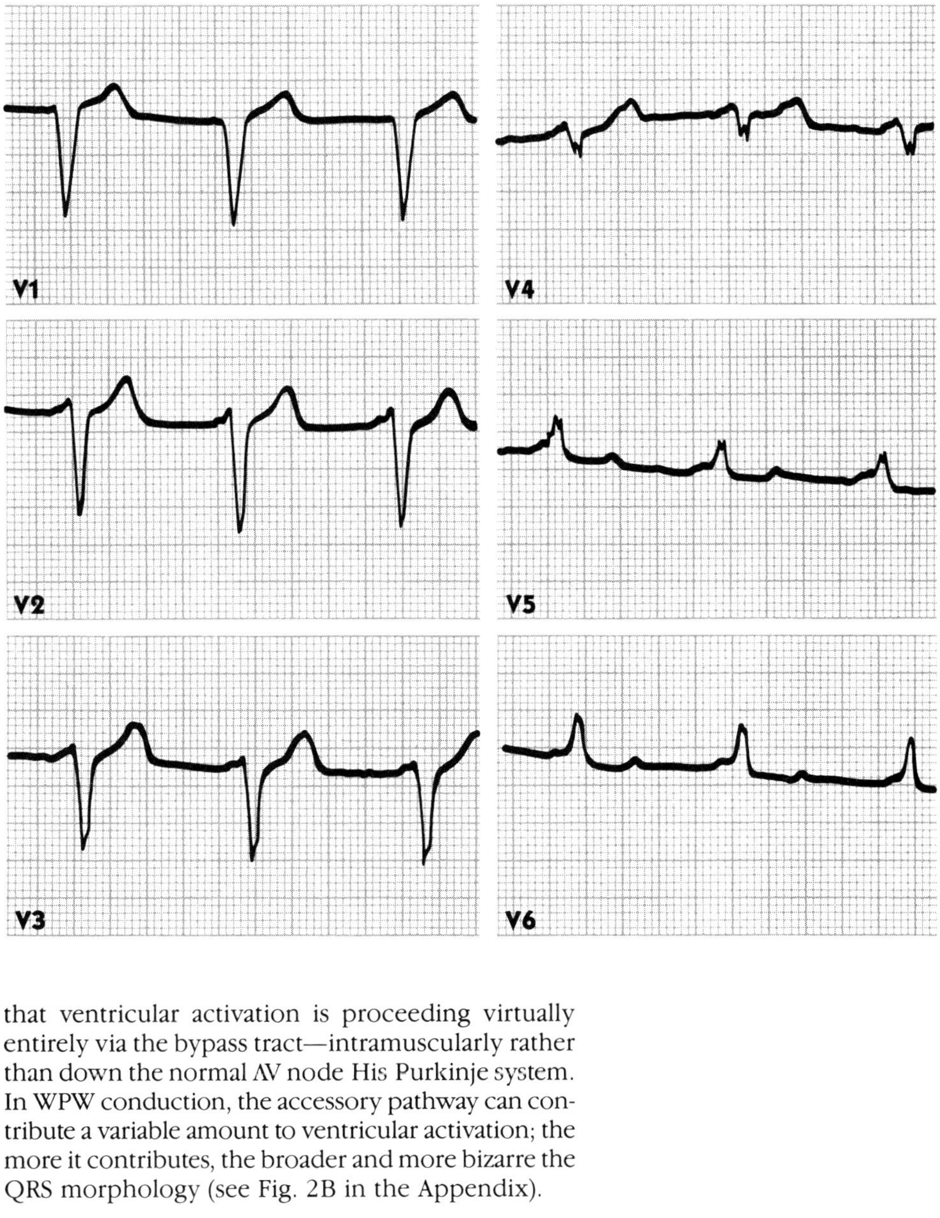

that ventricular activation is proceeding virtually entirely via the bypass tract—intramuscularly rather than down the normal AV node His Purkinje system. In WPW conduction, the accessory pathway can contribute a variable amount to ventricular activation; the more it contributes, the broader and more bizarre the QRS morphology (see Fig. 2B in the Appendix).

CASE 38

Mahaim Conduction

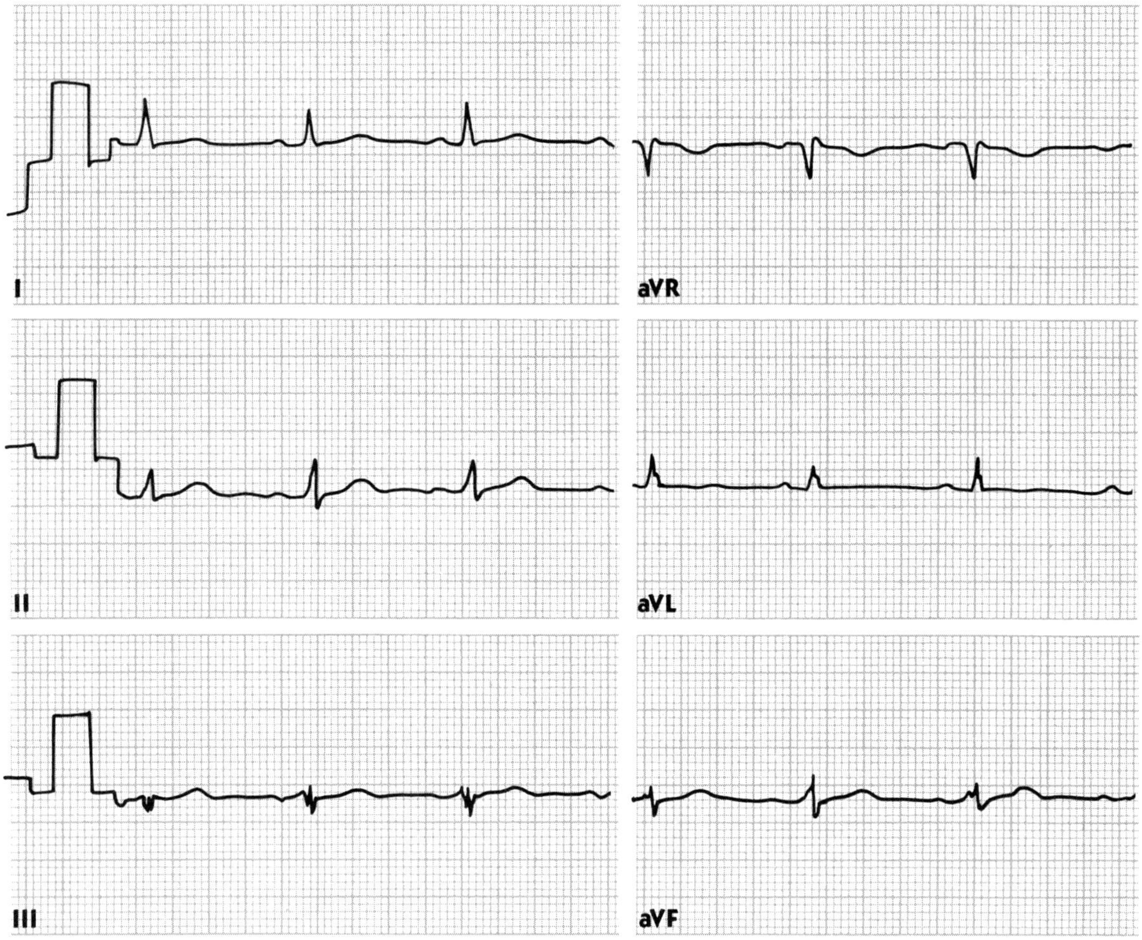

This 31-year-old man underwent electrophysiologic evaluation for tachycardias, revealing an accessory pathway of the Mahaim type. His ECG shows sinus rhythm, a normal PR interval of 0.18 second, and a QRS duration of 0.10 second. Delta waves are seen in leads II, aVL, aVF, and V4-5. The S waves in leads V2-3 are 32 mm deep, and there are nonspecific biphasic T waves in leads V4-5.

Pre-excitation of the Mahaim type is characterized on the ECG by the presence of delta waves with a *normal* PR interval. The accessory tract originates in the His bundle or the lower portion of the AV node in Mahaim conduction, *below* the site of AV nodal conduction delay. It inserts into ventricular myocardium or bundle branches. Since the AV node is not bypassed, the PR interval is normal (distinguishing Mahaim conduction from the Wolff-Parkinson-White syndrome).

Since the accessory pathway usually inserts directly into ventricular myocardium and initiates early ventricular activation, delta waves are inscribed as in the WPW syndrome (see Table 6 in the Appendix). Also as in the WPW syndrome, the degree of abnormal conduction can vary; i.e., ventricular activation may occur entirely via the accessory pathway, entirely via the AV node-His-Purkinje system, or via a combination of both. When Mahaim fibers terminate in a bundle branch, the opposite bundle branch is effectively bypassed, creating a bundle branch block pattern on the side opposite the Mahaim tract. As with the other pre-excitation syndromes, Mahaim conduction predisposes patients to reciprocating tachycardias.

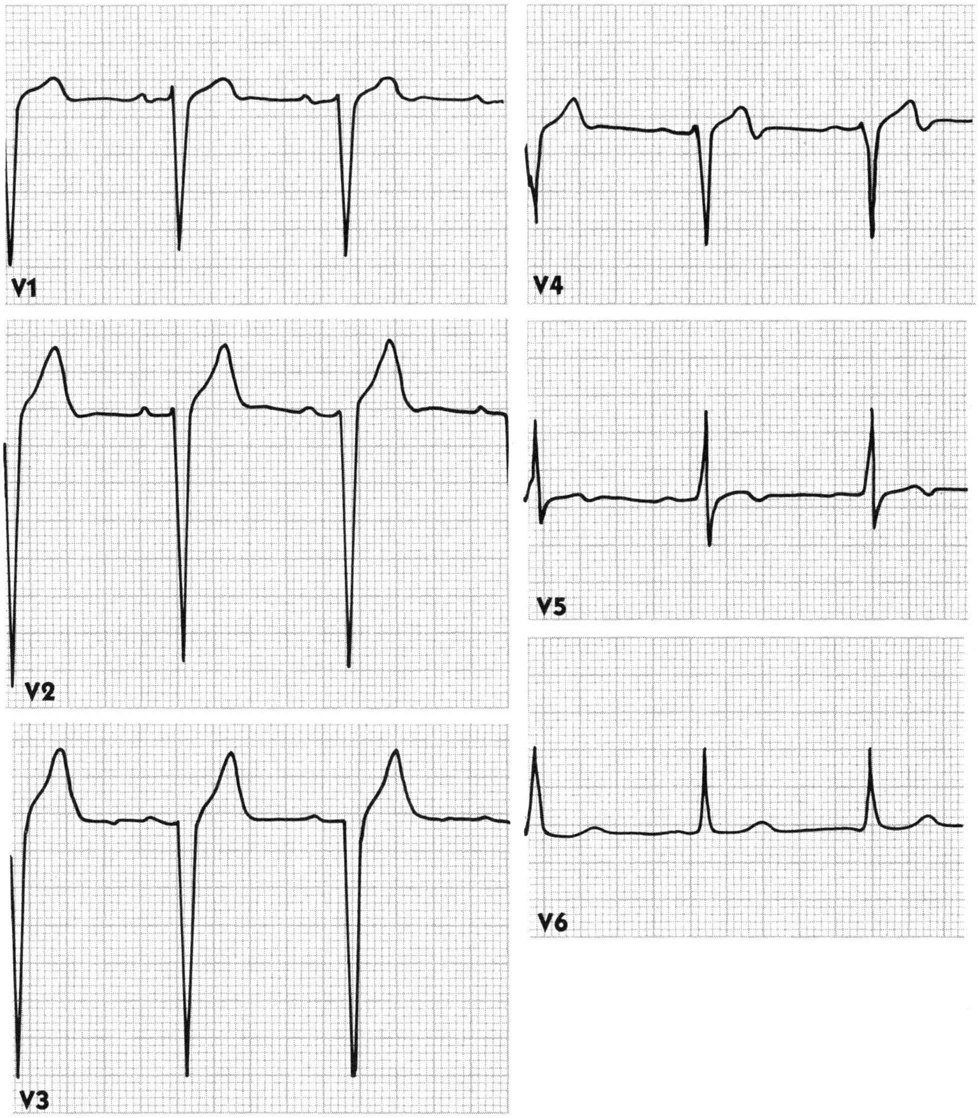
V1
V2
V3
V4
V5
V6

CASE 39

Lown-Ganong-Levine Conduction

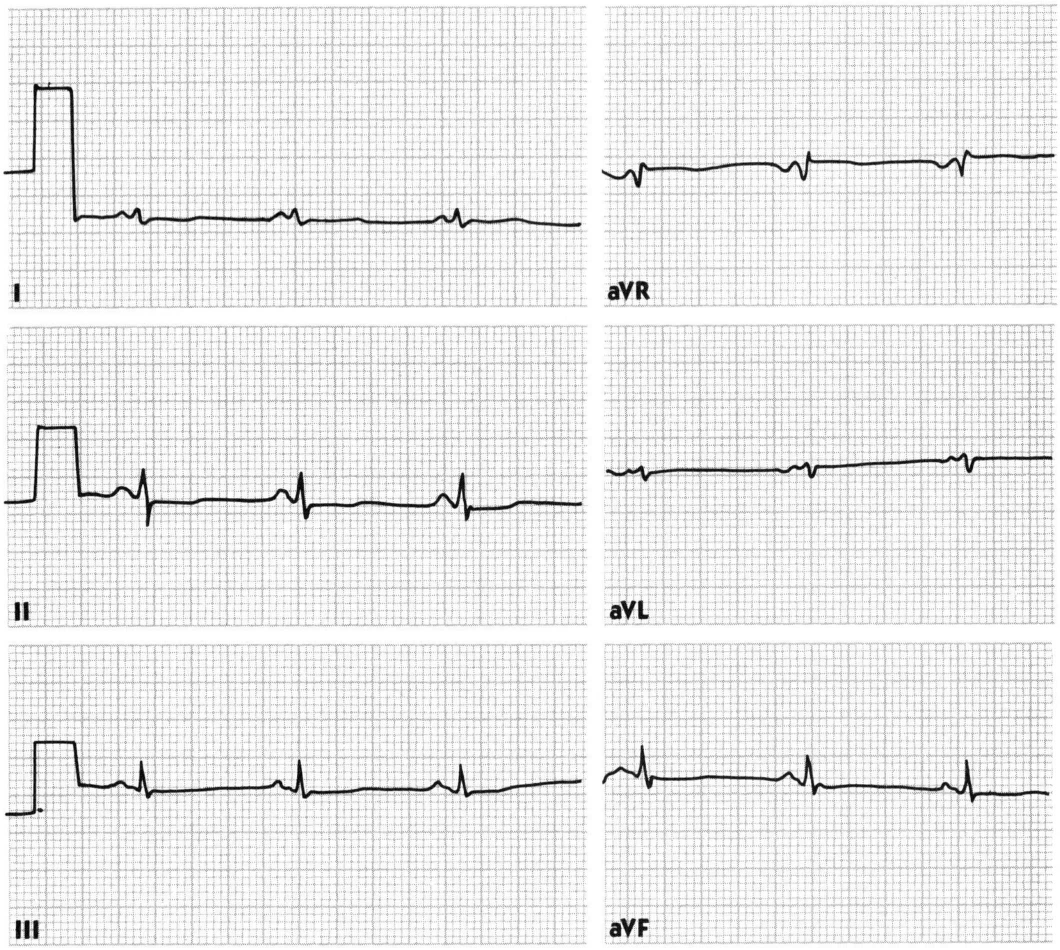

This ECG was recorded from a young man with a history of supraventricular tachyarrhythmias. It is notable for the short PR interval of 0.10 second; all other intervals, mean frontal plane QRS axis, and P wave and QRS morphology are normal. The limb leads show low QRS voltage and minor nonspecific T wave flattening.

The short PR interval is characteristic of, but not specific for, the Lown-Ganong-Levine (LGL) syndrome. In this syndrome, a form of pre-excitation, the PR interval is short, the QRS complexes are normal, and the patient experiences tachycardias. (If no tachycardias occur, the LGL syndrome, as originally described, is not present.) The short PR interval in the LGL syndrome (as well as in cases of short PR interval without tachycardias) may result from an anatomically short AV node or from an accessory tract. The accessory tract may originate within the AV node itself or proximal to it (James fibers), inserting into the His

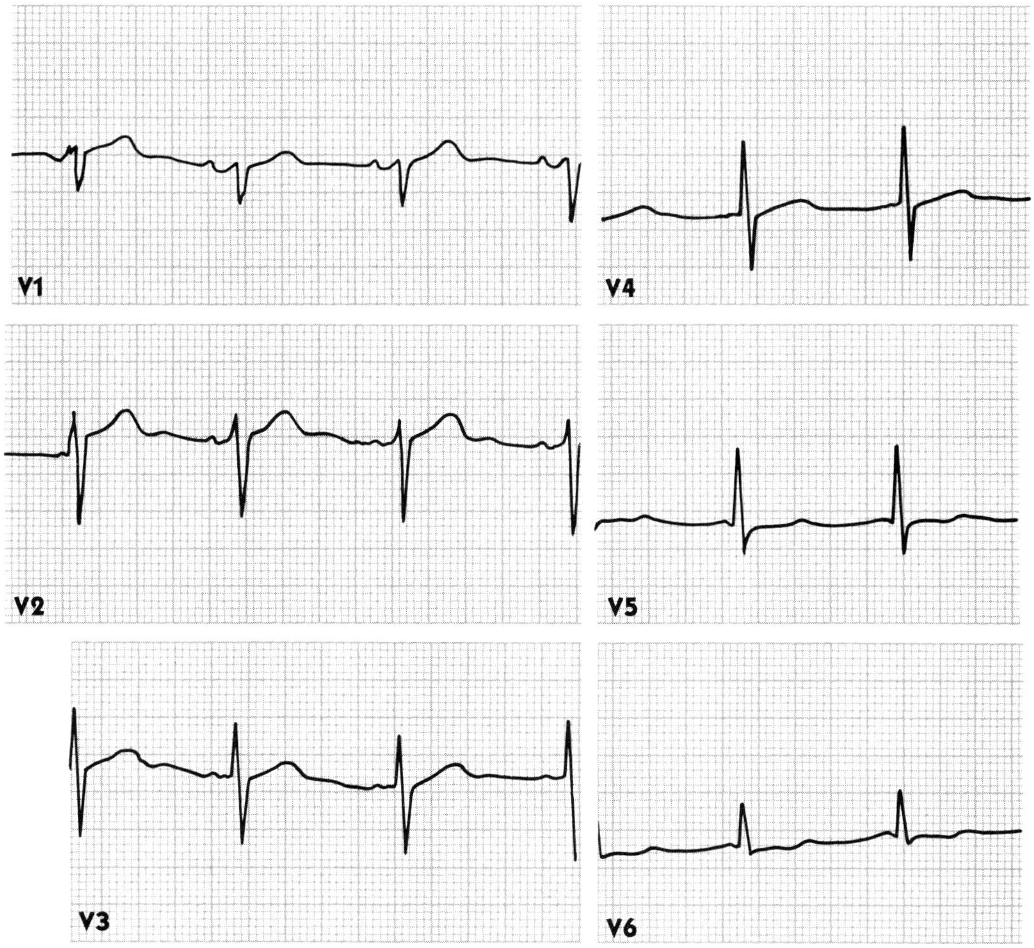

bundle or lower AV node, below the site of normal AV nodal conduction delay. The AV node is thus effectively bypassed; consequently, the PR interval is short. Because the accessory tract inserts into the normal infranodal-His conducting system (not directly into ventricular muscle), ventricular activation proceeds normally, no delta waves appear on the ECG, and the QRS configuration is normal. Unlike the Wolff-Parkinson-White and Mahaim syndromes, LGL does not mimic myocardial infarction, ventricular hypertrophy, or bundle branch block (see Table 6 in the Appendix).

SECTION VI Pericarditis

CASE 40

Acute Pericarditis

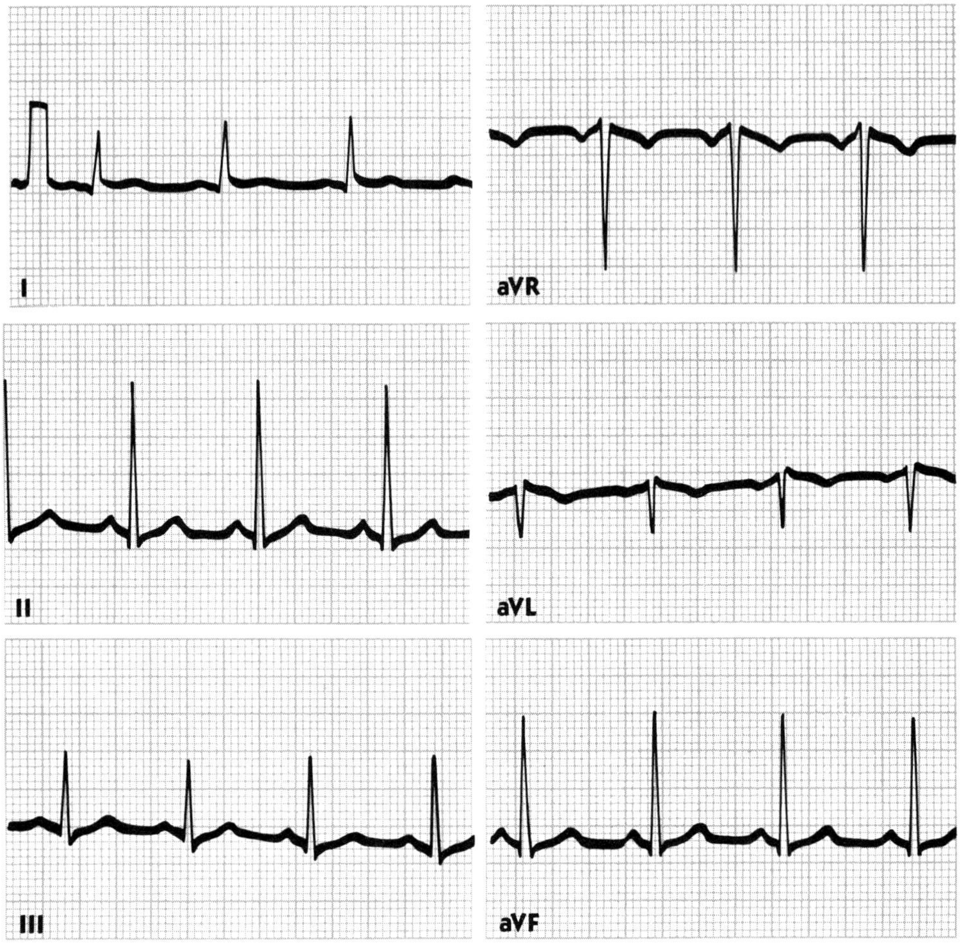

This ECG was recorded from a 34-year-old man with substernal discomfort during a flu-like illness. It shows a normal mean frontal plane QRS axis for his age, normal intervals, and normal P and QRS morphology. Marked J point elevation and upwardly concave ST segment elevation are present in all precordial leads. There is also mild ST elevation in lead I. The T waves are normal.

The differential diagnosis of this ECG includes acute myocardial infarction (MI) and early repolarization (see Case 61), in addition to pericarditis. The subsequently proved clinical diagnosis of pericarditis is, however, supported by this ECG in several ways:

First, the ST segment elevations are diffuse, occurring in all the precordial as well as one of the limb leads. In MI, they are usually more localized; in early repolarization, they tend to be seen primarily in the precordial leads. Second, the elevated ST segments are *concave* upward in this ECG. In early repolariza-

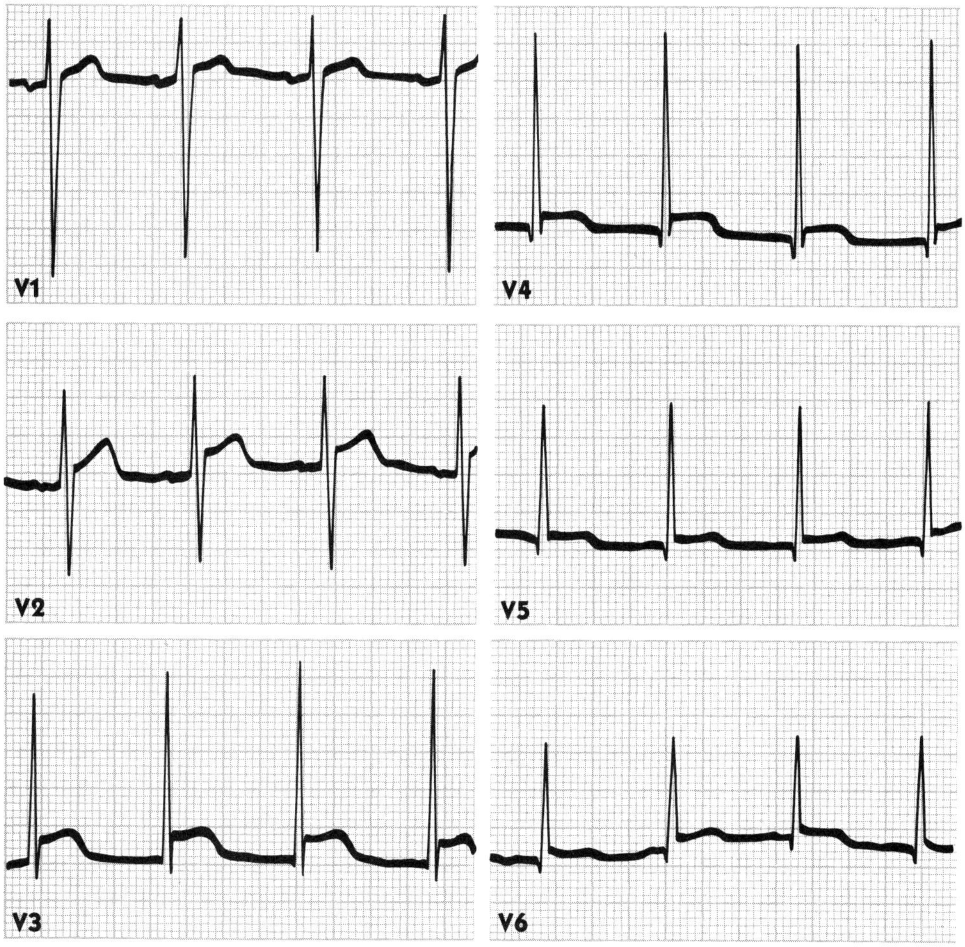

tion, they are also concave upward, but the clinical history and physical findings should suggest the correct diagnosis. In acute MI, the ST segments are generally *convex* upward. Third, in pericarditis and early repolarization, the ST segments are usually elevated less than 5 mm and do not obscure the terminal portions of the QRS complexes. In acute MI, the ST elevations frequently exceed 5 mm and do obscure the terminal QRSs. Fourth, the QT interval is expected to be normal in pericarditis and early repolarization, but is often prolonged in acute MI. Finally, exercise has no effect on ST abnormalities in pericarditis. However, in early repolarization, ST abnormalities normalize with exercise; in acute MI, they might worsen, as will the patient.

CASE 41

Evolving Pericarditis

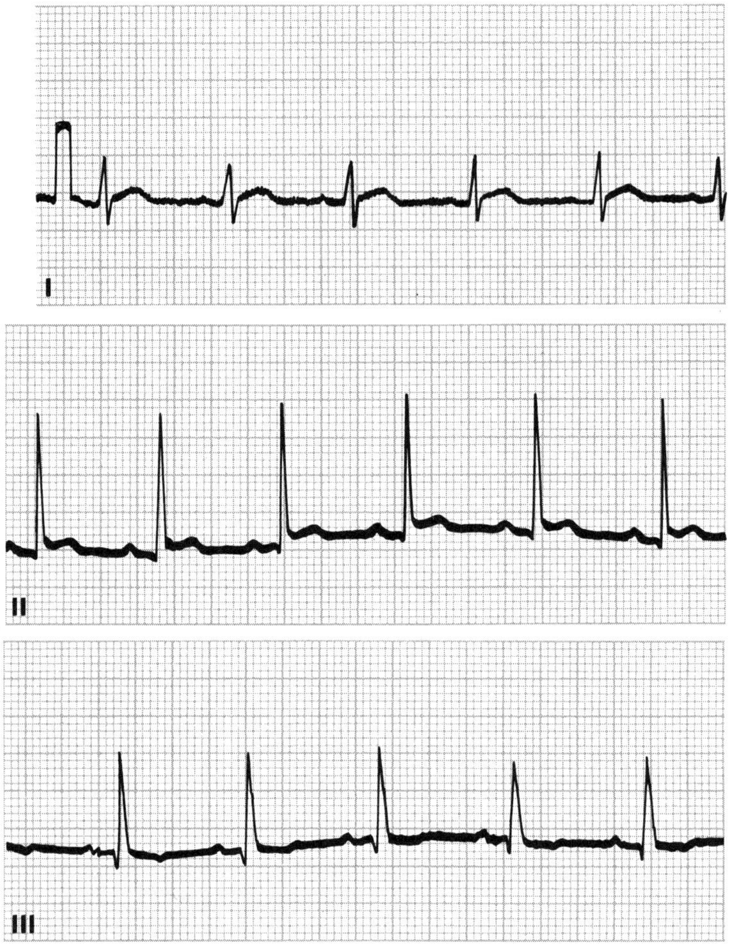

This 27-year-old man sustained a pericardial laceration from a stab wound to the chest, but no myocardial injury was demonstrated during operative repair. This ECG, recorded two days postoperatively, shows upwardly concave ST segment elevation in leads I, II, aVF, and V2-6. The T waves are biphasic in leads V3-4.

This patient has traumatic pericarditis. The ST segment elevations are diffuse, concave upward, less than 5 mm in height, do not obscure the terminal portions of the QRS complexes, and are associated with a normal QT interval. Compared with Case 40, this ECG illustrates a later phase in the evolution of pericarditis, with inverted T waves appearing in some leads. The early ST segment elevation of pericarditis persists for several hours to days and then resolves, followed by T wave inversion.

Coexisting ST elevation and T wave inversion, as seen in this case, raise the question of myocardial injury. But this pattern is not diagnostic of myocar-

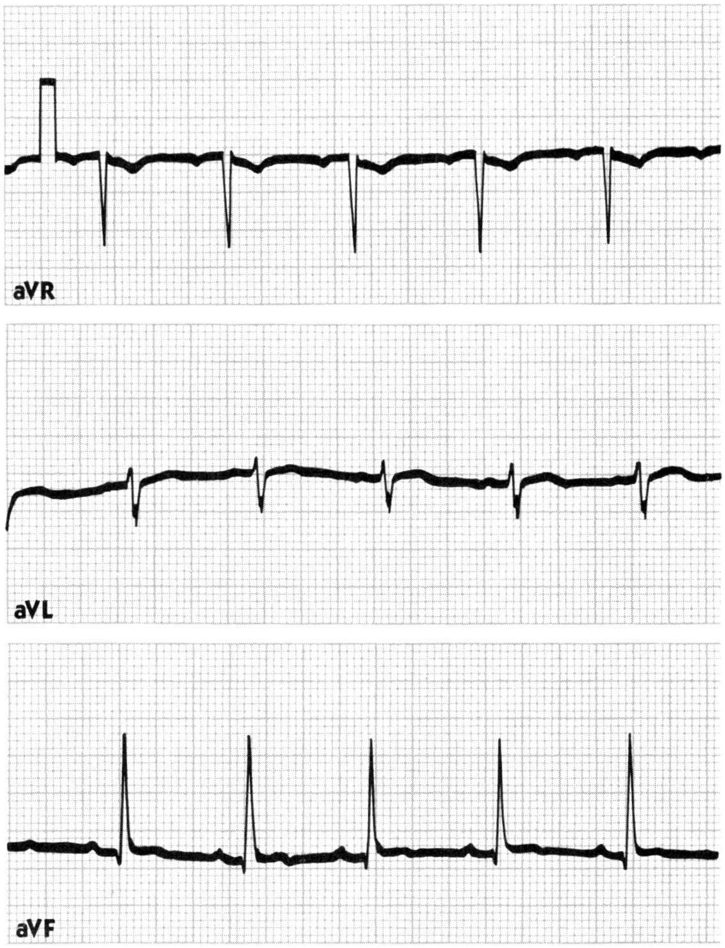

continued

dial injury, since it can occur in pericarditis alone as part of the evolutionary process. The epicardial irritation of pericarditis causes epimyocarditis, with the damaged myocardial tissue generating an injury current; this accounts for the similarity of some of the ECG features of pericarditis and myocardial infarction.

CASE 41 *(continued)*

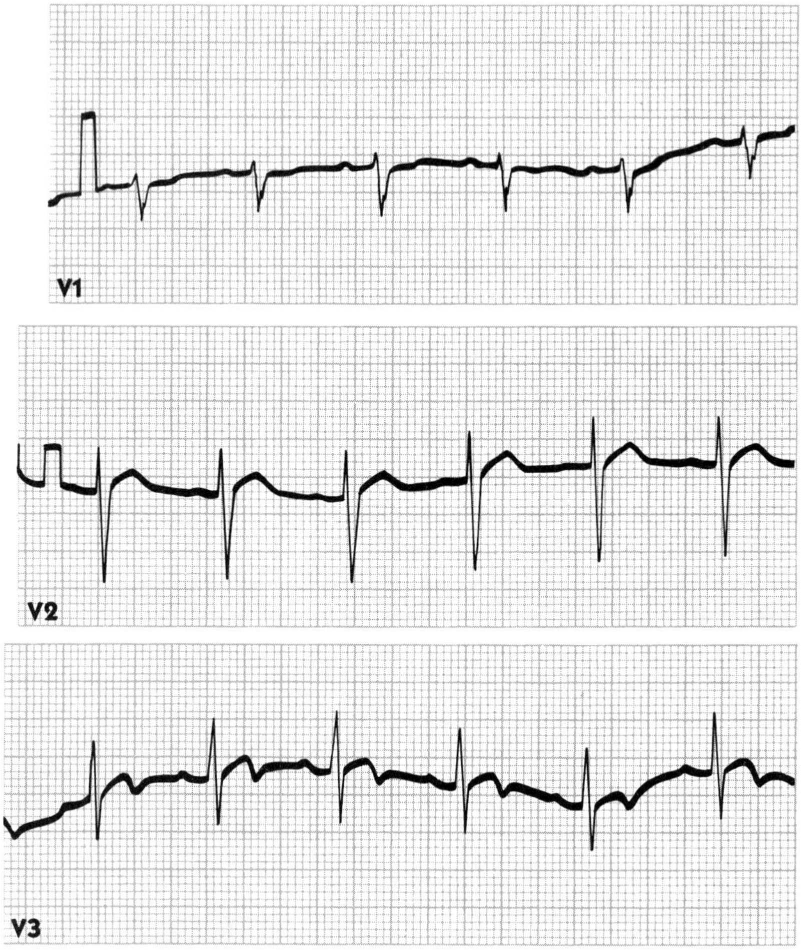

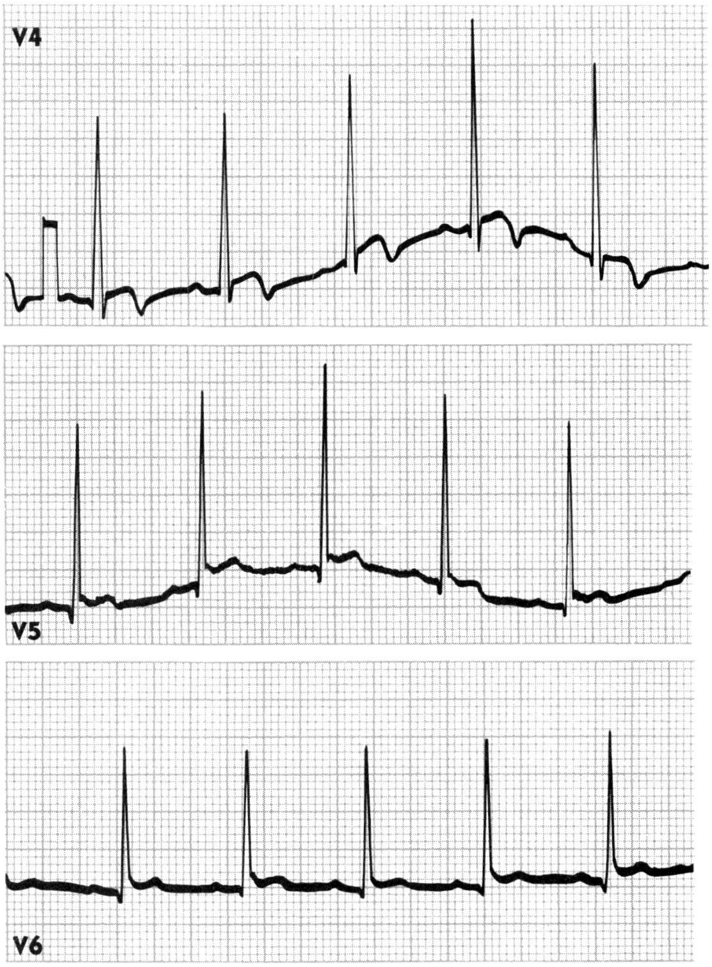
V4
V5
V6

CASE 42

Pericarditis

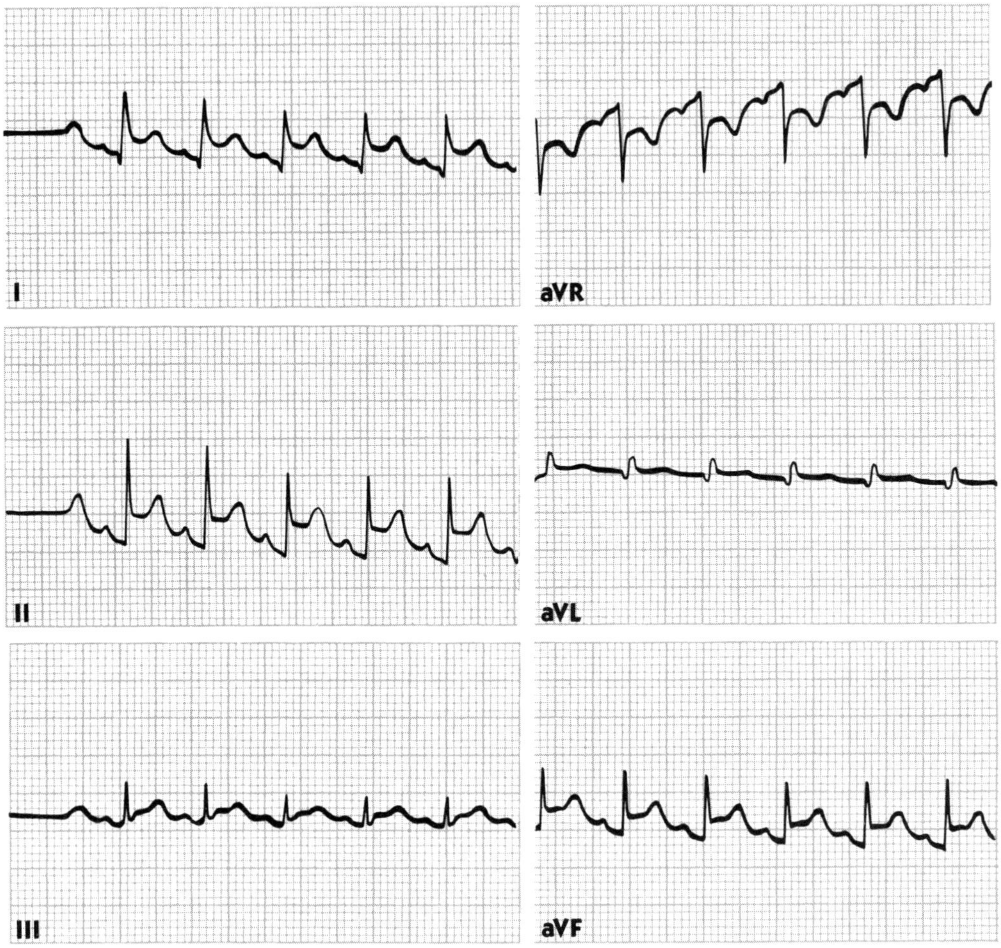

This 18-year-old man developed a sublingual abscess that extended into his mediastinum, resulting in empyema, purulent mediastinitis, and purulent pericarditis. This ECG, recorded two days after admission, shows sinus tachycardia, a normal mean frontal plane QRS axis, and normal intervals. The P waves are normal, but the PR segment (from the end of the P wave to the onset of the QRS complex) is depressed (best seen in lead II). The QRS complexes are normal, but ST segment elevation is present in every lead except aVR, which shows ST segment depression.

This ECG illustrates both typical and atypical features of pericarditis. The ST segments are diffusely elevated and concave upward. In contrast to the classic pattern of pericarditis, the ST elevation is marked (>5 mm) in many leads and obscures the terminal portions of some of the QRS complexes. PR segment depression, sensitive but not specific for pericarditis,

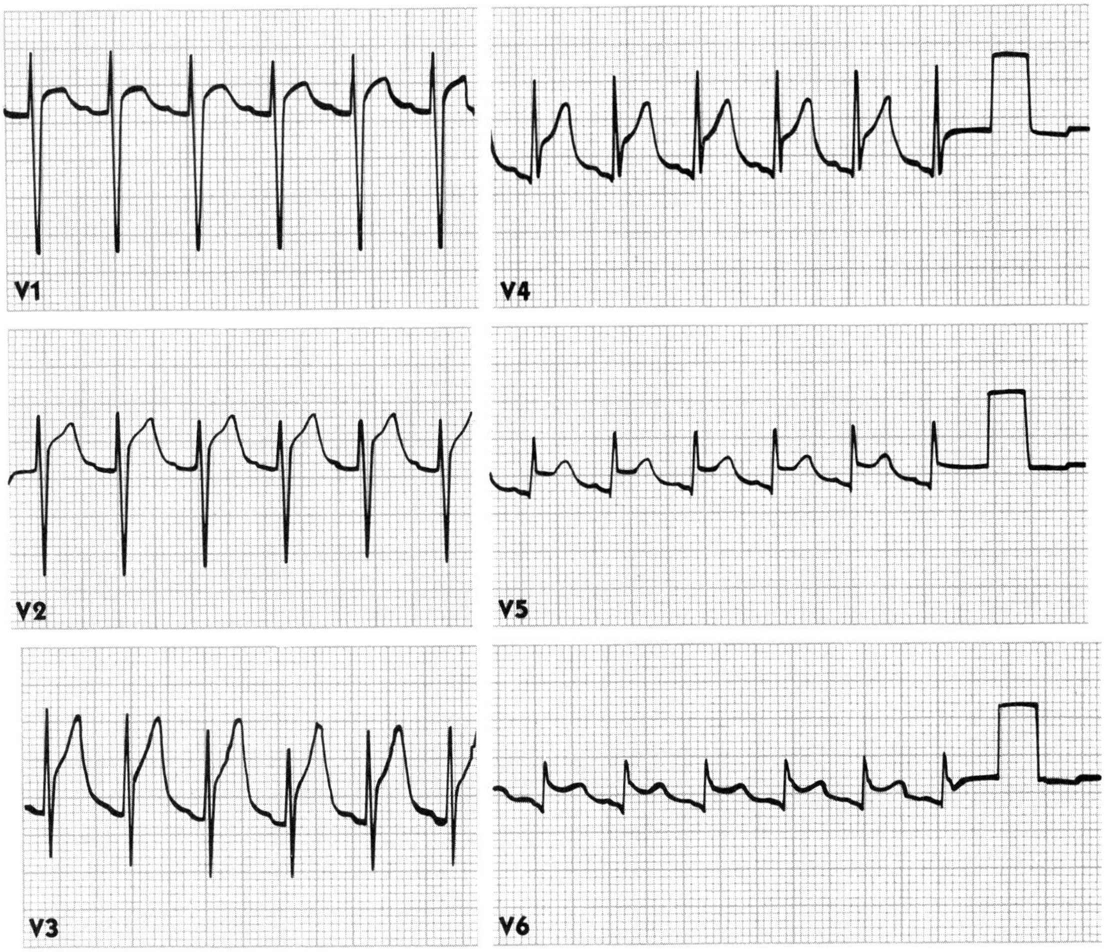

may precede the typical ST segment changes. A depressed PR segment may be seen in atrial infarction, but rarely without concomitant ECG and clinical evidence of ventricular infarction. This distinction is useful in the differential diagnosis.

CASE 43

Electrical Alternans Due to Large Pericardial Effusion

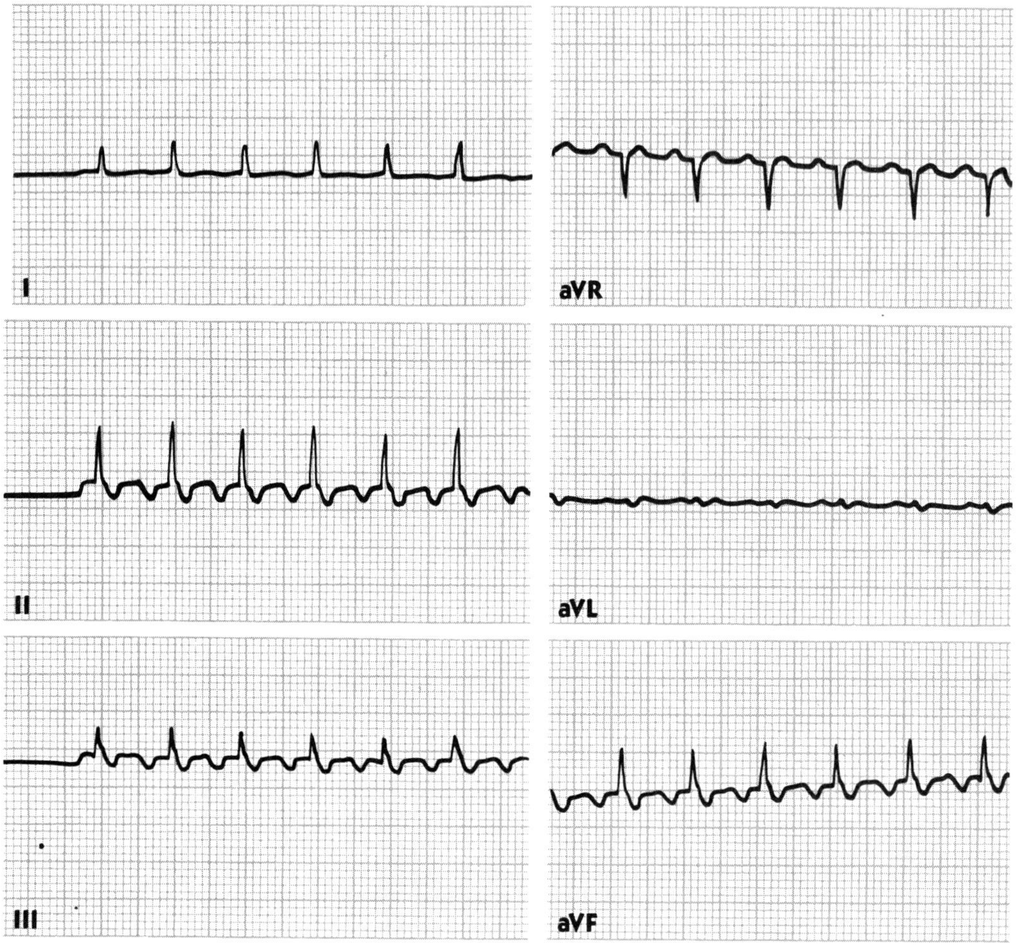

This patient has metastatic squamous-cell carcinoma. He was admitted with increasing cardiomegaly due to a large pericardial effusion. His ECG shows atrial flutter with 2:1 atrioventricular conduction and a ventricular rate of 150 per minute. The mean frontal plane QRS axis is normal at +60°. The QRS morphology is normal, but careful inspection reveals alternation of QRS amplitude (best seen in leads V4-5). This alternation (occasionally involving direction as well as amplitude) is termed "electrical alternans." It may involve not only QRS complexes but also P, T, and U waves, or any combination.

The electrical alternans pattern suggests a large pericardial effusion, with the heart swinging to and fro at each systole. Especially when tachycardia is present, the heart may not have enough time to return

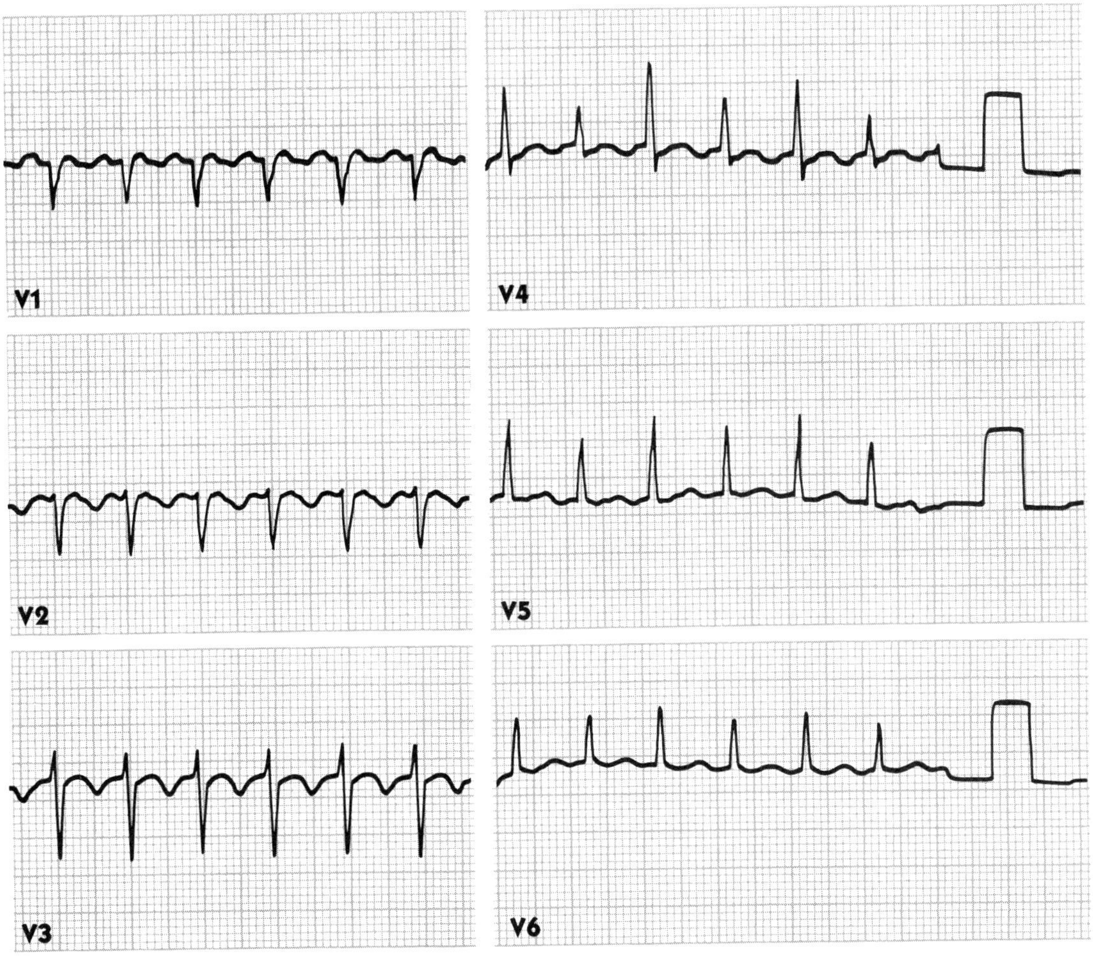

to its original position before the next systole. Ventricular activation occurring during this swinging motion is thought to contribute to electrical alternans.

Electrical alternans is also seen in the absence of pericardial effusion. It can occur in association with end-stage myocardial disease of various etiologies, myocarditis, hypocalcemia, lupus erythematosus, and after pneumonectomy. Its pathogenesis in these disorders is not well understood; thus the explanation above is still speculative.

CASE 44

ST-T Wave Alternation in Pericarditis With Effusion

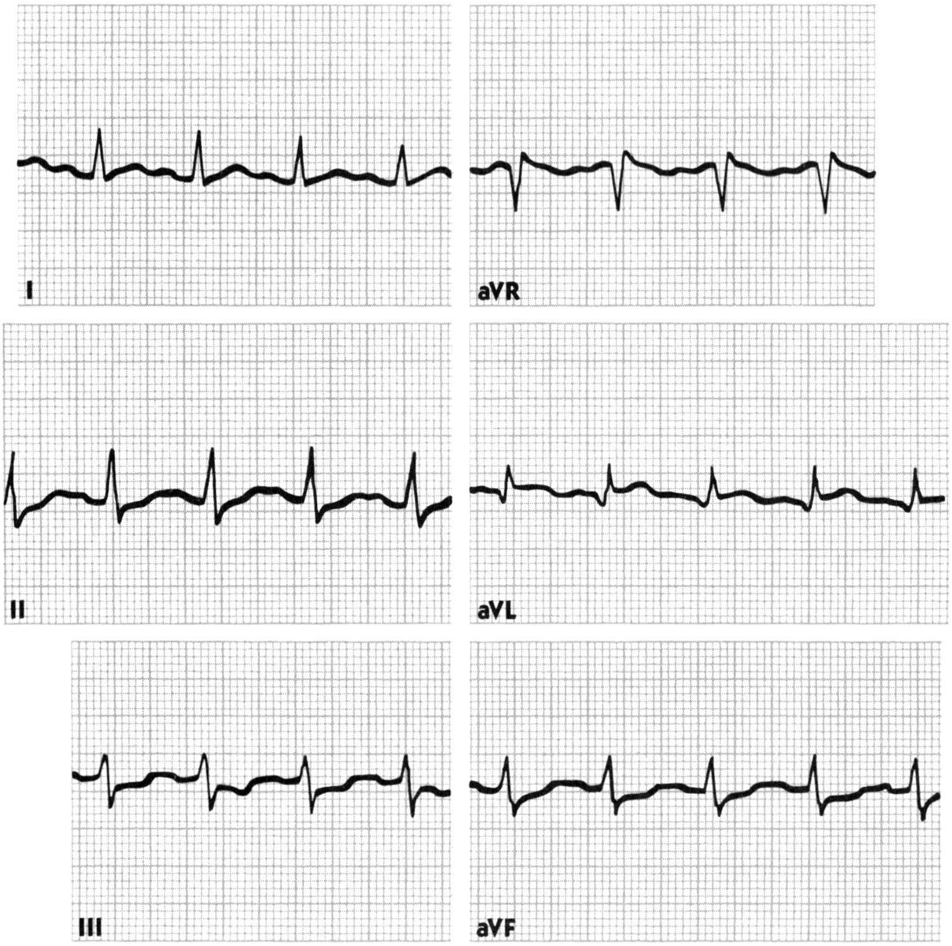

This ECG, recorded from a 37-year-old man with pericarditis and effusion, shows a QRS duration of 0.12 second, indicating slight intraventricular conduction delay. The QRS morphology is normal, but the ST segments are elevated in leads aVL and V1-4. There is alternation in both height and configuration of the ST-T waves (best seen in leads V2-3): (1) Upwardly convex, then downsloping ST segments with terminal T wave inversions alternate with (2) upwardly concave ST segments with tall, upright T waves. There is no alternation of the QRS complexes, as in Case 43.

This form of electrical alternans is called "ST-T wave alternans." Its genesis is unclear, but is thought to be similar to that of QRS alternation. The pattern is restricted to the ST-T waves for unknown reasons. ST-T wave alternans is much less common than QRS

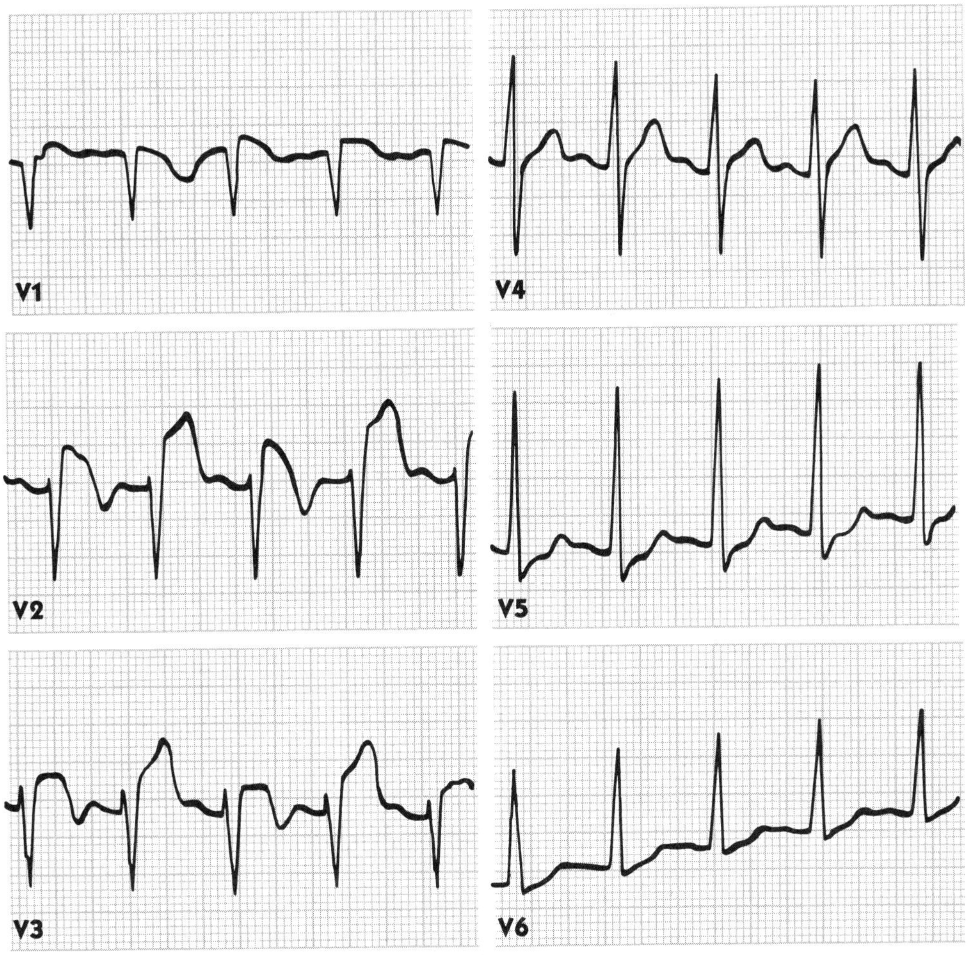

alternation in pericarditis with effusion. P and U wave alternation also may occur; P wave alternation is reportedly more frequent in malignant pericardial effusions. In this patient, the ST-T wave alternation spontaneously resolved one day later.

SECTION VII

The ECG in Lung Disease

CASE 45

Chronic Obstructive Pulmonary Disease With Right Atrial Abnormality

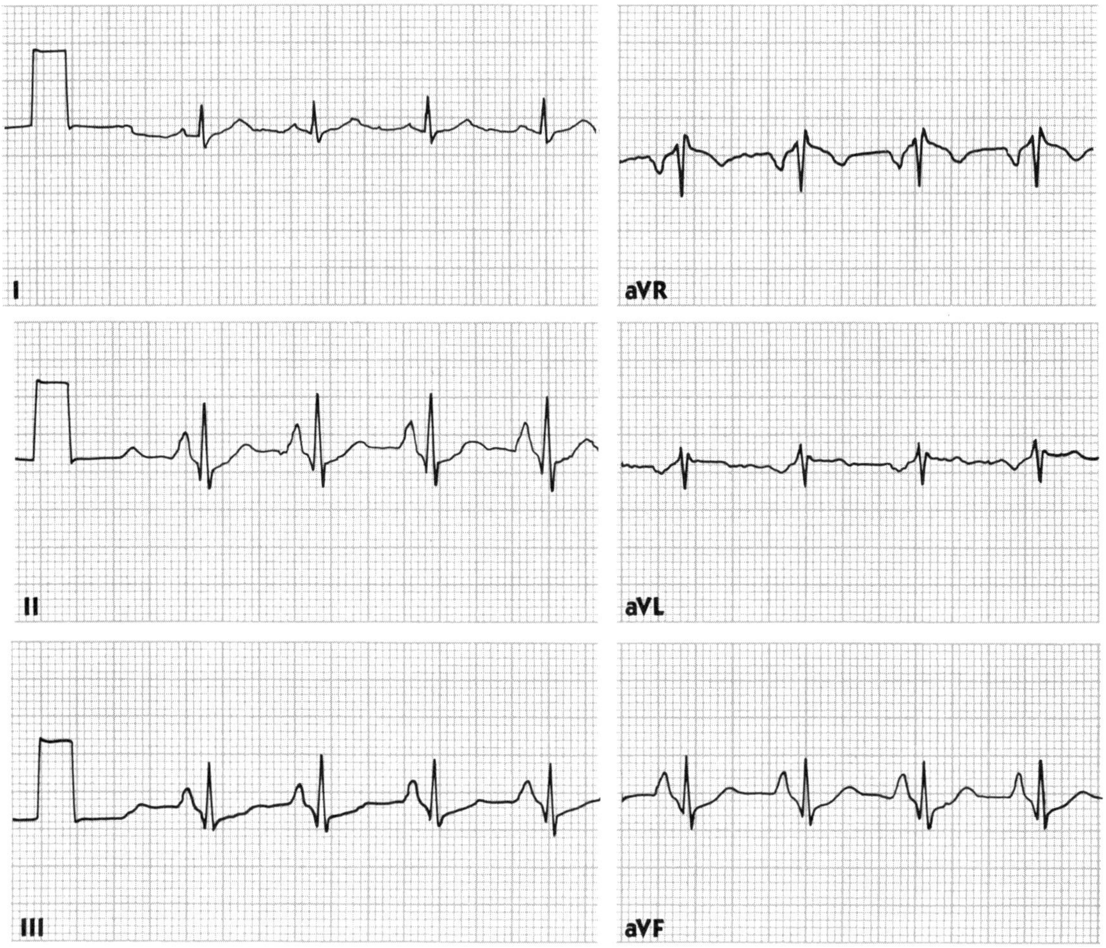

This patient has a long history of chronic obstructive pulmonary disease (COPD) with recurrent exacerbations. Her ECG shows a mean frontal plane QRS axis of about +75°, a P wave axis of about +75°, and normal intervals. There are tall, peaked P waves in leads II, III, and aVF, reaching 3.5 mm in height. Prominent, but not pathological, q waves are present in the inferior leads, and there is an rsr′ pattern in lead V1. The T wave morphology is normal.

A number of ECG abnormalities may be seen in COPD (see Table 8 in the Appendix). This case shows the classic pattern of P pulmonale: tall, peaked P waves of at least 2.5 mm in lead II. Pathological evidence does not confirm the traditional correlation between the P pulmonale pattern and right atrial enlargement and/or hypertrophy. A less misleading description of the pattern is "right atrial abnormality" (see Case 6).

The rsr′ pattern in lead V1 suggests right bundle branch block (RBBB), but the normal QRS duration excludes that diagnosis. The pattern must be considered to represent right ventricular conduction delay ("incomplete RBBB" in older, less precise terminology). It could also suggest early right ventricular hypertrophy (RVH), especially with the tall R waves in lead V2. Both right ventricular conduction disturbances and ECG evidence of RVH are frequent in COPD.

The q waves with upright T waves in the inferior leads may represent an old inferior wall myocardial infarction (MI). But in the presence of COPD, q waves do not necessarily connote MI. Septal q waves may

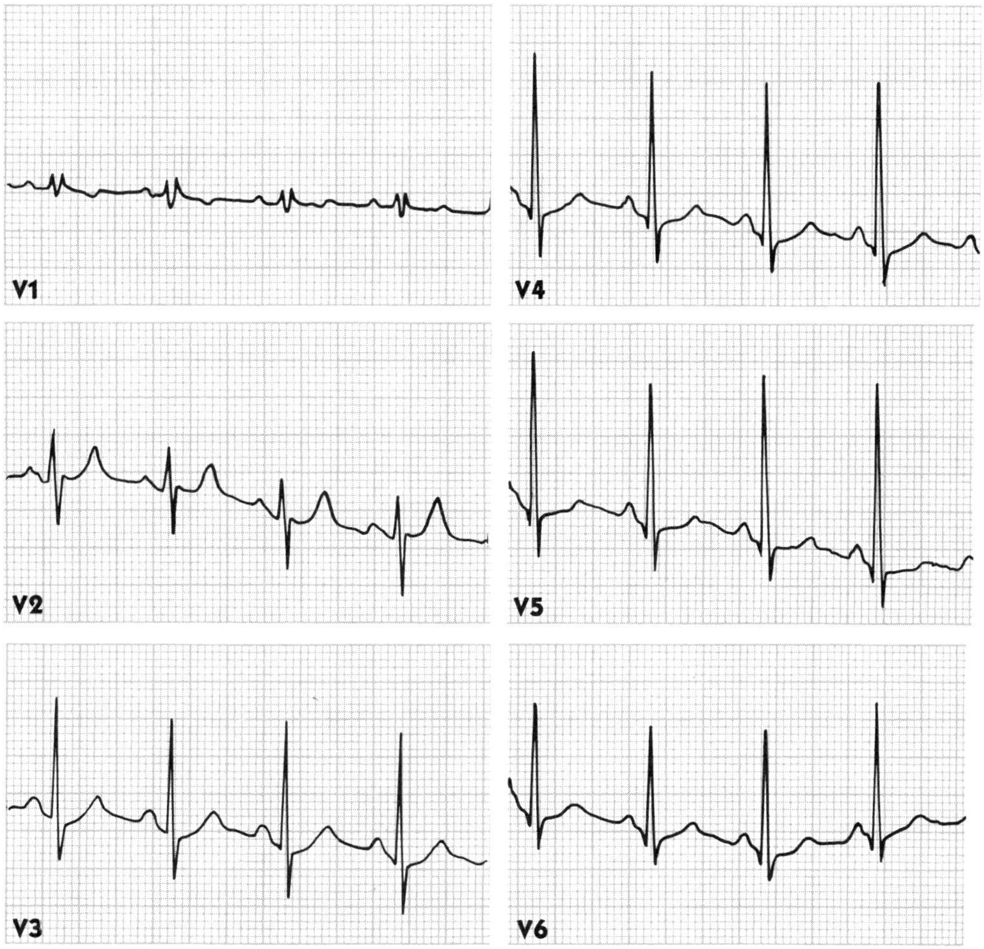

become pronounced in the inferior or lateral leads if RVH is present. In addition, an inferior qR or even QS pattern may result from hyperinflation of the lungs, which pulls the heart inferiorly and its apex more medially within the chest cavity (see Case 47).

CASE 46

Chronic Obstructive Pulmonary Disease Mimicking Lateral Wall Myocardial Infarction

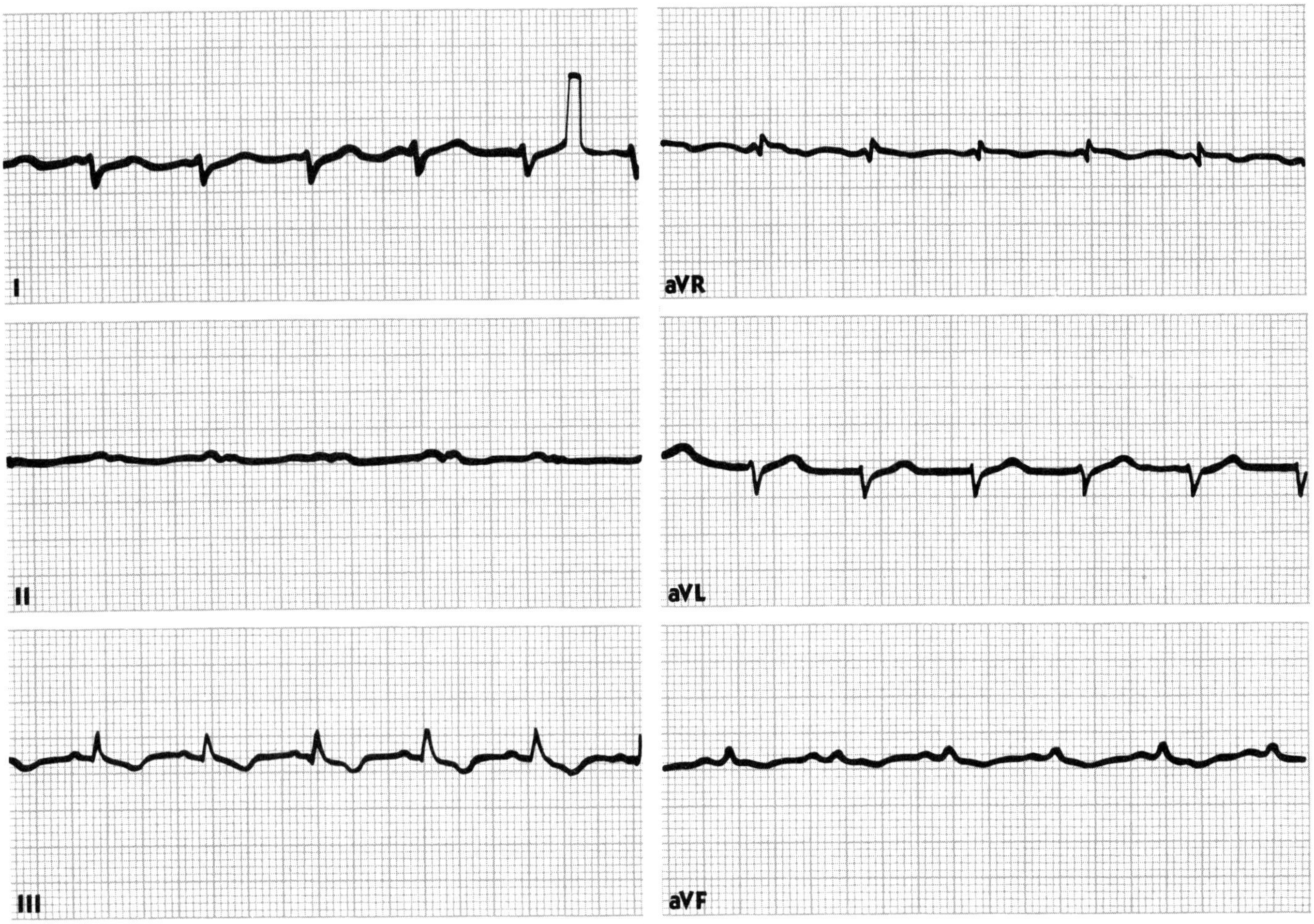

This ECG, recorded from a patient with severe chronic obstructive pulmonary disease (COPD), shows sinus rhythm and a mean frontal plane QRS axis of +140°. Unlike Case 45, the P waves here are normal in axis, amplitude, and configuration. This is despite the marked rightward deviation of the QRS axis indicating right ventricular hypertrophy (RVH). In the limb leads, the QRS voltage is diminished (see Table 9 in the Appendix); no complex exceeds 5 mm in height. Otherwise (except for the axis deviation), the QRS configuration in these leads is unremarkable. In the precordial leads, the QRS voltage is normal, but rS complexes appear in every lead but V1, which shows a qR pattern. There is T wave inversion in leads III, aVF, and V1-4.

This ECG illustrates several abnormalities commonly associated with COPD. The marked right axis deviation and the qR pattern in lead V1 indicate RVH (see Cases 5 and 6 and Table 3). Modest right axis deviation of +90° to +110° may not necessarily indicate RVH in patients with COPD, as the axis may result solely from inferior and rightward displacement of

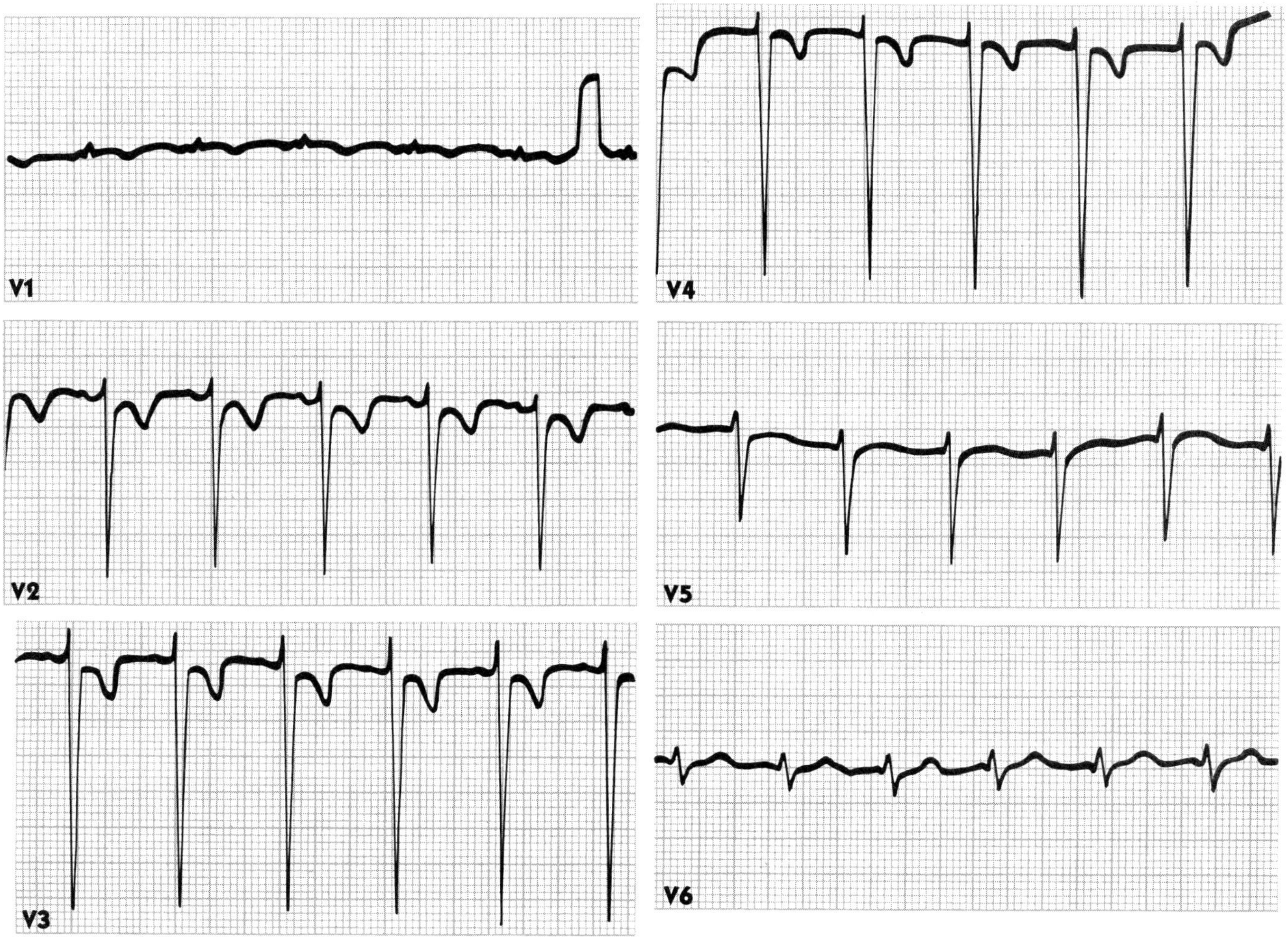

the heart. Anterior and inferior T wave inversions commonly accompany and tend to confirm the diagnosis of RVH.

The low QRS voltage in the limb leads results from hyperinflation of the lungs, with a consequent increase in distance between the heart and surface ECG leads. Lung hyperinflation, with concomitant flattening of the diaphragm, also pulls the heart inferiorly and its apex medially and away from the lateral wall, resulting in loss of R wave voltage (poor R wave progression) in the lateral leads.

Poor R wave progression may occur in many conditions (see Table 2 in the Appendix), including COPD without RVH, RVH alone, and lateral wall myocardial infarction (MI). In COPD without RVH, poor R wave progression results from inferior and medial displacement of the heart. In RVH alone, it is explained by posterior displacement of the left ventricle, away from the anterior leads. (Appropriate R waves will appear in posterior leads V7-10.) In lateral wall MI, actual loss of lateral forces due to infarcted myocardium is responsible for the abnormal R waves.

CASE 47

Chronic Obstructive Pulmonary Disease Mimicking Inferior and Anterior Wall Myocardial Infarction

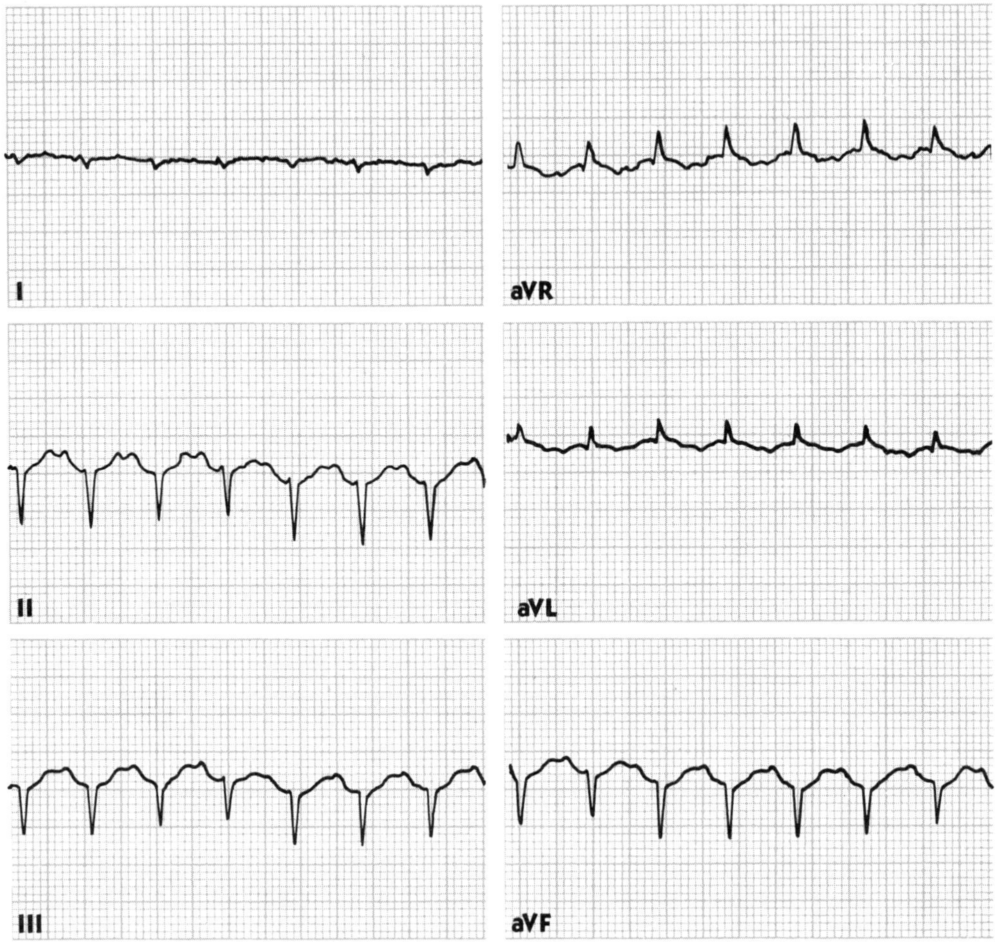

This ECG was recorded from a patient with severe chronic obstructive pulmonary disease (COPD). The mean frontal plane QRS axis is shifted leftward and superiorly to about −90°. Leads aVR and aVL show a qR pattern. In the inferior leads, the P waves are superimposed on the T waves, but do not appear to be tall or peaked. There are QS complexes in leads V1-3 and rS complexes in leads V4-6, as well as in II, III, and aVF. The T waves are somewhat flattened laterally.

The superior axis deviation with inferior rS complexes might suggest left anterior fascicular block (see Case 16) and thus left-sided conduction system disease. However, considering how frequently inferior rS or QS patterns occur in COPD and the absence of fibrosis of the left ventricular conduction system at autopsies, another explanation is possible: As the heart is pulled inferiorly by hyperinflation of the lungs, the mean vector of left ventricular depolarization swings inferoposteriorly. But in some patients, there may be sufficient downward displacement to redirect the mean vector superiorly as well as posteriorly, explaining the deep inferior S waves. Although the exact mechanism of left axis deviation remains ill-defined, it is important to remember that inferior QS complexes appear frequently in severe COPD, representing a pseudoinfarction pattern (see Table 7 in the Appendix).

The QS complexes in the anterior leads could represent old anterior wall myocardial infarction (MI) or yet another pseudoinfarction pattern. In Case 46,

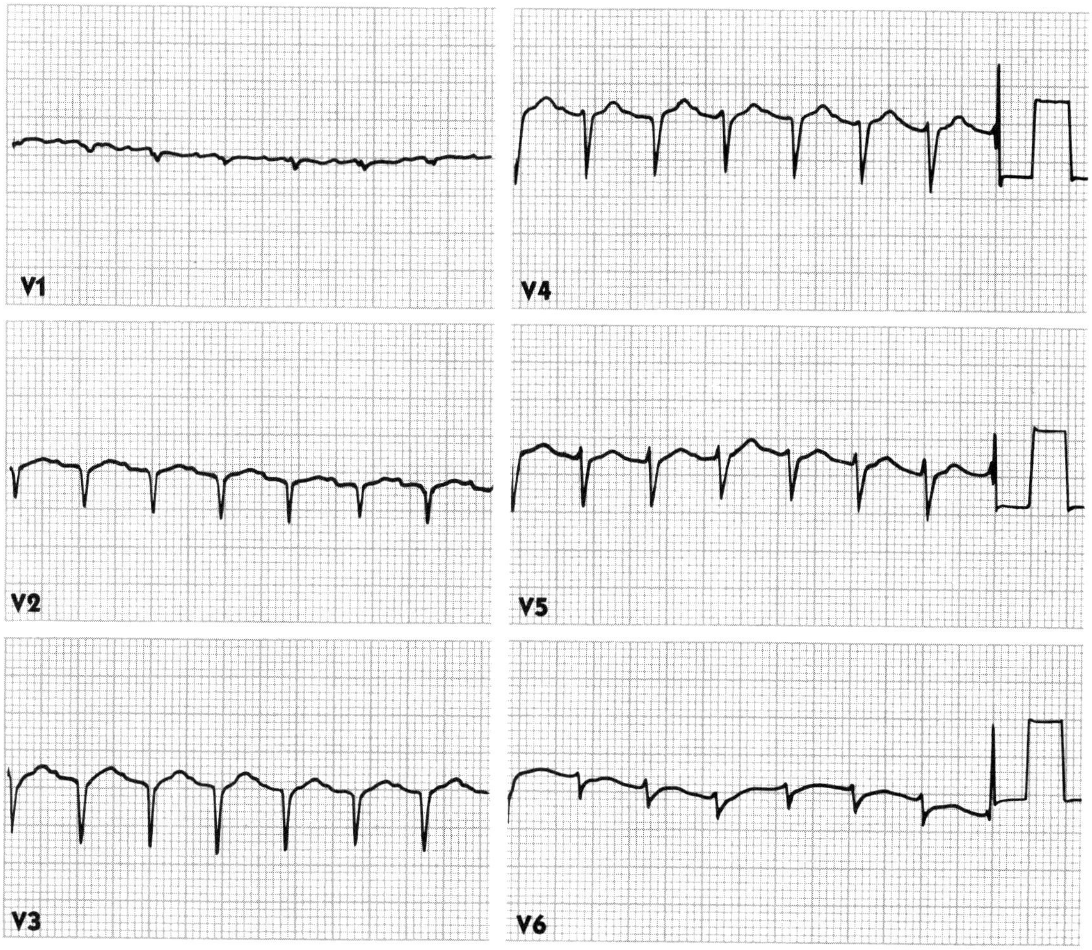

it was seen that COPD can be associated with deep S waves and poor R wave progression in the anterior leads. Anterior QS complexes may represent the extreme of this pattern, and the differential diagnosis discussed in Case 46 applies here also. The genesis of the anterior QS pattern in this case can best be explained by posterior displacement of the mean QRS vector or by increased distance between the high anterior leads and the inferiorly displaced heart. Either possibility can result from hyperinflated lungs.

CASE 48A

Acute Pulmonary Embolism

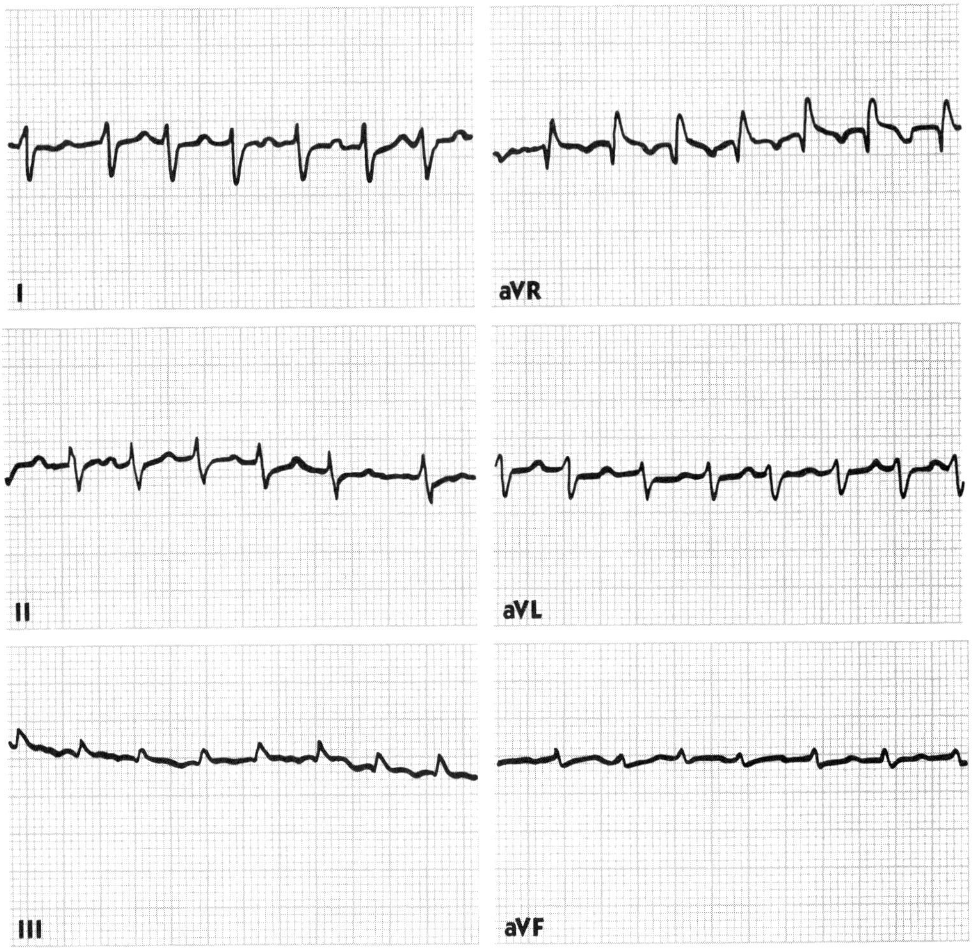

This 67-year-old woman with previously normal ECGs had an abrupt onset of dyspnea and pleuritic chest pain. This ECG shows atrial fibrillation with a rapid ventricular rate. The mean frontal plane QRS axis is shifted rightward to about +130°. The QRS duration is 0.09 second, and an rSR'S' pattern appears in lead V1, indicating right intraventricular conduction delay. The QT interval is prolonged (0.30 second). There is an rS pattern in lead I and a qR pattern in lead III. The ST segments and T waves show nonspecific abnormalities.

The newly present right axis deviation and right intraventricular conduction delay suggest acute pulmonary embolism (PE). These findings are thought to be due to acute right heart strain produced by an abrupt increase in pulmonary artery pressure. Another characteristic ECG finding is the $S_1Q_3T_3$ (or S_1Q_3 as seen here) pattern. It consists of a deep S wave in lead I, a significant Q wave in lead III, and an

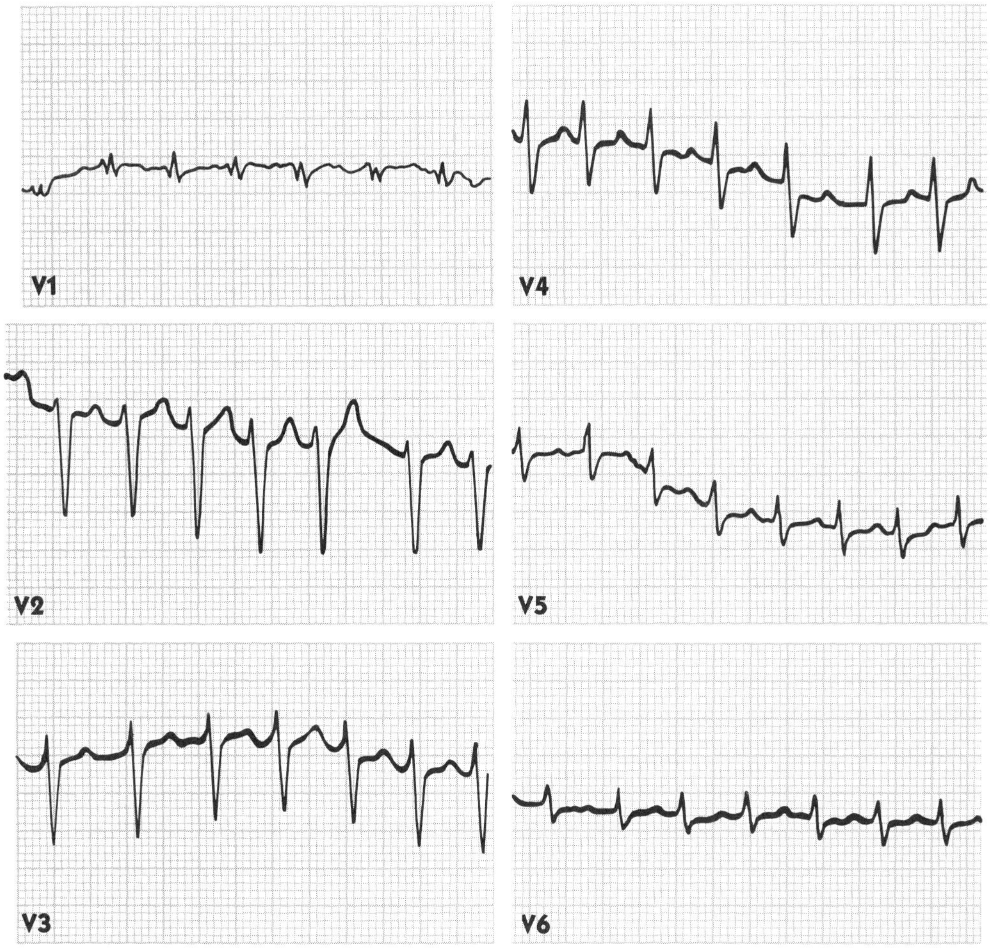

inverted T wave in lead III. These changes might suggest acute inferior wall myocardial infarction (MI) and right axis deviation. However, the absence of Q waves in leads II and/or aVF and of noteworthy ST segment changes militates against the diagnosis of MI.

While PE is often difficult to distinguish from acute MI on clinical grounds, correlation of the history, physical examination, and ECG (see Table 10 in the Appendix) are often sufficient to direct attention to the correct diagnosis.

CASE 48B

Evolution of the ECG in Acute PE

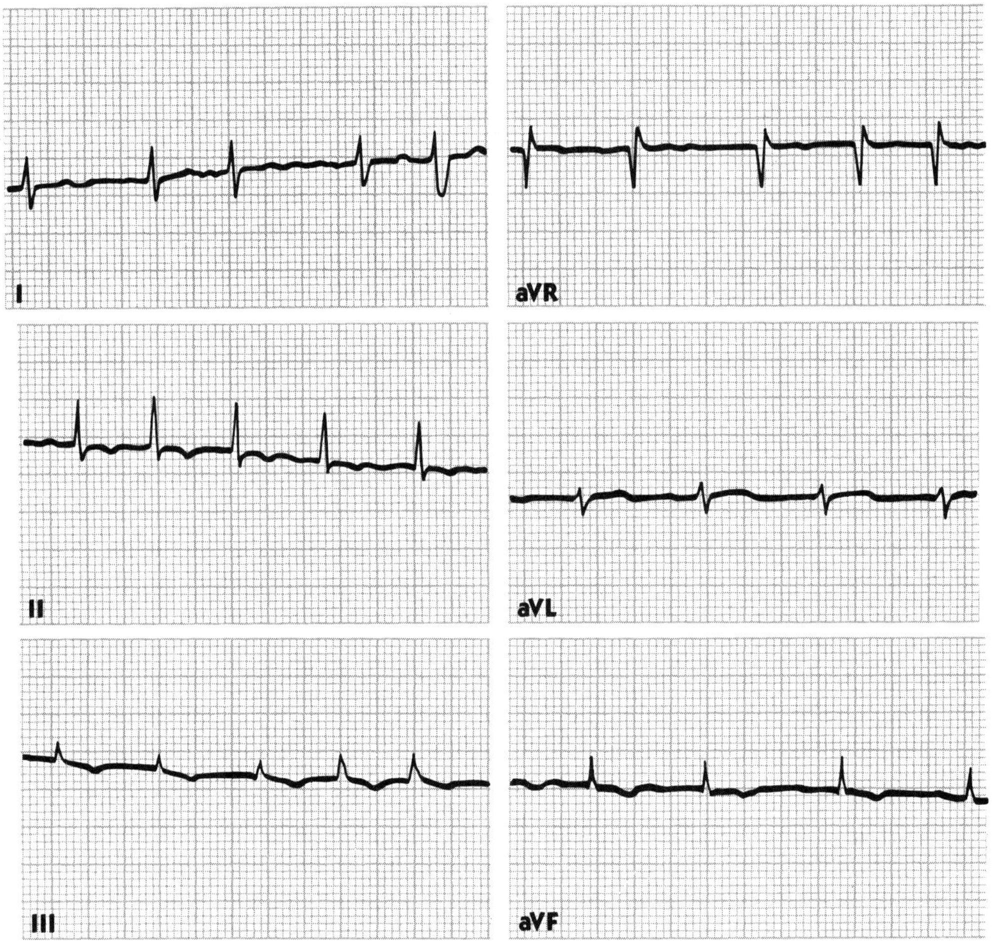

Three days later, the ECG still shows atrial fibrillation, but with a slower ventricular rate than before (about 90 per minute). The mean frontal plane QRS axis is now less rightward (about +60°), the QRS duration is 0.08 second, and the right intraventricular conduction delay is no longer present. The Q wave in lead III is now barely discernible. There are diffuse T wave inversions involving the inferior and precordial leads.

The resolution of the right axis deviation, right-sided conduction delay, and Q wave in lead III most likely reflects normalization of the pulmonary artery pressures. The only significant ECG findings remaining are the atrial fibrillation and the nonspecific ST-T abnormalities. Although the most common cardiac rhythm in acute PE is sinus tachycardia, a number of atrial arrhythmias can occur. Atrial fibrillation is the most frequent of these. The diagnosis of PE should always be considered when there is atrial fibrillation

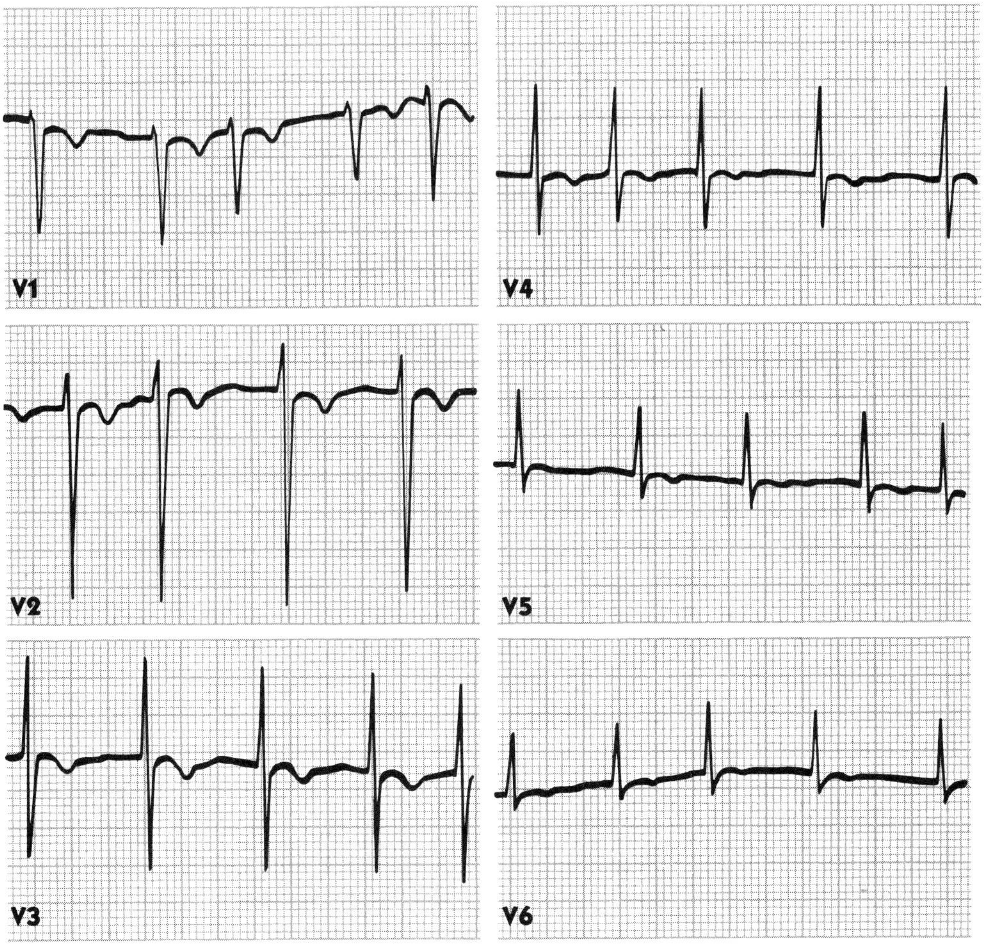

of new onset, but this rhythm is neither a specific nor a sensitive indicator of PE.

Nonspecific ST segment and T wave abnormalities are common in PE, but by definition they are nondiagnostic and thus not helpful clues. Such ST-T abnormalities in PE might reflect alterations in repolarization due to the acute changes in right-sided pressures. The diffuse T wave inversions in this ECG might suggest anteroinferior ischemia or nontransmural myocardial infarction, but such changes also occur in several noncardiac conditions (see Table 5 in the Appendix).

CASE 49—A, B, and C

Acute Pulmonary Embolism

CASE 49A Emergency Room

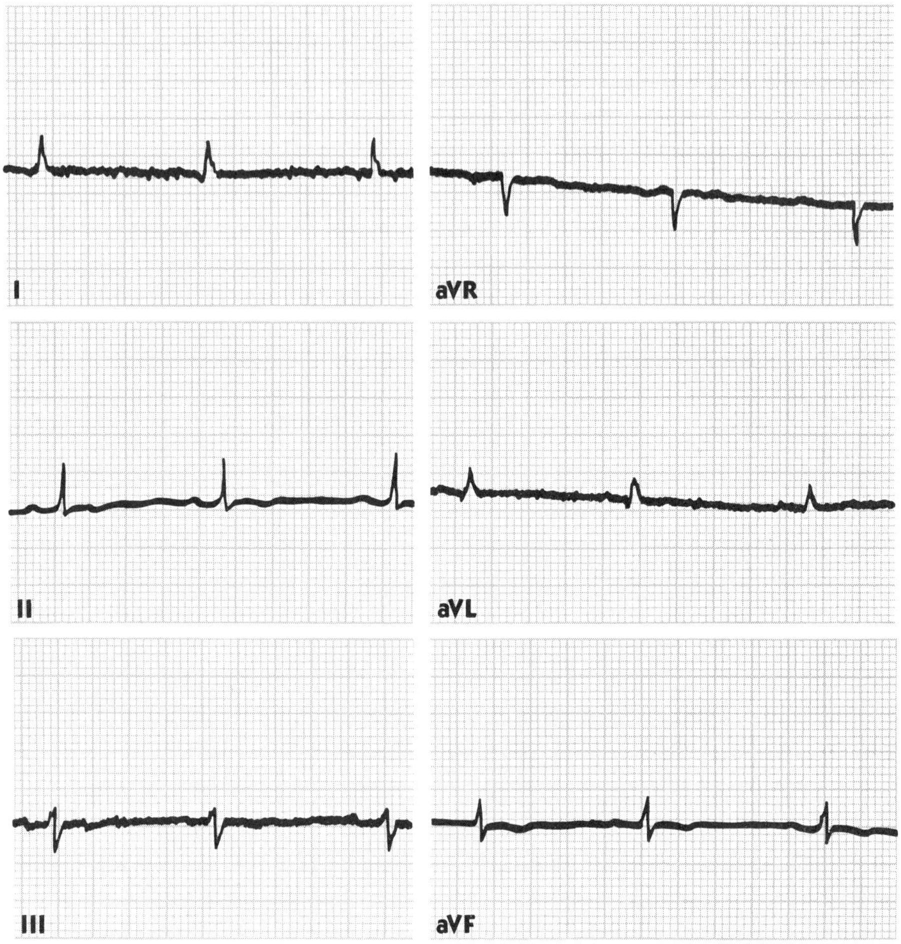

This series of ECGs was recorded from a 55-year-old woman who developed atypical substernal chest pain and was admitted to the hospital to exclude myocardial infarction. Her ECG recorded in the Emergency Room (A) shows T wave flattening in the limb and early precordial leads and T wave inversion in leads V3-6.

Two days later, a second ECG was recorded during an episode of severe pleuritic chest pain (B). It shows a mean frontal plane QRS axis of about −20°, very low voltage in the limb leads, poorly discernible P waves, and a prolonged QRS duration of 0.12 second. There is an rS pattern in lead III and an rsR′ pattern in lead V1, and there are notched R waves in leads V2-3. The T waves are inverted in leads II, III, aVF, and V1-5. ST segment depression is present in leads V4-5 and possibly also in lead I.

As the clinical course suggests, the patient had an acute pulmonary embolus while in the hospital. This is consistent with her second ECG, which shows a new right bundle branch block (RBBB) pattern and a leftward and superior shift of the QRS axis (from about +20° to about −20°). The ST-T abnormalities in the inferior and lateral leads suggest myocardial ischemia, but are nondiagnostic. The T wave inversions in the anterior precordial leads are probably due to delay in right ventricular depolarization (RBBB pattern).

The major ECG finding suggestive of pulmonary embolism (PE) in this case is the acute onset of the RBBB pattern. It could be due to RBBB per se, to acute right ventricular (RV) dilatation with consequent prolongation of RV activation, or to RV ischemia. The leftward and superior axis shift, while not expected,

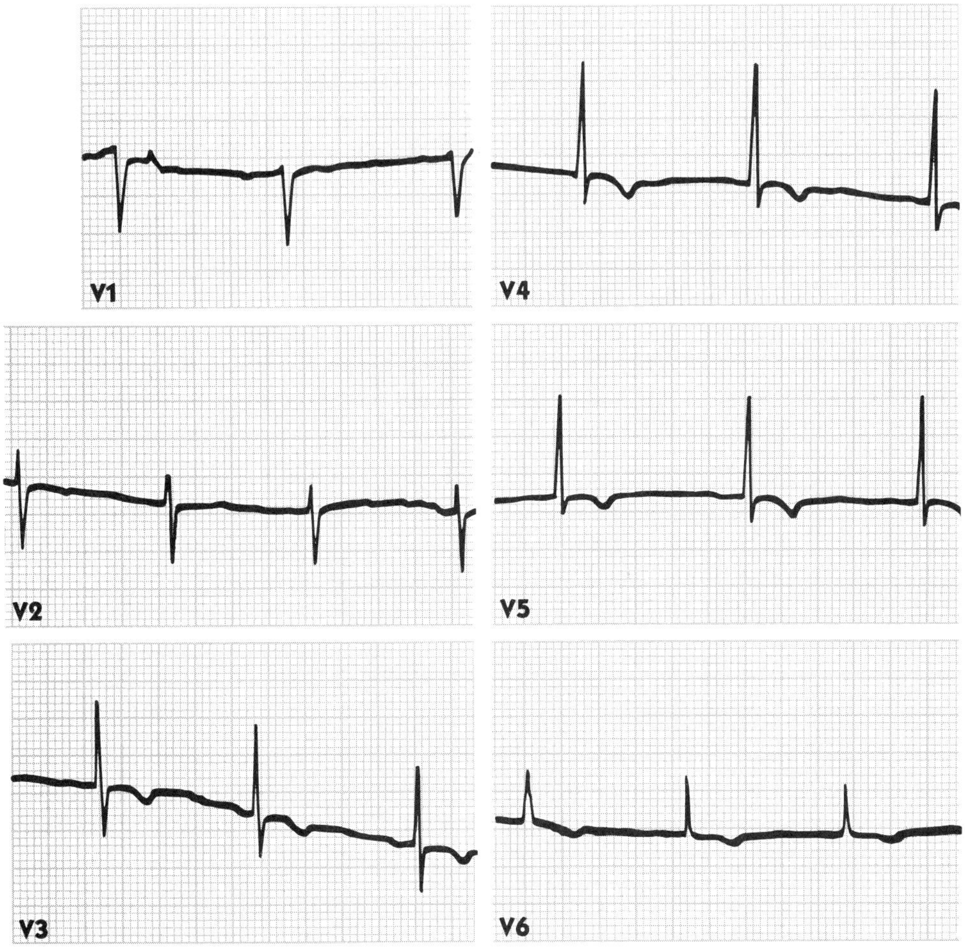

continued

is occasionally seen in PE; in this clinical circumstance, it does not represent left anterior fascicular block. In fact, sometimes an $S_1S_2S_3$ pattern (deep S waves in leads I, II, and III) is present, along with extreme left axis deviation. The genesis of this pattern is not entirely clear, but may involve the leftward and posterior shift of the mean QRS vector generated by the left ventricle due to acute RV dilatation. Low voltage in the limb leads is a fairly common ECG finding in PE, but is not specific for this diagnosis (see Table 9 in the Appendix). No ECG findings are actually specific for PE, and 15% of patients with acute PE have a normal ECG.

Two hours after this patient's acute pulmonary embolus, the third ECG (C) was recorded. Further changes are noticeable. The axis is still leftward at about −20°. However, the QRS duration is now normal and the RBBB pattern has disappeared. As in the initial ECG, there are nondiagnostic T wave inversions in the inferior and anterolateral leads.

This series illustrates the fleeting nature of some of the ECG findings in PE. If an ECG had not been recorded promptly with the onset of pleuritic chest pain, the abnormalities would not have been observed.

CASE 49B **With severe pleuritic chest pain**

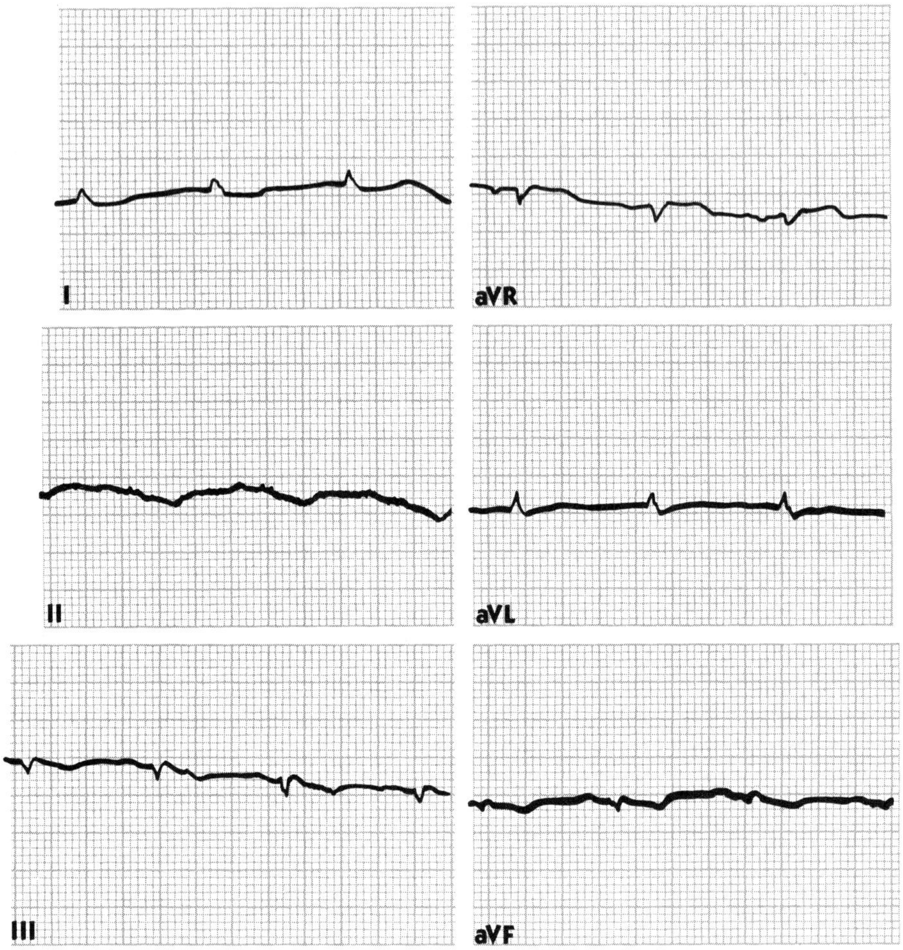

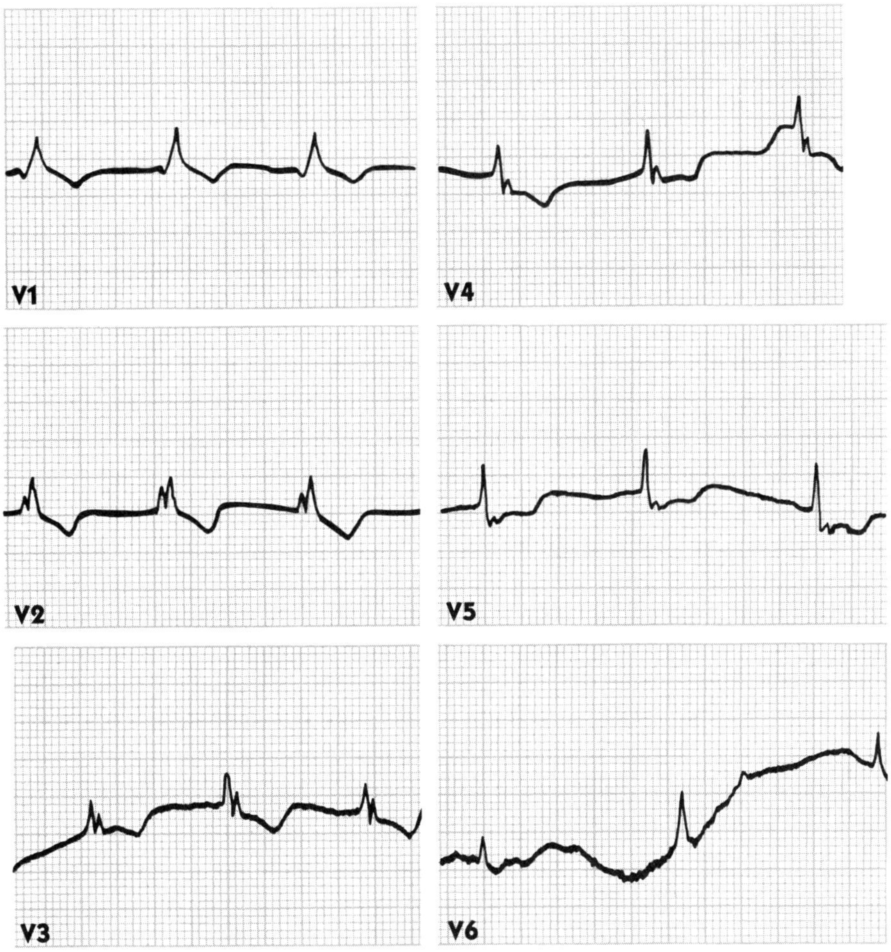

continued

CASE 49C Two hours later

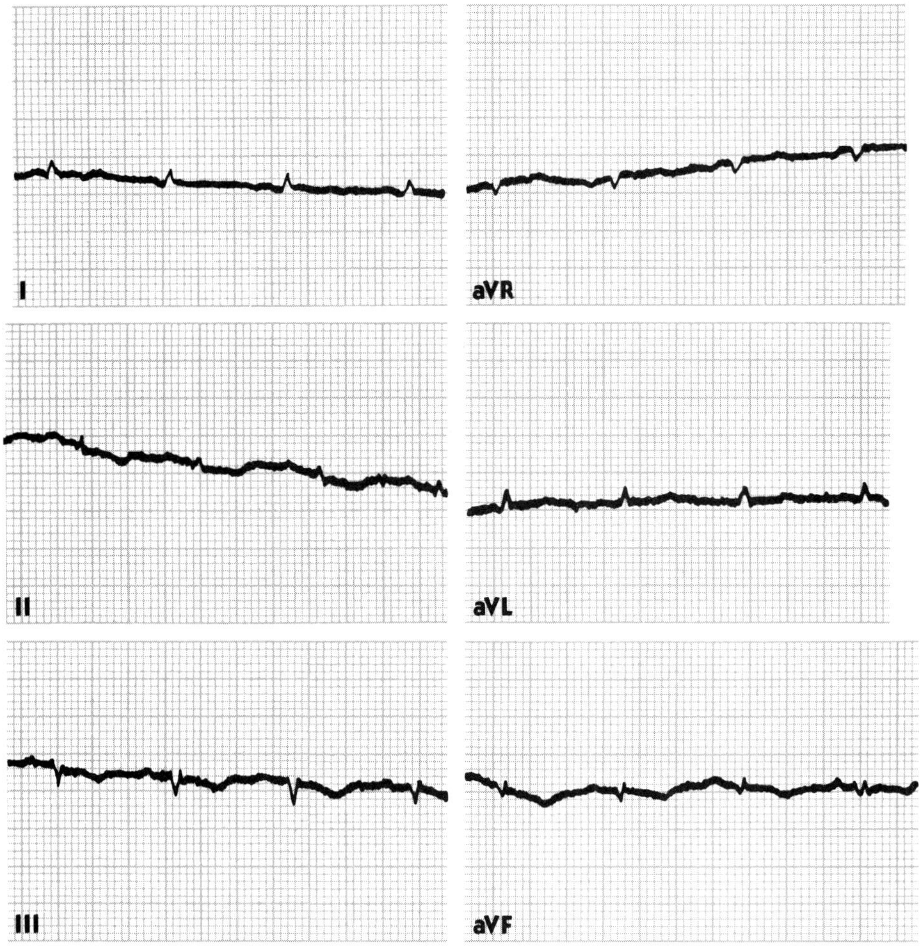

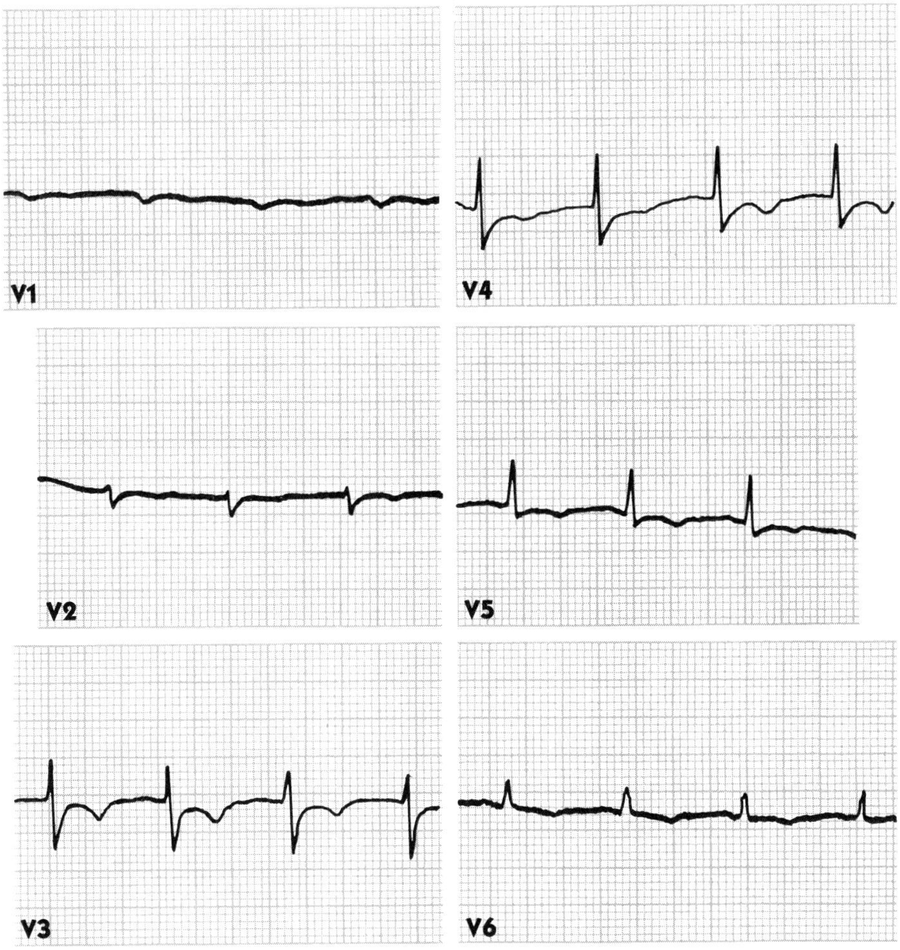
V1
V4
V2
V5
V3
V6

SECTION VIII

The ECG in Electrolyte and Metabolic Disturbances

CASE 50—A and B

Hyperkalemia

CASE 50A Serum K^+ = 7.6 mEq/l

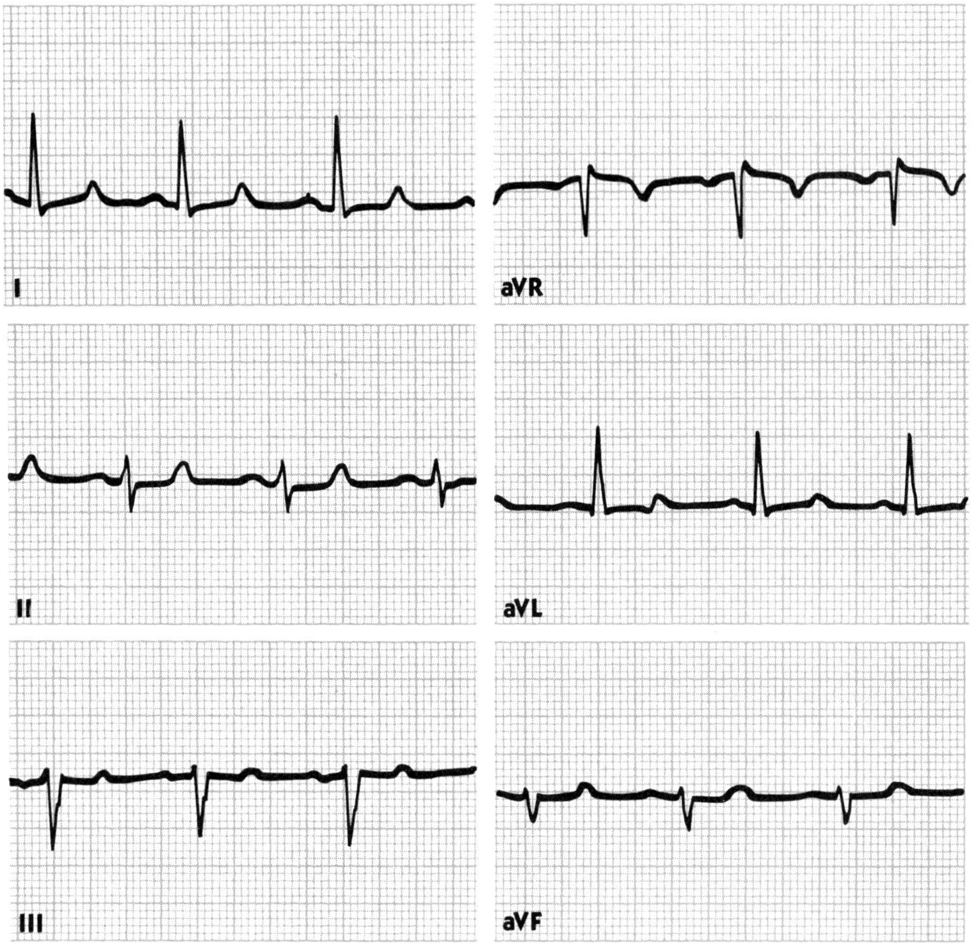

These two tracings were obtained from a 57-year-old woman who had received excessive potassium during increasing renal failure. The first ECG (A) shows a mean frontal plane QRS axis of −30° and normal P and QRS durations. The QT interval is 0.44 second, abnormally long for the rate. The T waves are tall in the anterior leads and definitely peaked and "tented" in leads I, aVL, and V5-6. Although the ST segment is straightened and prolonged in leads I, aVL, and V5-6, suggesting hypocalcemia, the serum calcium level was normal.

The patient's potassium level was well above normal at 7.6 mEq/l. Her ECG shows the classic "tombstone" T waves of hyperkalemia—narrow-based and peaked or tented. The height of the anterior precordial T waves may be substantial, dwarfing the QRS complexes preceding them, but tall T waves alone without peaking or tenting do not suggest hyperkalemia. Similar-appearing, hyperacute T waves occur during the very early stages of acute myocardial infarction (MI) or transmural ischemia (see Cases 24 and 31). In fact, the hyperacute T wave changes of MI and ischemia may be due to potassium release from ischemic or necrotic cells, with local extracellular hyperkalemia surrounding surviving myocardium. As the local increase in potassium equilibrates with total body potassium, the ECG abnormalities resolve.

Further increases in the serum potassium level lead to PR interval prolongation, ST segment depression, and loss of atrial muscle activation with loss of P wave voltage or even total absence of P waves.

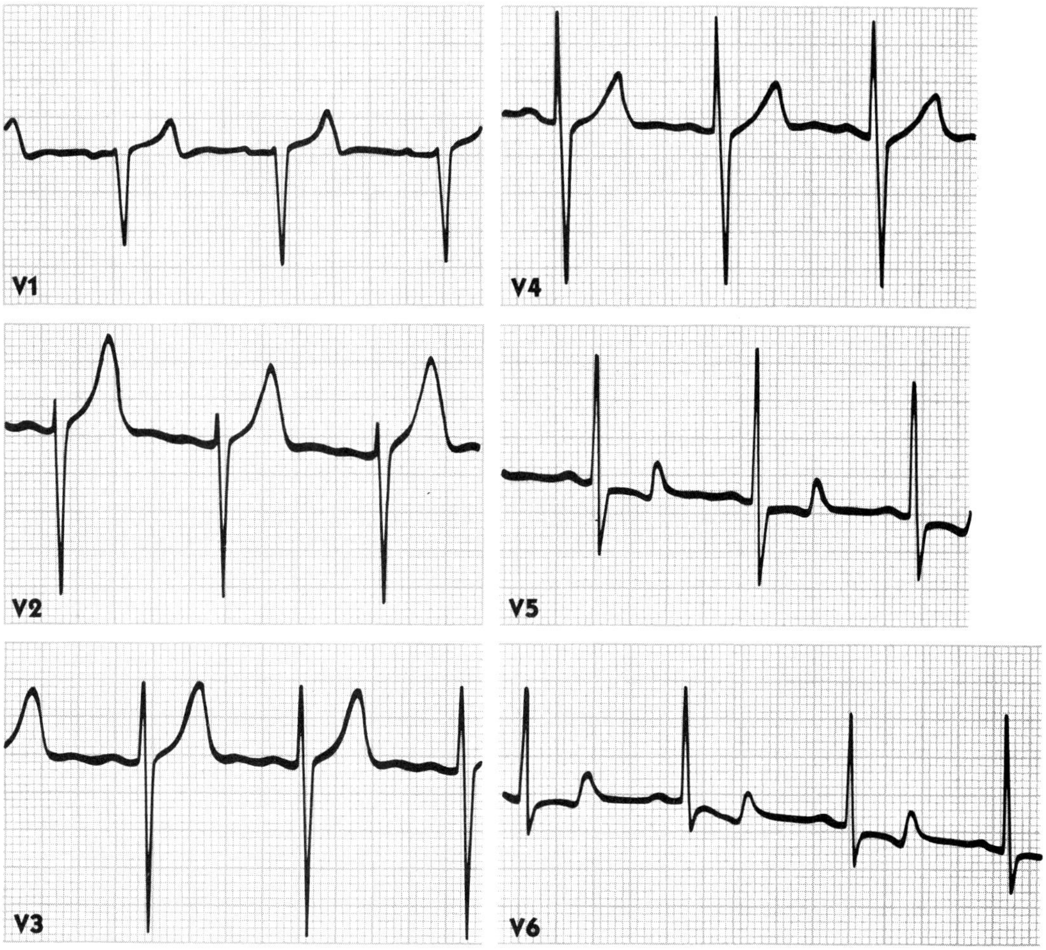

continued

Eventually, progressive prolongation of the QRS duration, leading to a sine wave configuration, and ventricular asystole can occur.

The patient was given intravenous glucose sodium bicarbonate, and insulin, with prompt resolution of her hyperkalemia. The second ECG (B), recorded one hour later, shows resolution of the T wave abnormalities.

CASE 50B **After glucose and insulin**

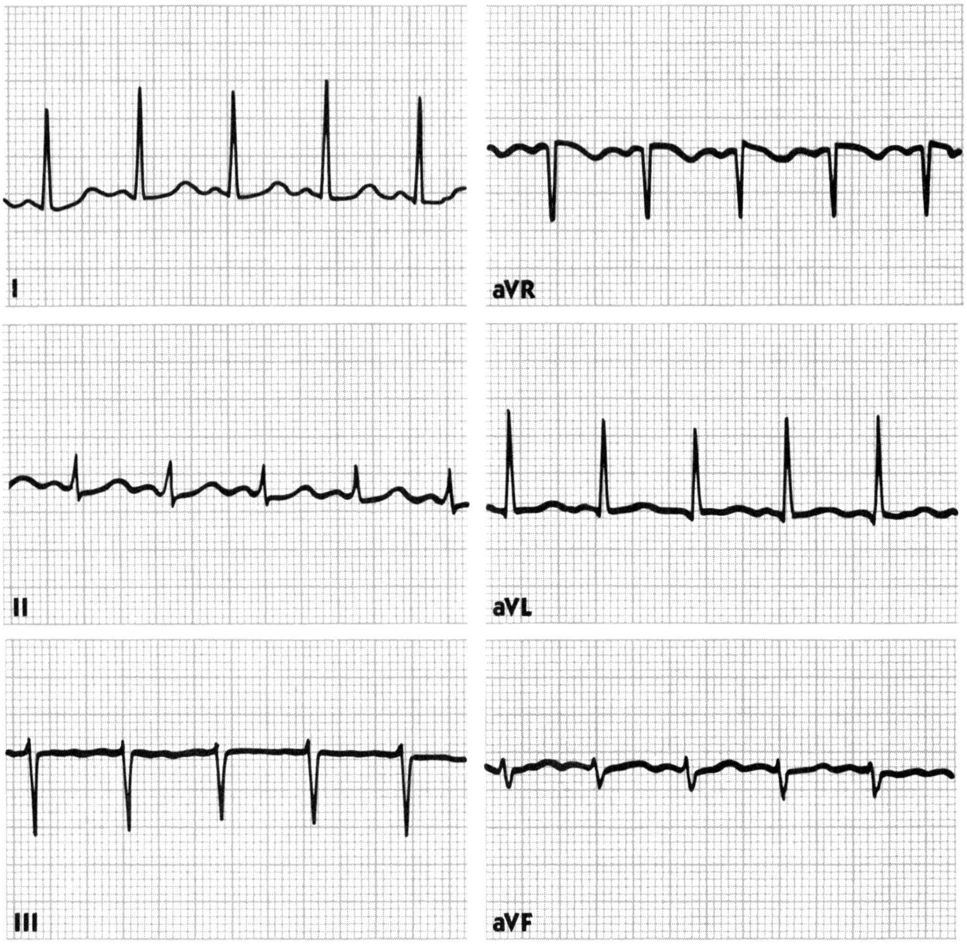

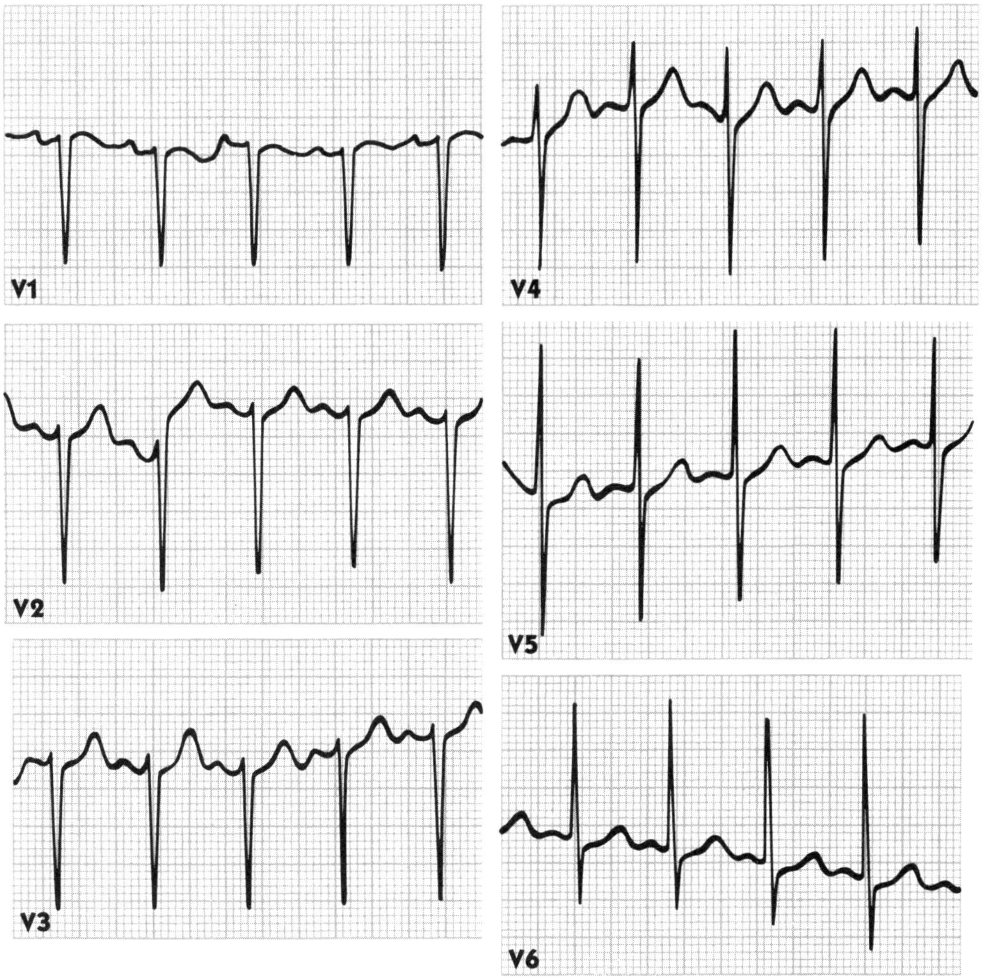
V1
V2
V3
V4
V5
V6

CASE 51

Hypokalemia

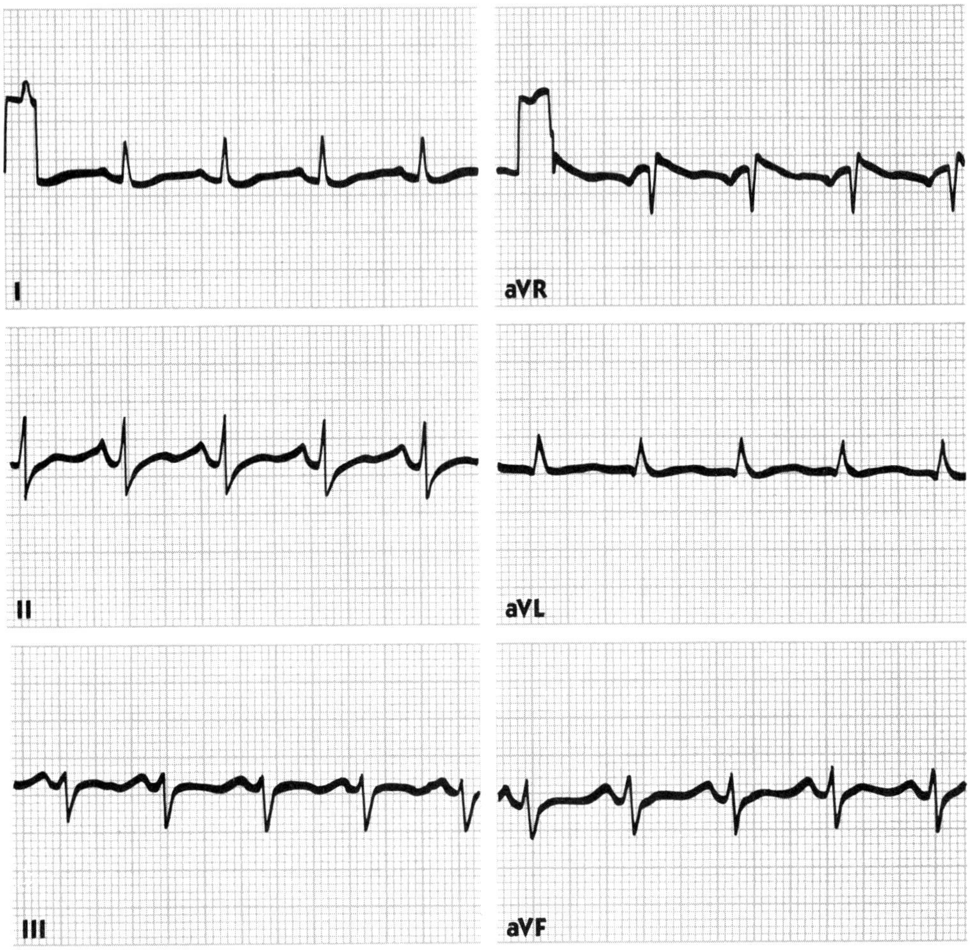

This 35-year-old malnourished man on diuretic therapy for mild hypertension was admitted to the hospital complaining of generalized weakness and malaise. His ECG shows a mean frontal plane QRS axis of 0°. The QT interval, measured in lead I, is prolonged at 0.42 second. The P waves are somewhat peaked, but not tall, in the inferior leads. The PR interval, measured in the limb leads, is 0.12 second. There is diffuse T wave flattening. In leads V2-6 (especially marked in V2-4), a tall wave is superimposed on the latter portion of the T wave. This is a giant U wave. In the leads with the most readily apparent U wave, not only is the T wave dwarfed, but the P wave is also obscured. It is not uncommon for giant U waves to be mistaken for P waves. But if the PR interval can be accurately assessed, it will allow distinction of P and U waves in leads where they are not clearly separated.

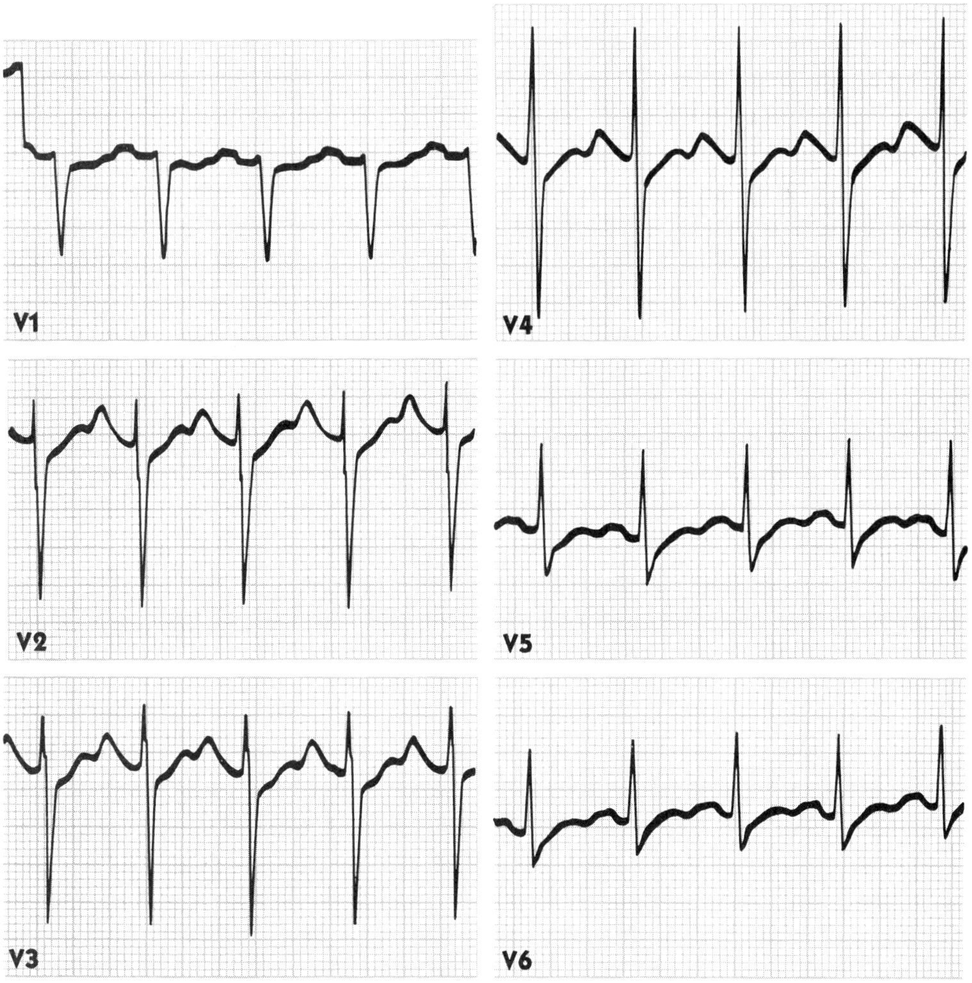

U waves occur in normal individuals and in patients with left ventricular hypertrophy, left bundle branch block, and acute myocardial infarction. But when they are *very* prominent—and particularly when they dwarf the T wave, as in this case—they are usually due to severe hypokalemia or type I antiarrhythmic (quinidine, procainamide, or disopyramide) therapy. This patient had a serum potassium level of 1.8 mEq/l. When his hypokalemia was corrected with supplemental potassium, his giant U waves disappeared.

The major ECG findings in hypokalemia are: large, sometimes giant, U waves; prolongation of the QT (actually QTU) interval due to the presence of the U wave; and flat T waves.

CASE 52

Hypercalcemia

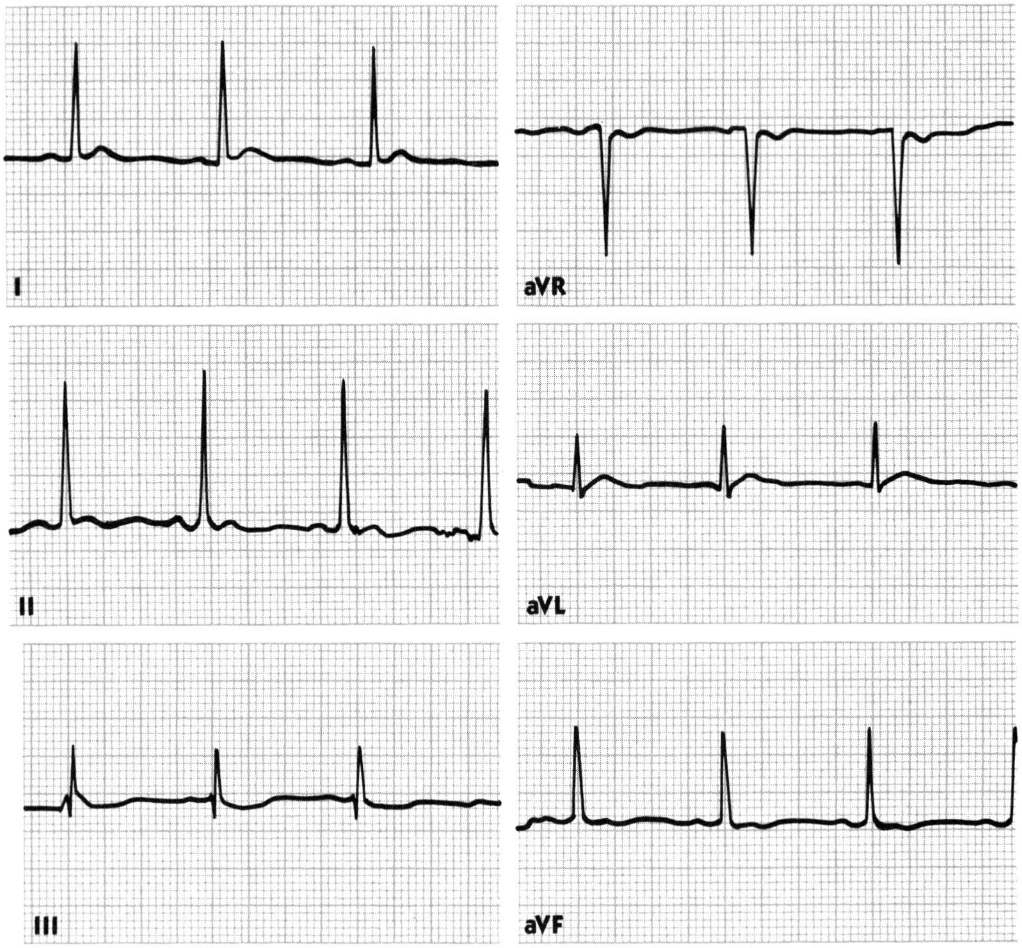

This ECG was recorded from a patient with hyperparathyroidism who regularly took more than 2 grams of calcium carbonate and drank more than 6 glasses of milk daily. Her serum calcium on admission to the hospital was 20 mg/dl. The ECG is characteristic of hypercalcemia: There is marked shortening of the QT interval due to virtual absence of the ST segment. In severe hypercalcemia, the T wave configuration is usually characterized by a rapid ascent to the peak with a more gradual descent. Thus, in many leads in this ECG, the QT interval appears to be even shorter than 0.32 second, since the T wave's rapid ascent makes it appear to hug the base of the QRS complex.

In general, only marked elevations in serum calcium cause these ECG changes; modest increases do not alter the surface ECG appreciably. Unlike prolongation of the QT interval, which has a number of pos-

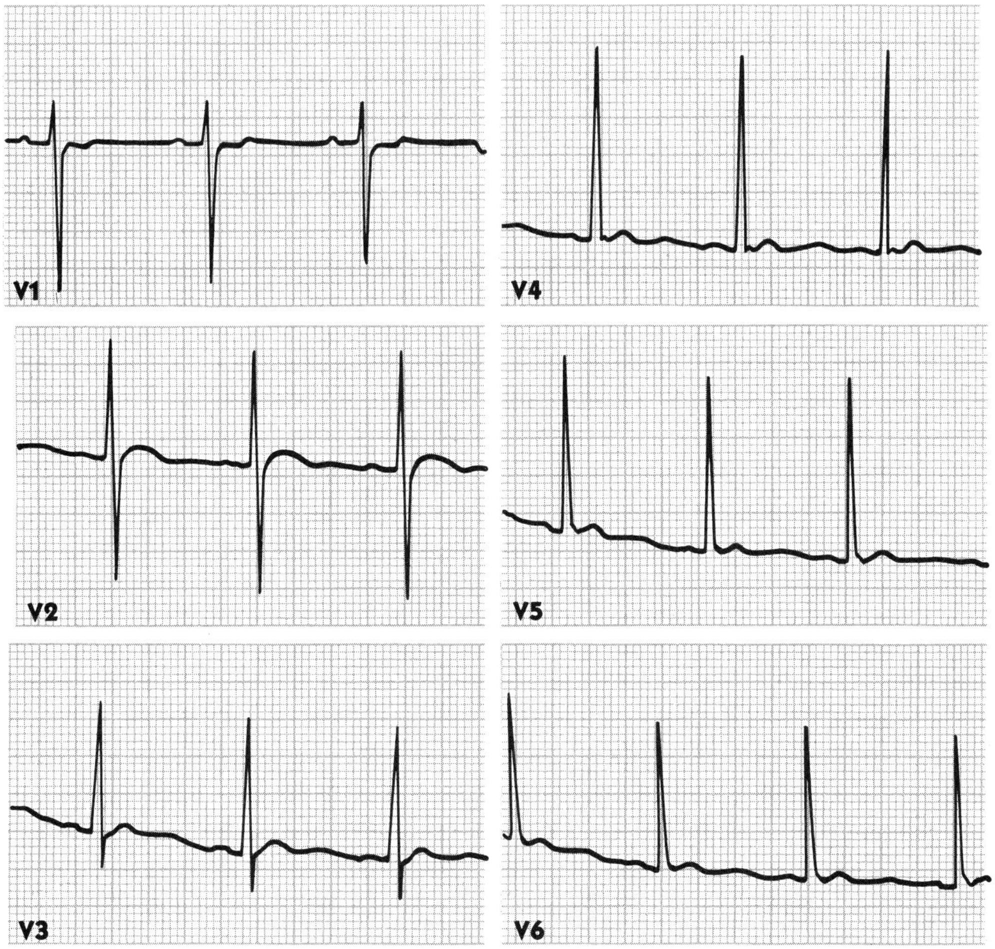

sible causes, very few conditions other than hypercalcemia produce QT shortening. Hyperkalemia and digitalis therapy may occasionally result in a measurably shortened QT interval, but associated diagnostic changes are usually present.

CASE 53

Hypocalcemia

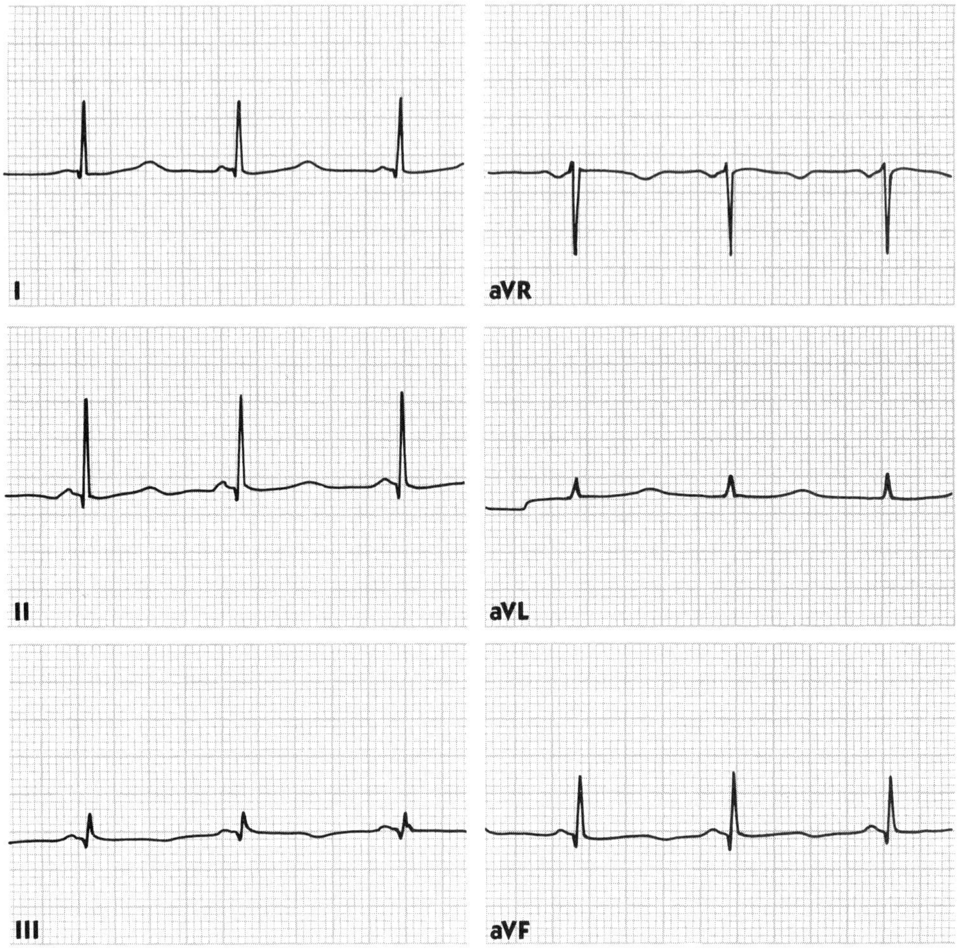

This ECG was recorded from a 26-year-old man with renal failure and nephrotic syndrome. It shows mild T wave flattening and a prolonged QT interval of 0.48 second (upper limit of normal for rate = 0.40).

The differential diagnosis of QT prolongation is lengthy. It includes electrolyte disturbances, drug effects, metabolic alterations, and myocardial infarction (see Table 11 in the Appendix). In this patient, the QT interval is prolonged due to prolongation of the ST segment, the classic ECG finding in hypocalcemia. The T wave itself is of normal duration. The serum calcium was measured at 4.1 mg/dl; the potassium level was normal at 4.2 mEq/l.

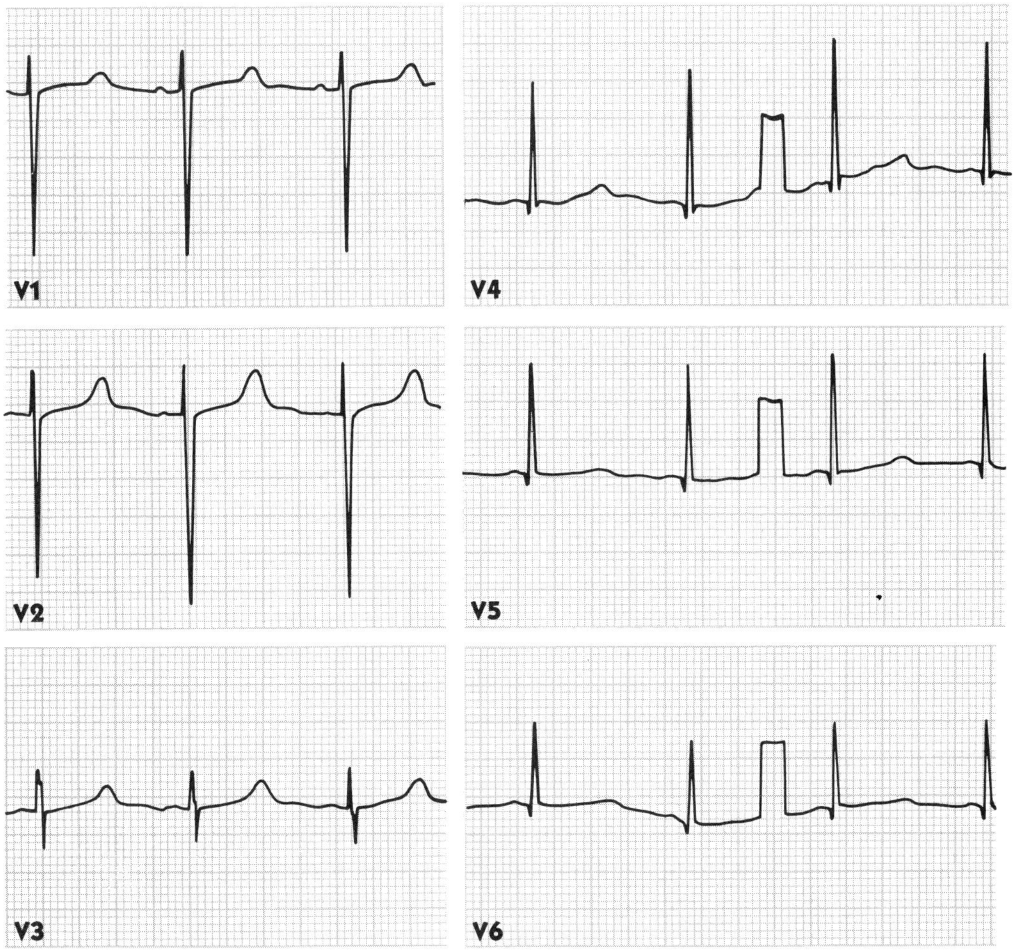
V1
V4
V2
V5
V3
V6

CASE 54

Hypothyroidism

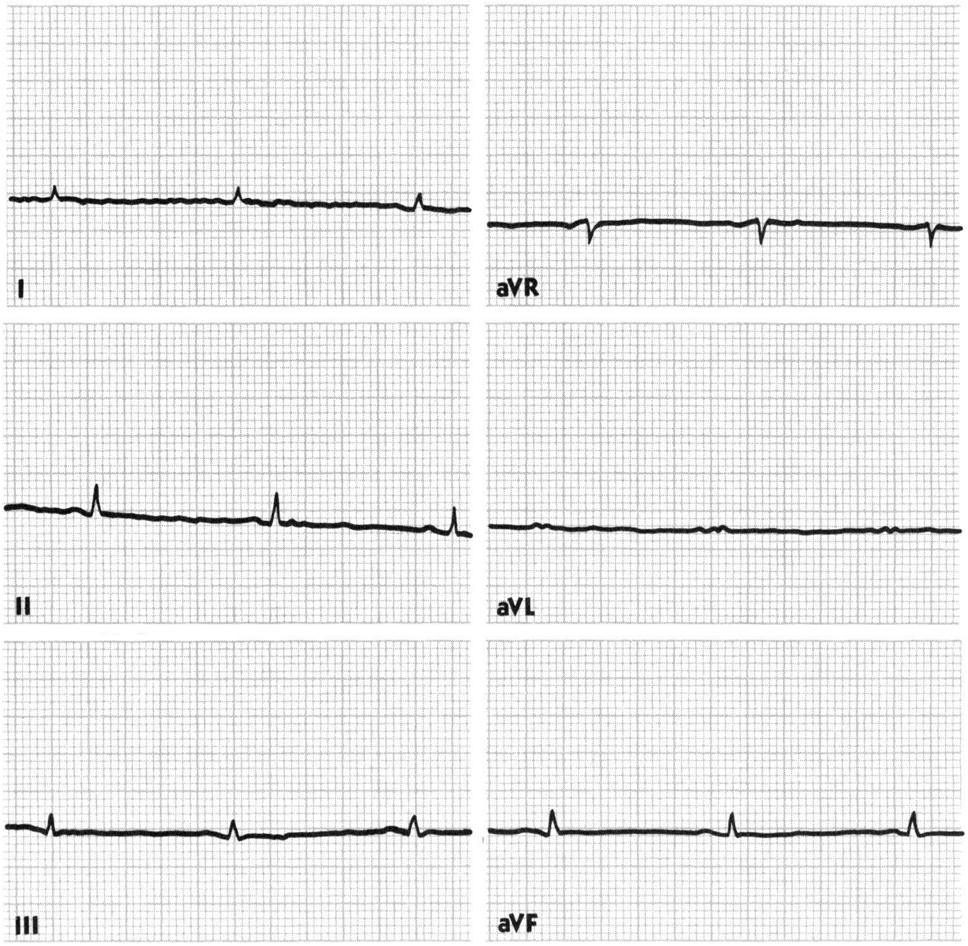

A 57-year-old woman was seen because of lethargy, cold intolerance, and alteration in mental status. Her ECG shows sinus rhythm at a rate of 60. The mean frontal plane QRS axis is +60°, and the intervals are normal; however, the QT interval cannot be measured accurately since there is profound T wave flattening. The T waves are slightly inverted in leads V1-3. The ST segments appear normal.

This patient's ECG, like her history, suggests severe hypothyroidism. The most common ECG findings in hypothyroidism are nonspecific low voltage (see Table 9 in the Appendix) and/or T wave inversion. In *severe* hypothyroidism, the ECG hallmark is T wave flattening producing virtual absence of T waves. This ECG shows essentially straight lines between R waves, with minimal anterior T wave inversion.

Low voltage of both QRS complexes and P waves is apparent here. Low voltage often occurs in the pres-

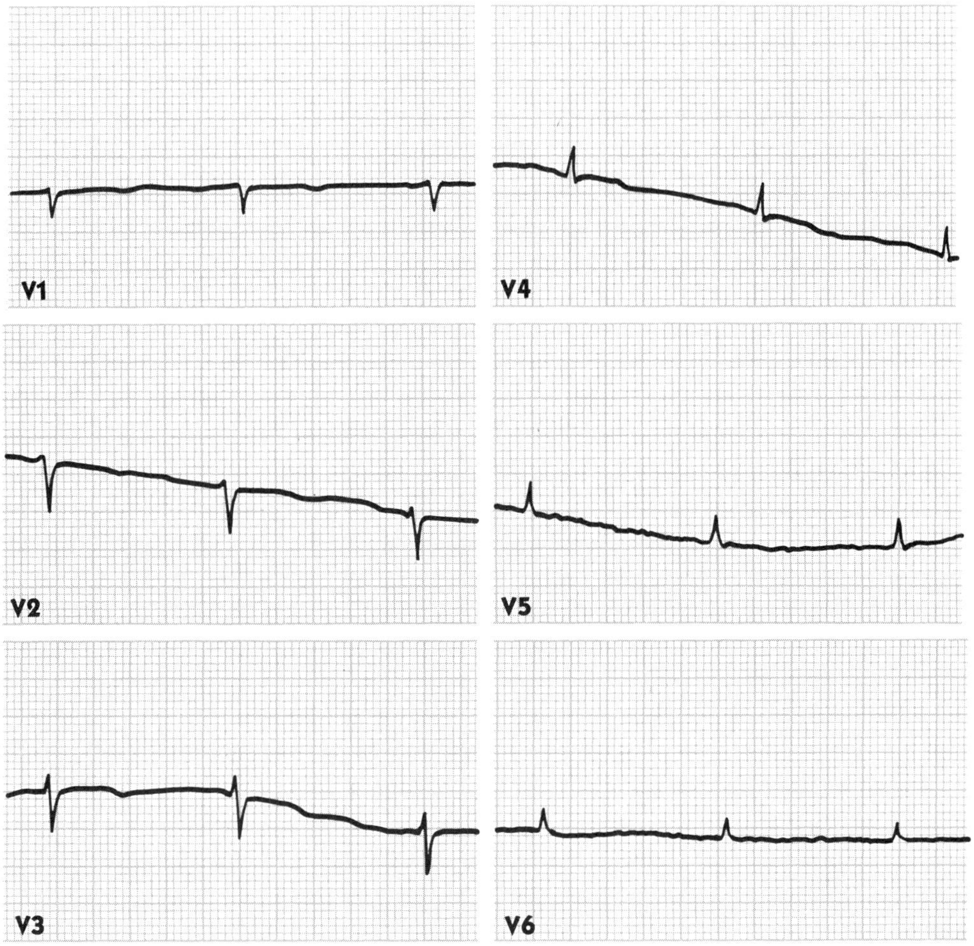

ence of pericardial effusion associated with hypothyroidism, but may also occur in its absence, presumably due to myocardial infiltrative processes.

Sinus bradycardia is common in this disorder. Occasionally, if the P waves are not discernible due to low voltage, the rhythm will appear to be junctional bradycardia. Prolongation of the QT interval is also reported to occur, but in most cases the T wave flattening makes it difficult to assess. There is an increased incidence of intraventricular conduction delay and bundle branch block patterns. In summary, the triad of findings that most strongly suggest hypothyroidism consists of: low voltage, flat and/or inverted T waves, and sinus bradycardia.

CASE 55

Cerebrovascular Accident

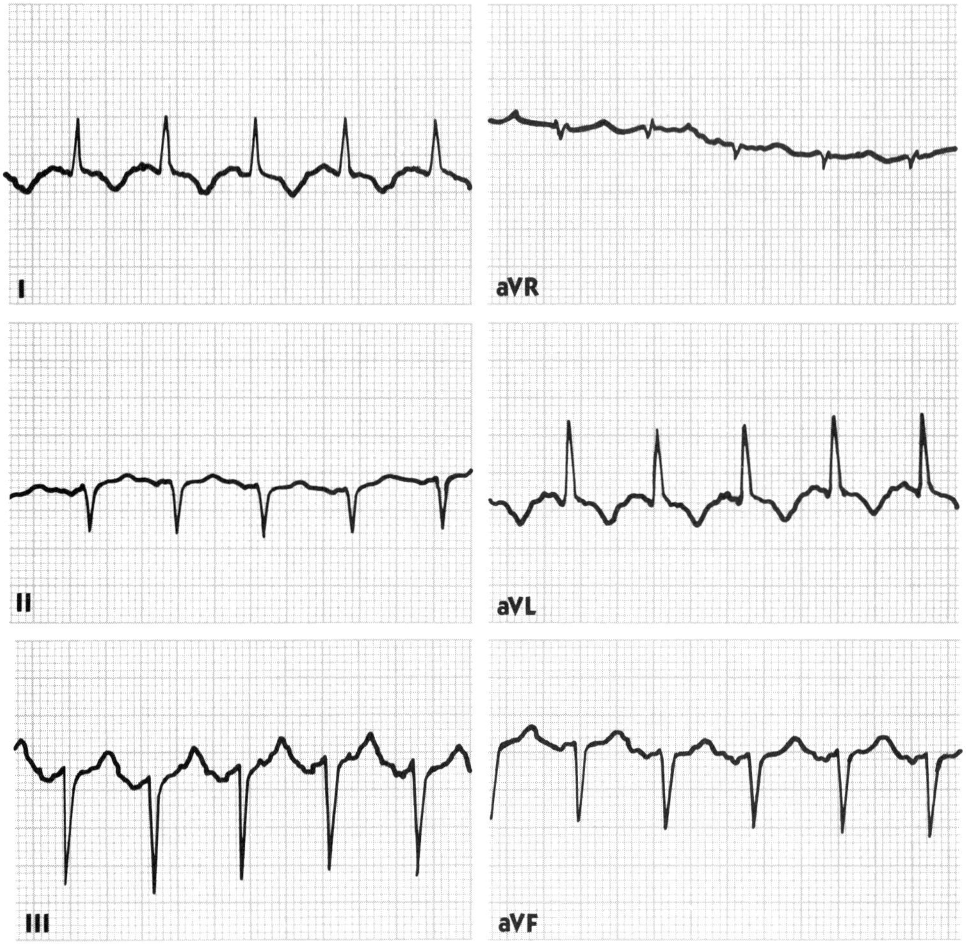

This patient suffered a large hemispheric cerebrovascular accident. Her ECG shows sinus tachycardia, normal PR and QRS intervals, and modest prolongation of the QT interval (0.35 second) for the rate. The mean frontal plane QRS axis is −60°. The left axis deviation, qR complexes in leads I and aVL, rS complexes in lead III, and S waves laterally all suggest left anterior fascicular block (see Case 16). The most notable finding in this ECG is the diffuse, symmetrical T wave inversion in leads I, aVL, and V2-6. Although this finding is compatible with the diagnosis of anterolateral ischemia or infarction, a large stroke was the only clinical event in this patient.

A number of ECG alterations occur with major central nervous system events—classically with subarachnoid hemorrhage, but also with other types of stroke. The most common are QT interval prolongation and ST-T alterations, including T wave inver-

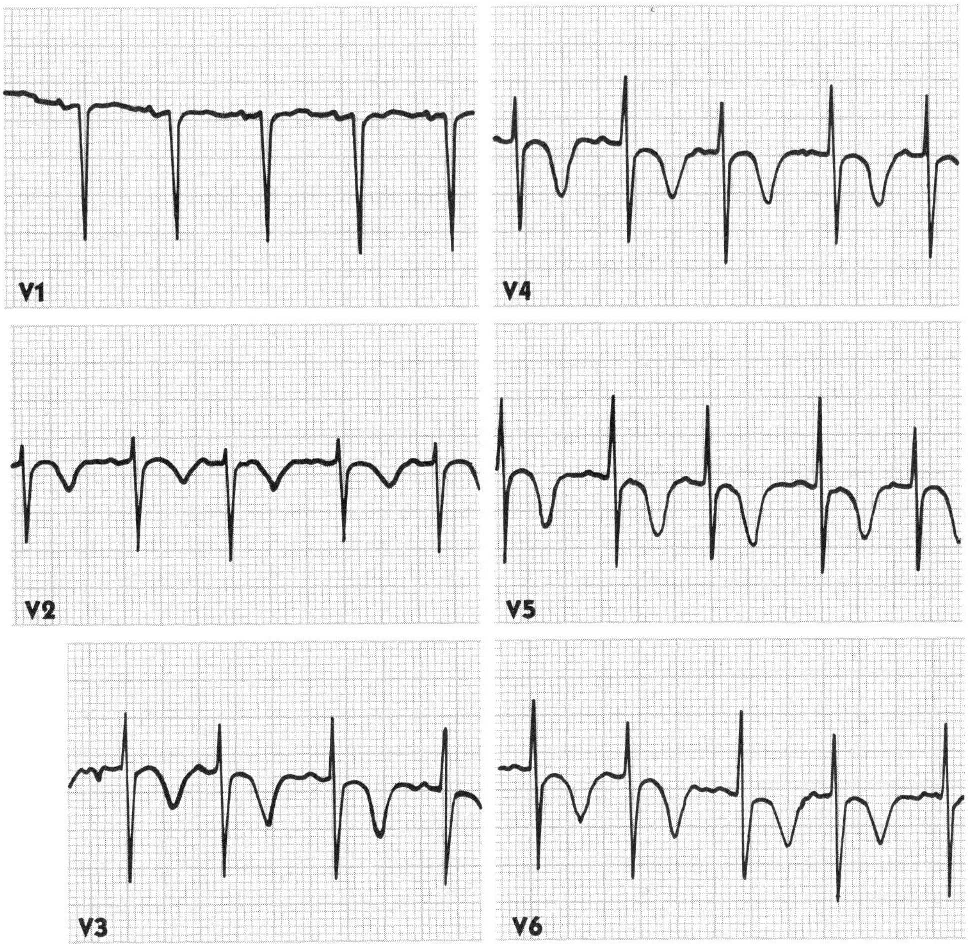

sion and peaking, ST segment depression and elevation, and prominent upright or inverted U waves. These findings are not specific and are seen in other conditions (see Table 5 in the Appendix). Less frequently, fascicular and bundle branch block patterns and supraventricular and ventricular arrhythmias occur. Stroke-related ECG changes illustrate the poorly understood influences of the central nervous system upon the heart.

SECTION IX The ECG and Drug Toxicity

CASE 56

Effect of Digitalis on the ECG

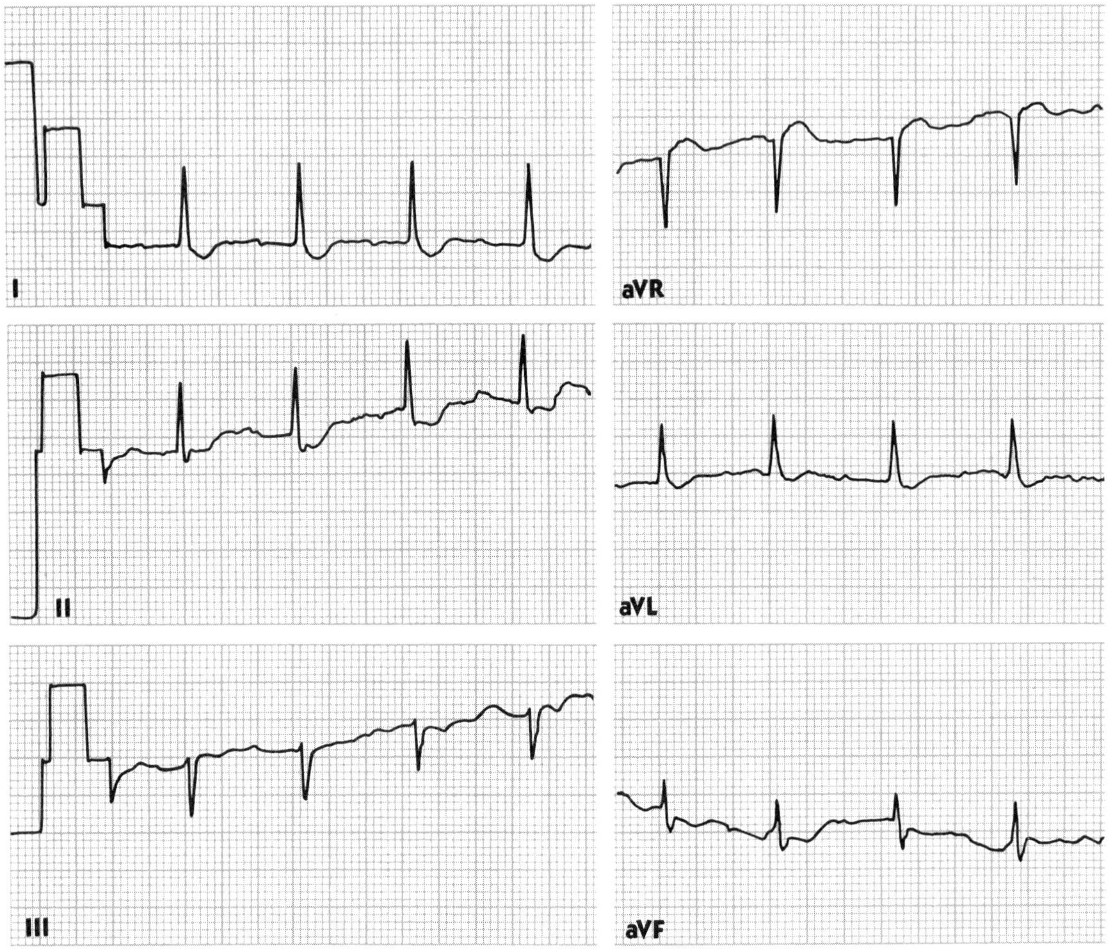

This ECG was recorded from an 85-year-old woman receiving digoxin and furosemide for congestive heart failure, who complained of nausea, vomiting, and palpitations. It shows sinus rhythm with first degree atrioventricular (AV) block (PR interval = 0.27 second). The QRS morphology is normal, and the QT interval is somewhat short (0.34 second) for the rate (98). Asymmetric, upwardly concave ST segment depression is present, primarily in leads I, II, aVL, and V3-6. There is ST segment elevation in lead aVR.

This ECG shows the classic changes characteristic of the digitalis *effect* on the PR interval and ST-T configuration and, combined with the patient's symptoms, suggests the diagnosis of digoxin *toxicity*. The patient's serum digoxin level was 3.2 ng/ml. The digitalis effect on the ECG, which is seen at therapeutic levels, comprises three major findings: PR interval prolongation, asymmetric ST-T depression, and QT interval shortening (which may be difficult to measure). Digoxin can also cause prominent (but not giant) U waves.

The PR prolongation is due to delayed conduction at the AV node caused by both vagotonic and direct effects of digitalis. Prolongation beyond 0.28 second suggests digitalis toxicity, rather than effect. The short QT interval is considered to be due to enhanced repolarization of ventricular tissue associated with therapeutic digoxin levels.

The ST-T depression is a classic finding in patients on digitalis and occurs even in subjects with normal hearts who receive the drug. Usually, a straight, downsloping ST segment merges with an inverted, foreshortened T wave, yielding asymmetrically inverted T waves. This differs from the more symmetrically inverted T waves of ischemia or infarction. The ST-T changes occur primarily in leads show-

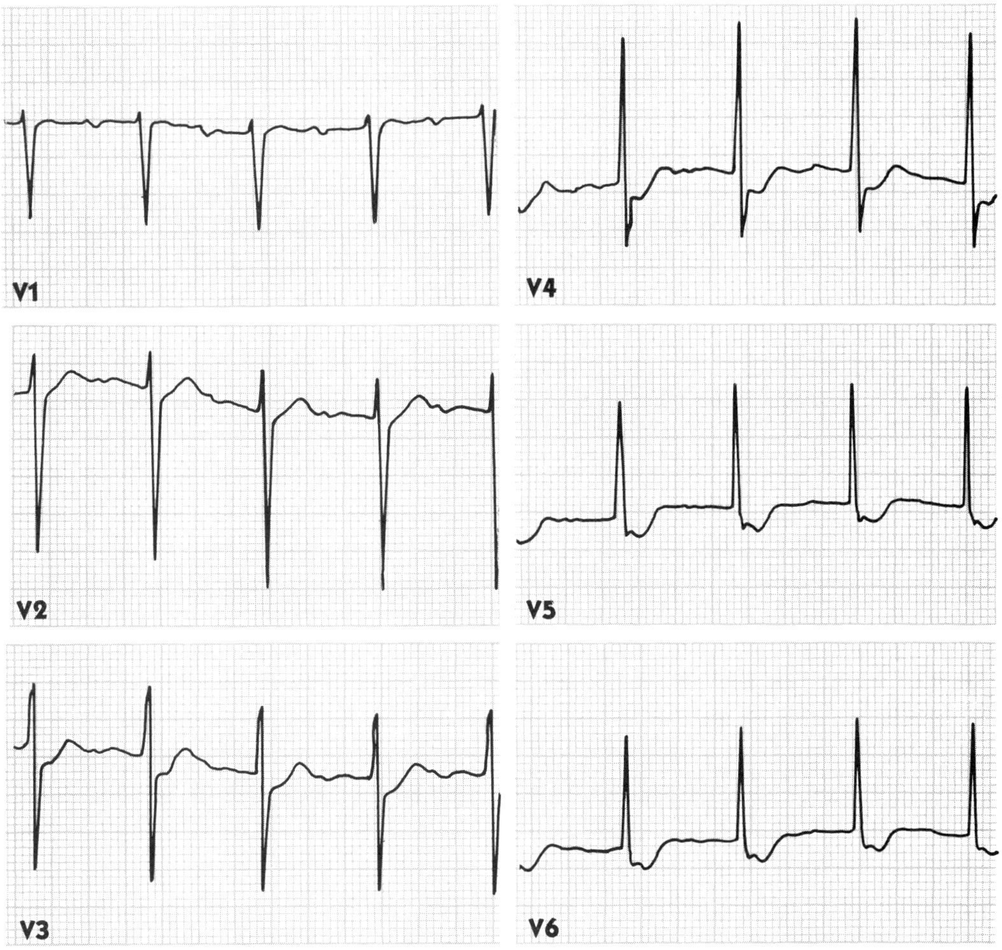

ing a dominant R wave (I, aVL, and V5-6). When they are seen in leads with dominant S waves (such as lead V3 in this case), digitalis toxicity or myocardial ischemia should be suspected. It is important to note that the ST-T alterations produced by digitalis preparations can obscure those associated with other conditions—such as ventricular hypertrophy, myocardial ischemia, nontransmural infarction, and bundle branch block. The digoxin effect can also lead to pseudonormalization of ST segment elevation in lateral myocardial infarction.

Cardiac arrhythmias, rather than morphologic ECG changes, are the hallmark of digitalis toxicity. Toxic digitalis levels have been implicated in the genesis of almost every arrhythmia, especially premature ventricular beats, ventricular bigeminy, AV junctional tachycardia, ectopic atrial tachycardia (with or without AV block), ventricular tachycardia, sinoatrial block and sinus arrest, and second degree and complete AV block. The atrial arrhythmias, such as atrial premature beats, atrial flutter and fibrillation, and multifocal atrial tachycardia, are usually not seen in digitalis toxicity.

CASE 57

Quinidine Effect

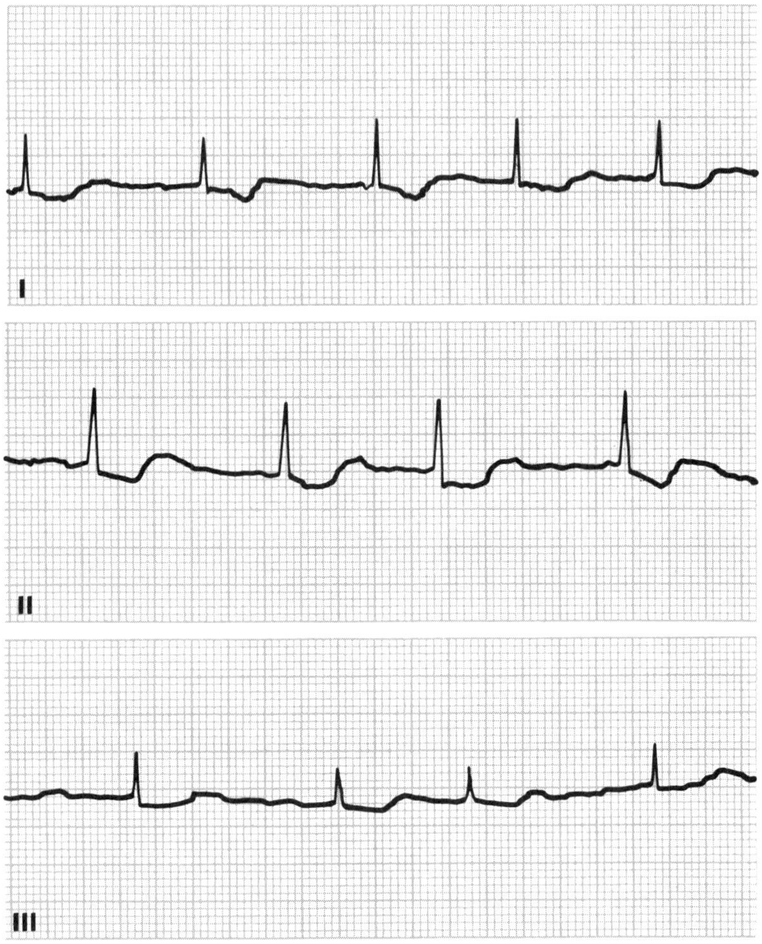

This ECG was recorded from a 69-year-old woman taking quinidine and digoxin for supraventricular arrhythmias. Serum levels of both quinidine and digoxin were normal at the time of this tracing. The rhythm is atrial fibrillation with a moderate ventricular response of 60-80 per minute. The QRS duration is normal, but the QT interval is markedly prolonged (0.52 second). The mean frontal plane QRS axis is normal. Leads I, II, III, aVF, and V3-6 show downsloping ST segment depression with upright T waves. Prominent U waves are best seen in leads I and V2-3.

Quinidine at therapeutic serum levels causes a number of alterations in the ECG. Prolongation of the QT interval and prominent U waves are the most common, along with nonspecific ST-T abnormalities. These include ST segment depression and T wave flattening or inversion. The changes caused by quinidine resemble almost exactly those seen in hypokalemia.

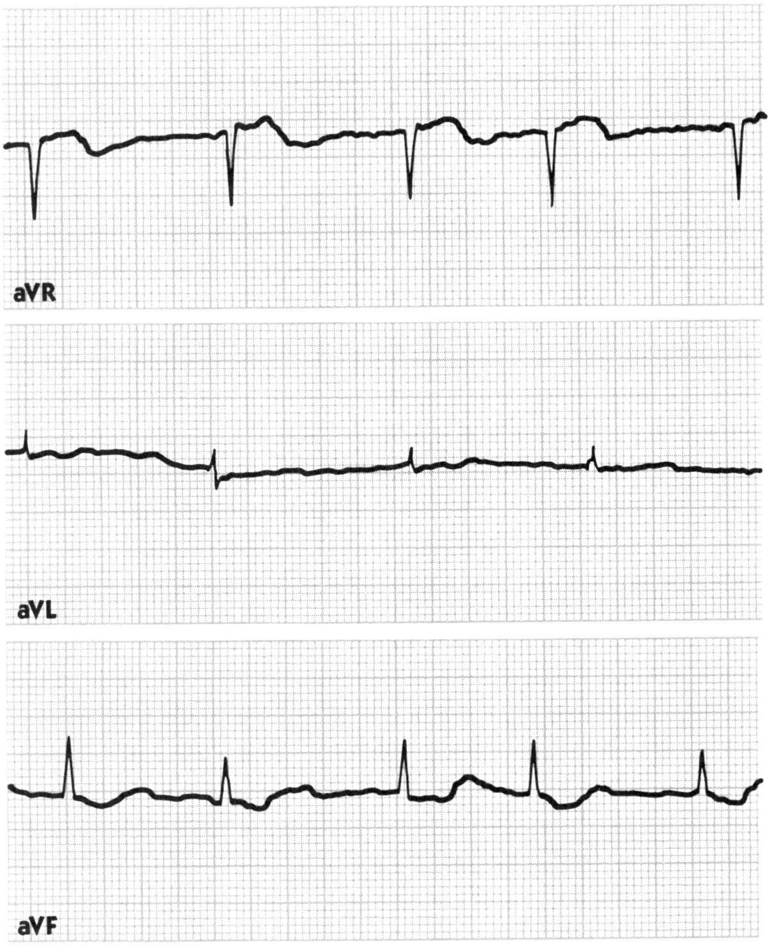

continued

The distinction must be made on clinical grounds. In this patient, the digitalis effect undoubtedly contributes to the downsloping ST segment depression (see Case 56).

The QT interval prolongation, prominent U waves, and ST segment and T wave abnormalities seen with quinidine therapy are also caused by the other type I antiarrhythmic agents, procainamide and disopyramide. Type II antiarrhythmics (lidocaine and phenytoin) and Type III antiarrhythmics (the beta-blockers) have little appreciable effect on the intervals or morphology of the surface ECG when given in nontoxic doses.

CASE 57 *(continued)*

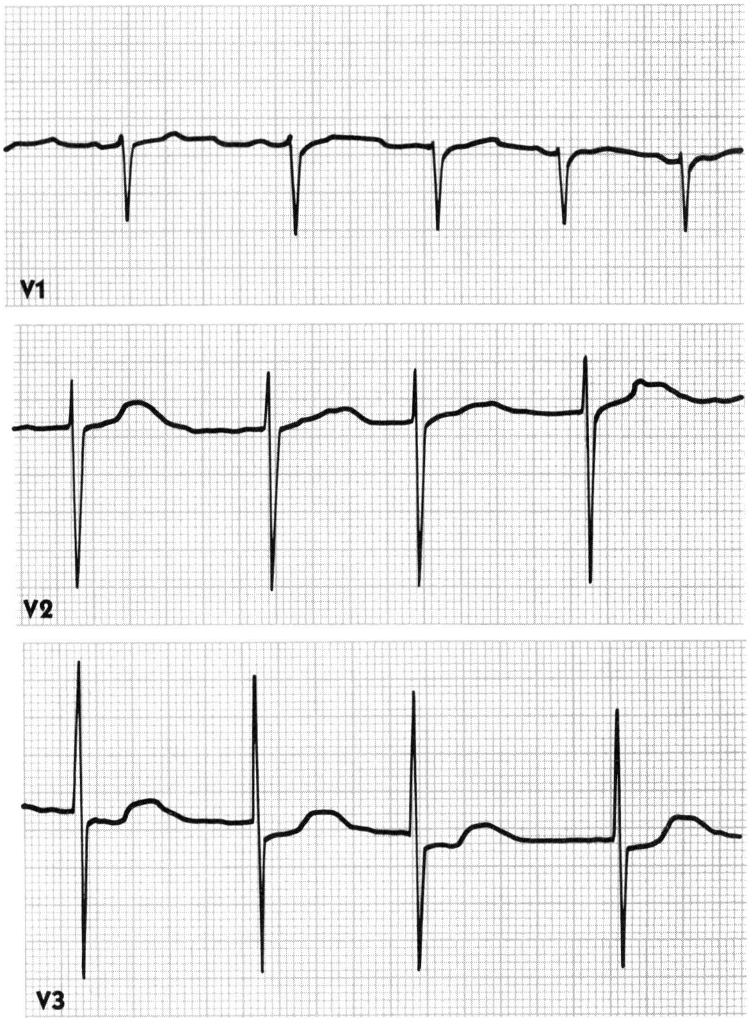

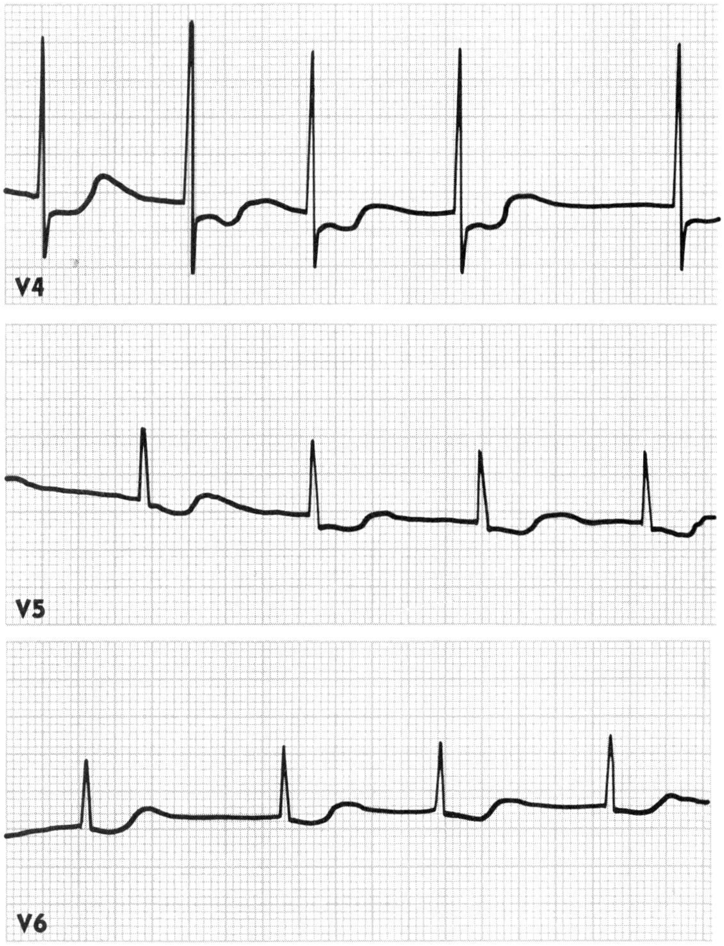
V4
V5
V6

CASE 58

Quinidine Toxicity

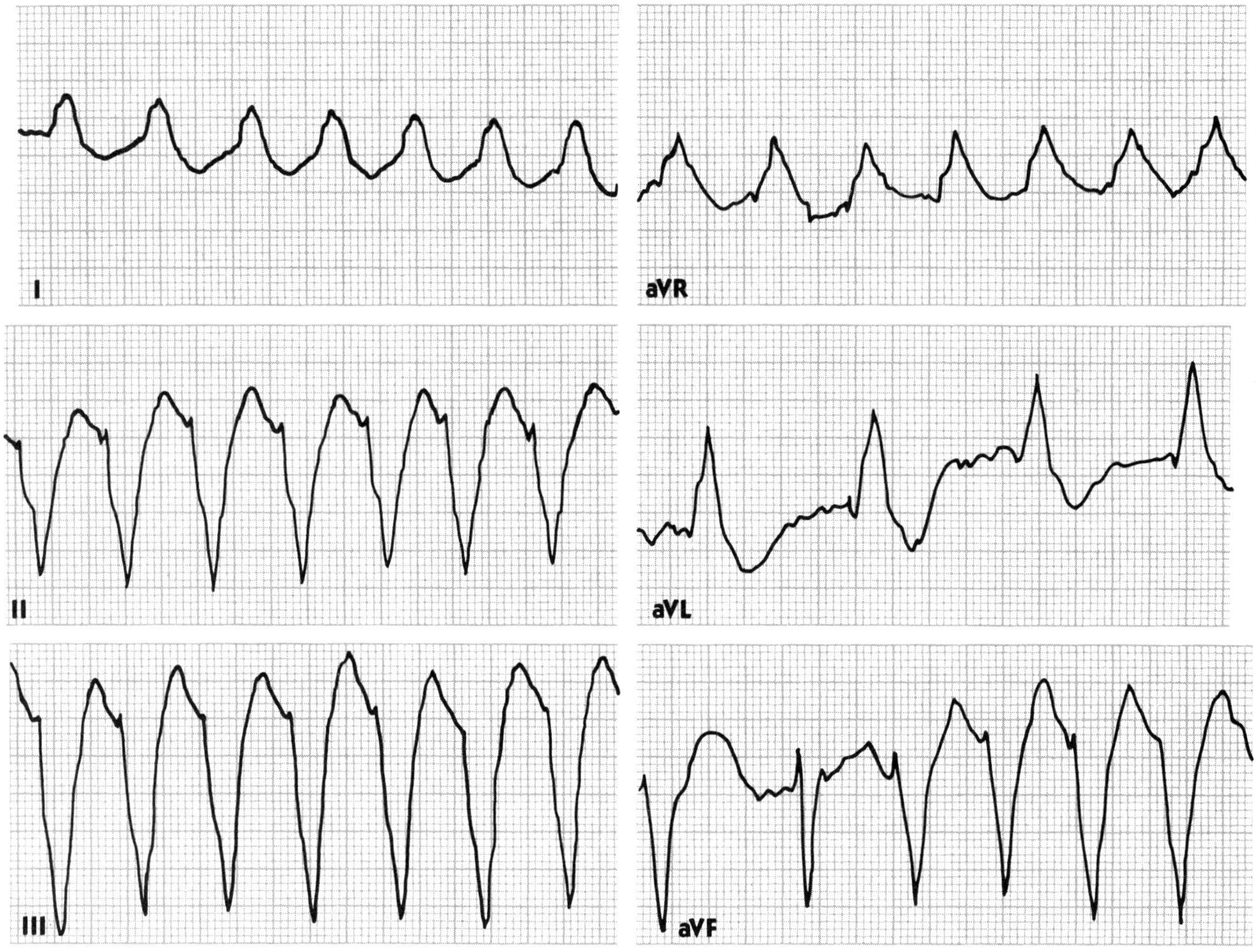

This 19-year-old woman took toxic doses of quinidine. Her ECG shows an irregular, wide-complex tachycardia at rates of 70 to 130 per minute. There is no clearly discernible atrial activity. The QRS duration is at least 0.22 second, and the QT interval is so prolonged that it extends to the onset of the next QRS complex. There is a qR pattern in lead aVL and an rS pattern in lead III, with a mean frontal plane QRS axis of about −90°. Lead V1 shows an RR′ pattern. The T waves are generally opposite in direction to the QRS complexes, thus representing secondary T wave changes.

The QRS morphology is compatible with drug-induced, diffuse conduction system delay involving the left and right bundle branches and the anterior division of the left bundle branch. The major question in this case is whether the arrhythmia is supraventricular (with intraventricular aberration) or ventricular in origin. In the absence of drug therapy, some

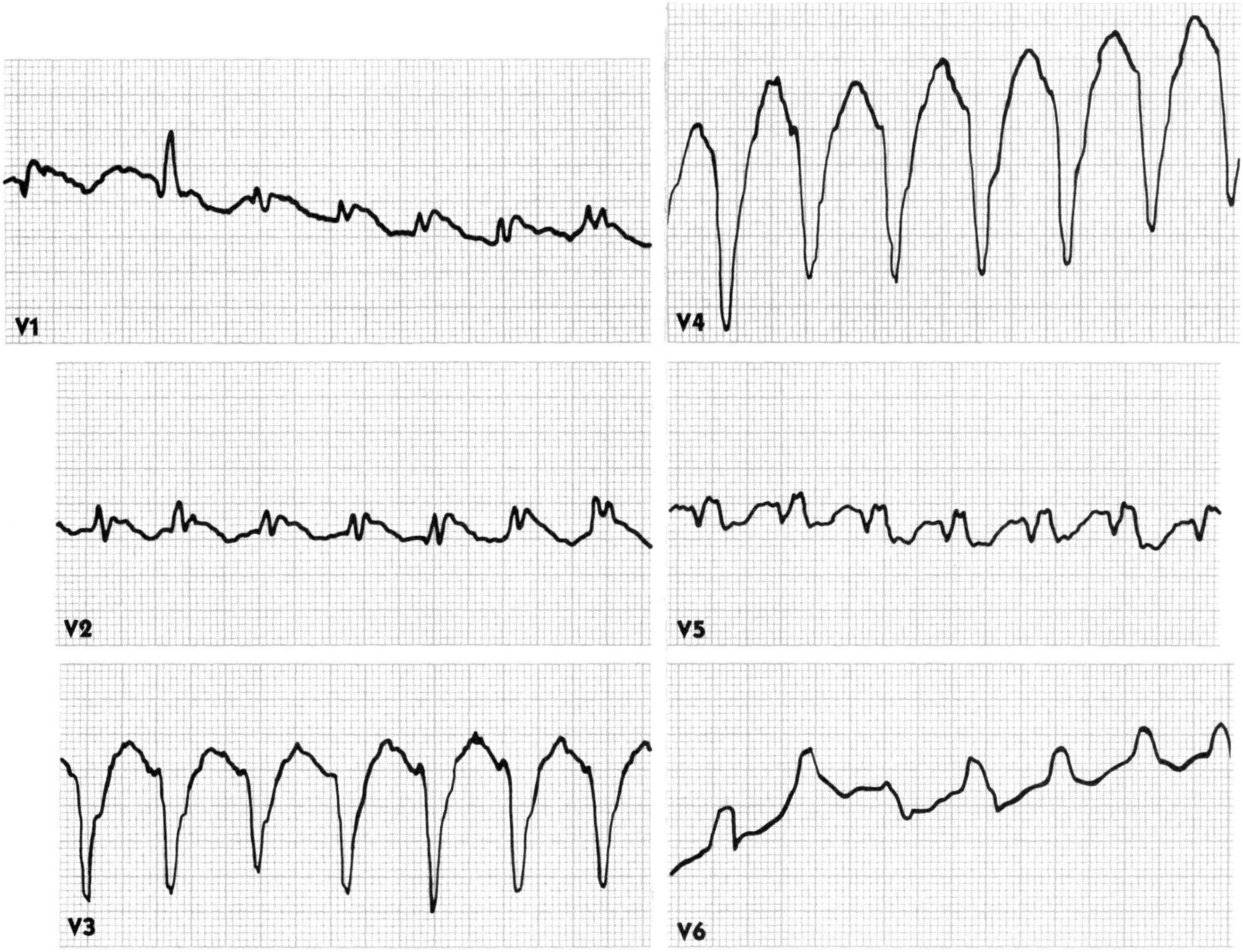

ECG criteria have been found to be useful in making the distinction; however, in drug-related wide-complex rhythms, these criteria may not be valid.

The patient tolerated this tachycardia well. With conservative management, the wide-complex rhythm resolved after several hours. On the following day, her ECG was normal except for a prolonged QT interval.

CASE 59

Procainamide Toxicity

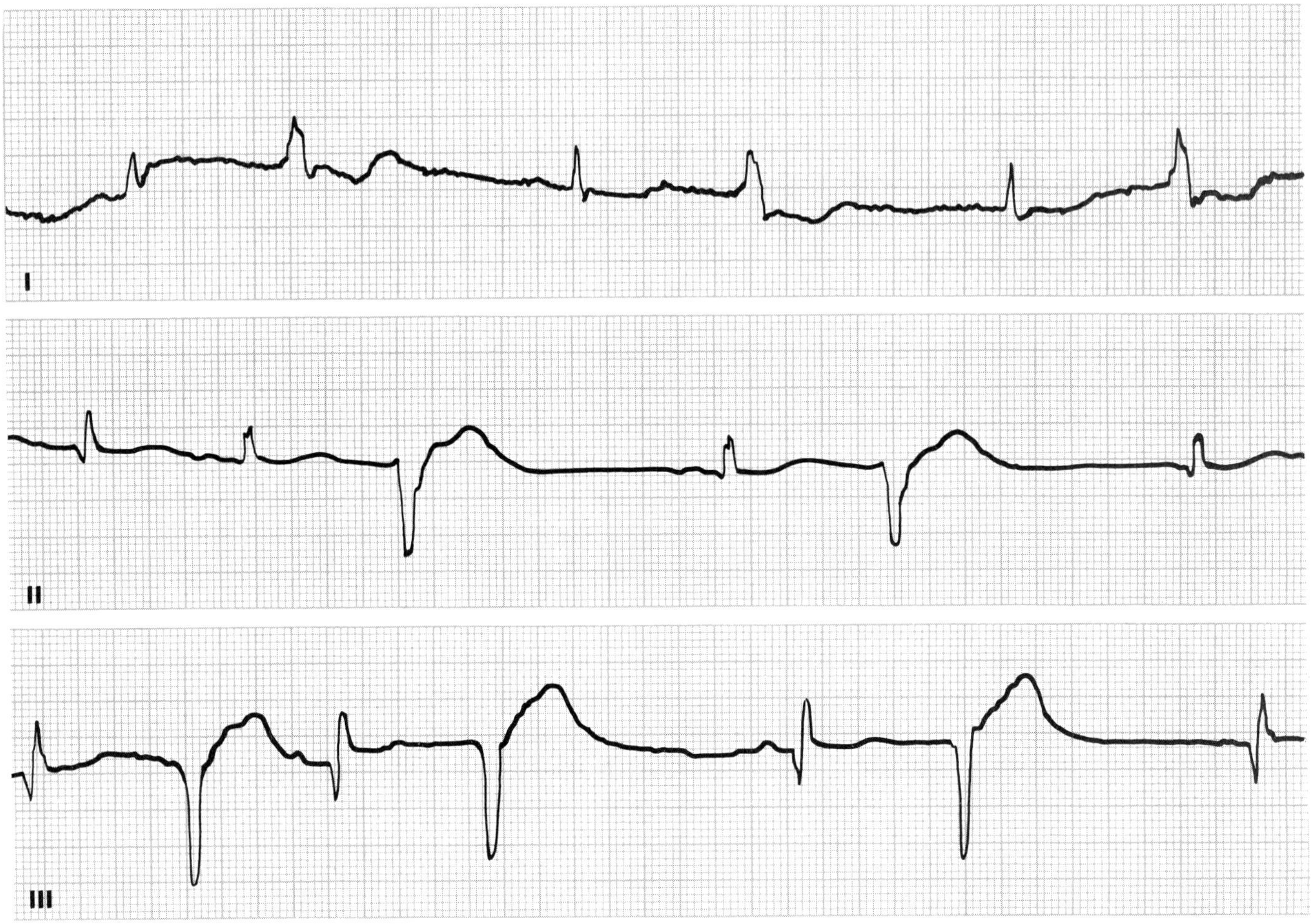

This 52-year-old woman was taking a long-acting procainamide preparation for frequent premature ventricular beats. Her serum level of procainamide at the time of this ECG was 14.7 μg/ml (therapeutic range = 4-8 μg/ml).

The rhythm is sinus with ventricular bigeminy. The P waves and PR intervals are normal. The sinus-stimulated QRS complexes are 0.11 second in duration and have a qR pattern in leads II, III, and aVF, consistent with past inferior wall myocardial infarction. The QT interval is markedly prolonged at 0.80 second (best seen in the lateral precordial leads) and appears to be symmetrical in configuration. However, a change in slope of the T wave is discernible in lead V3, and two waves (a T wave and a giant U wave) are discernible in lead II. Thus the U wave is contributing to the measured QT (actually QTU) interval. The ventricular premature beats are 0.20 second in dura-

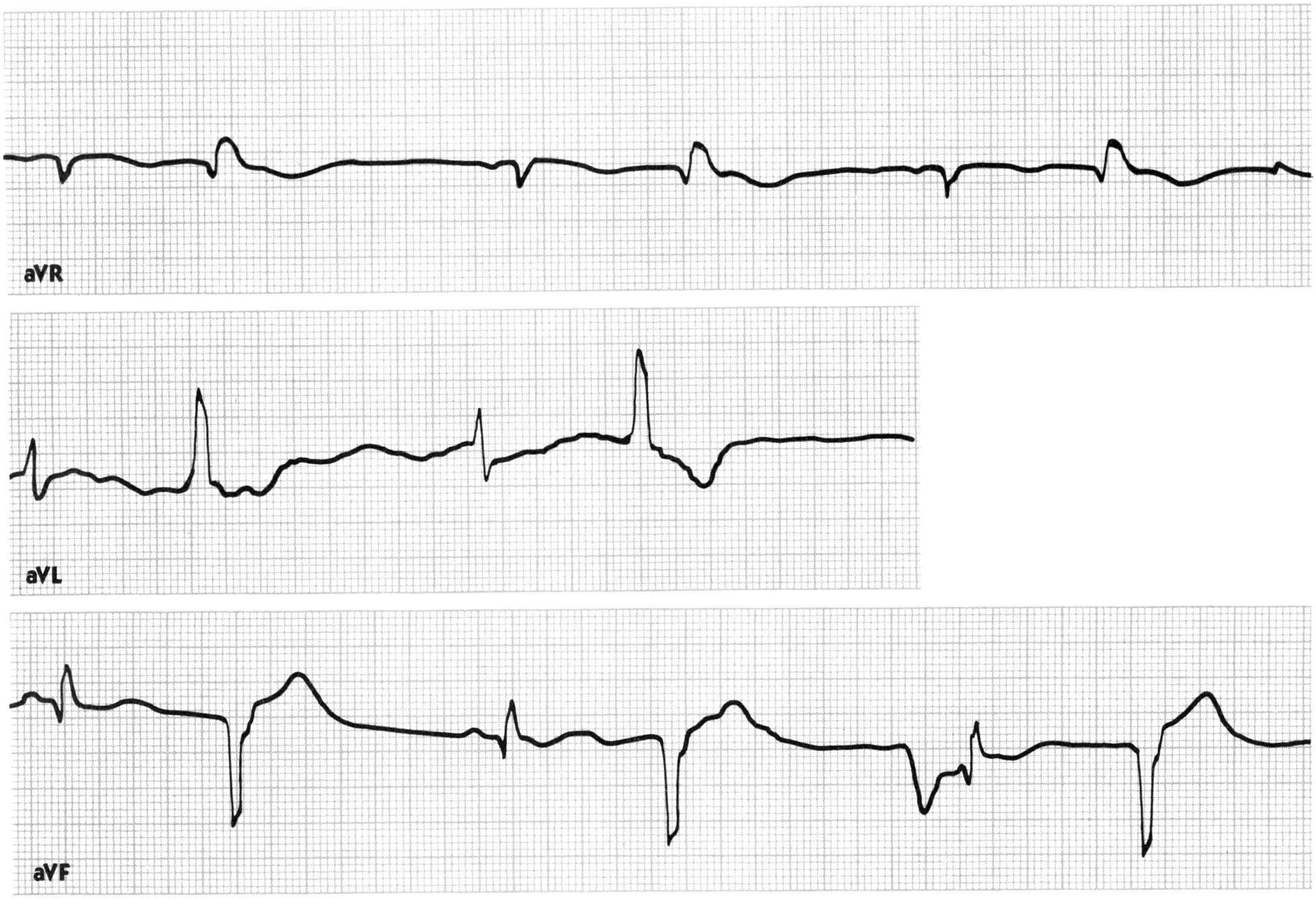

continued

tion and also associated with a markedly prolonged QT interval.

Discontinuation of the procainamide resulted, over a period of several days, in resolution of the abnormally prolonged QTU interval, along with disappearance of the ventricular ectopic activity.

CASE 59 *(continued)*

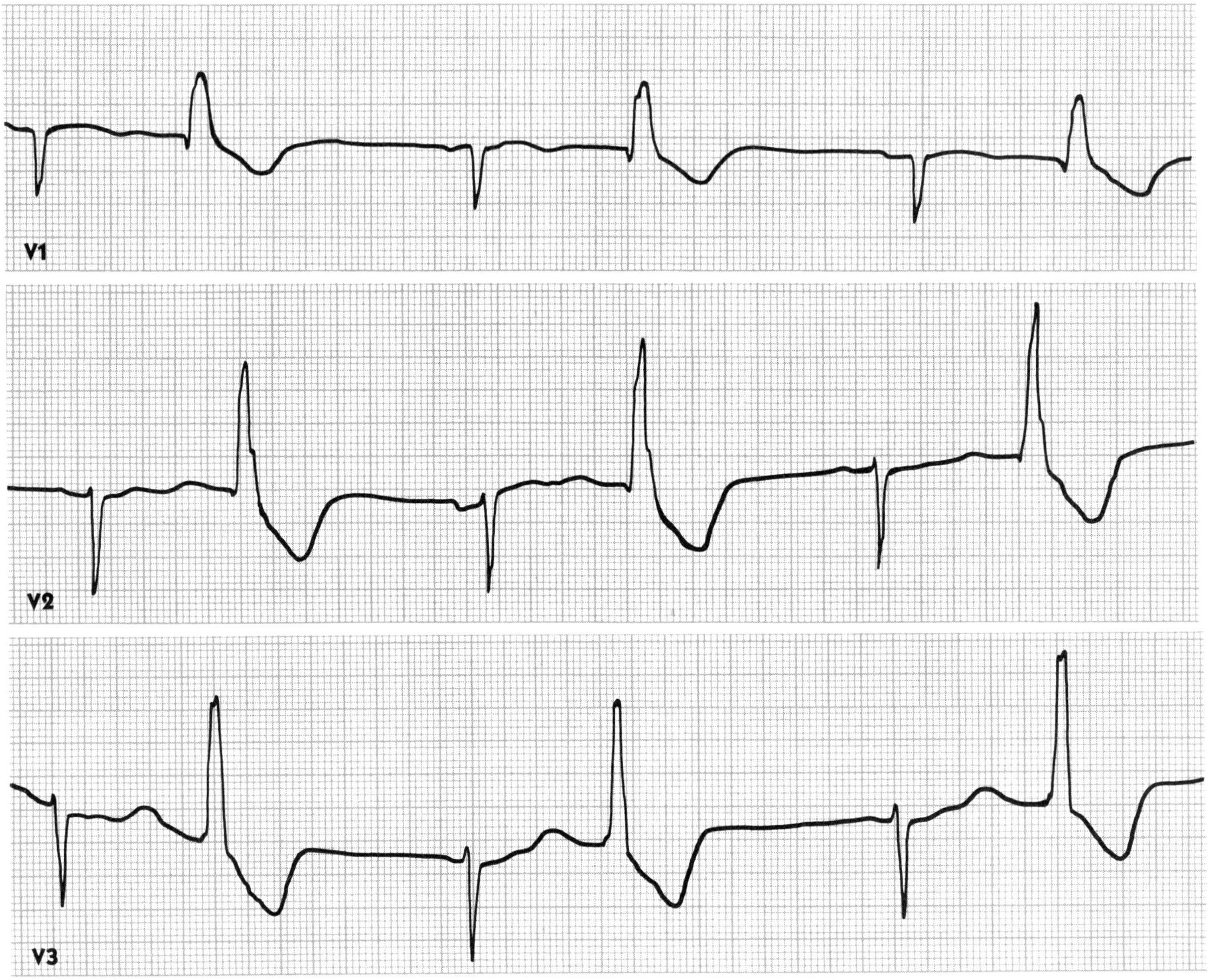

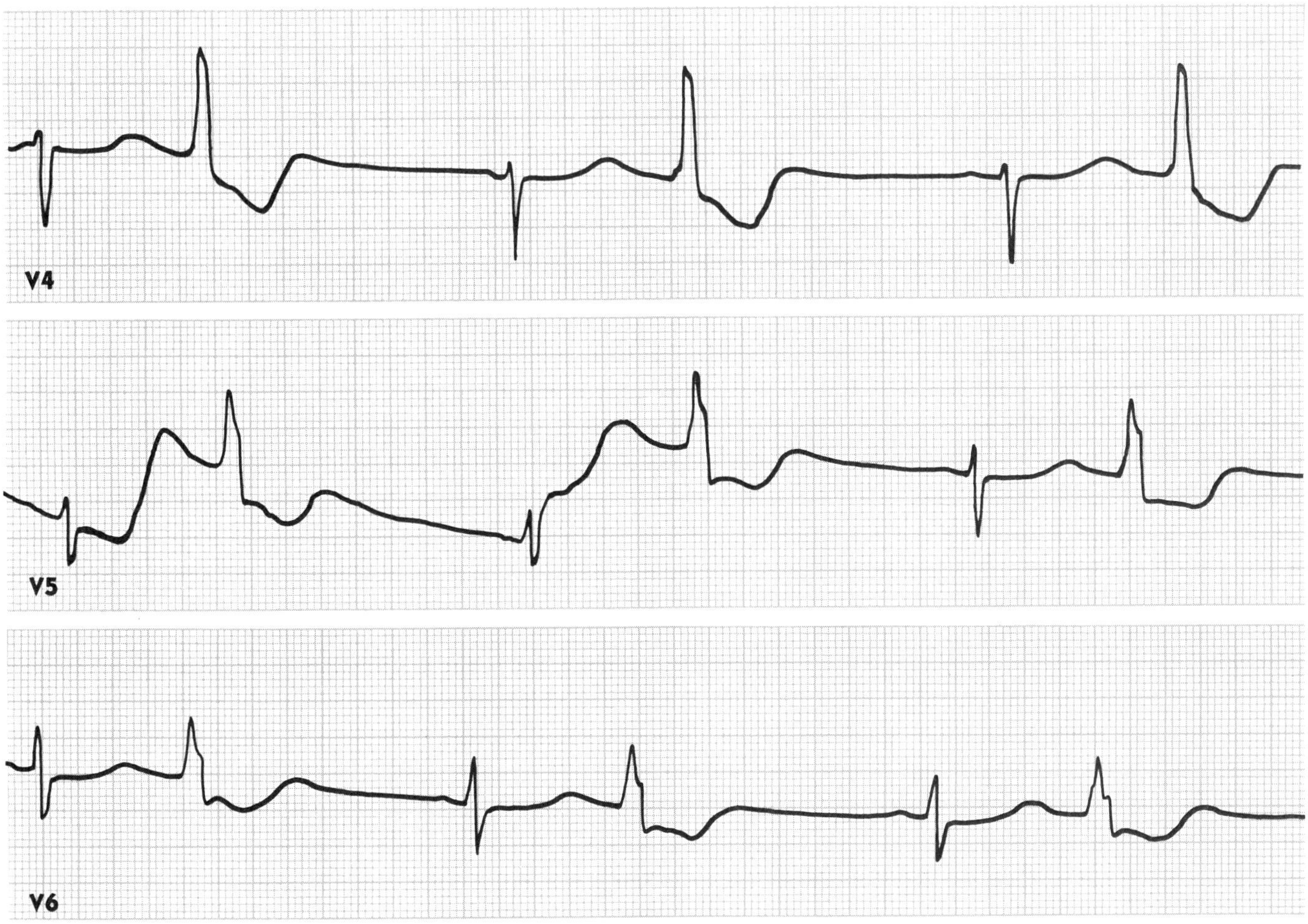
V4
V5
V6

CASE 60

Tricyclic Antidepressant Overdose

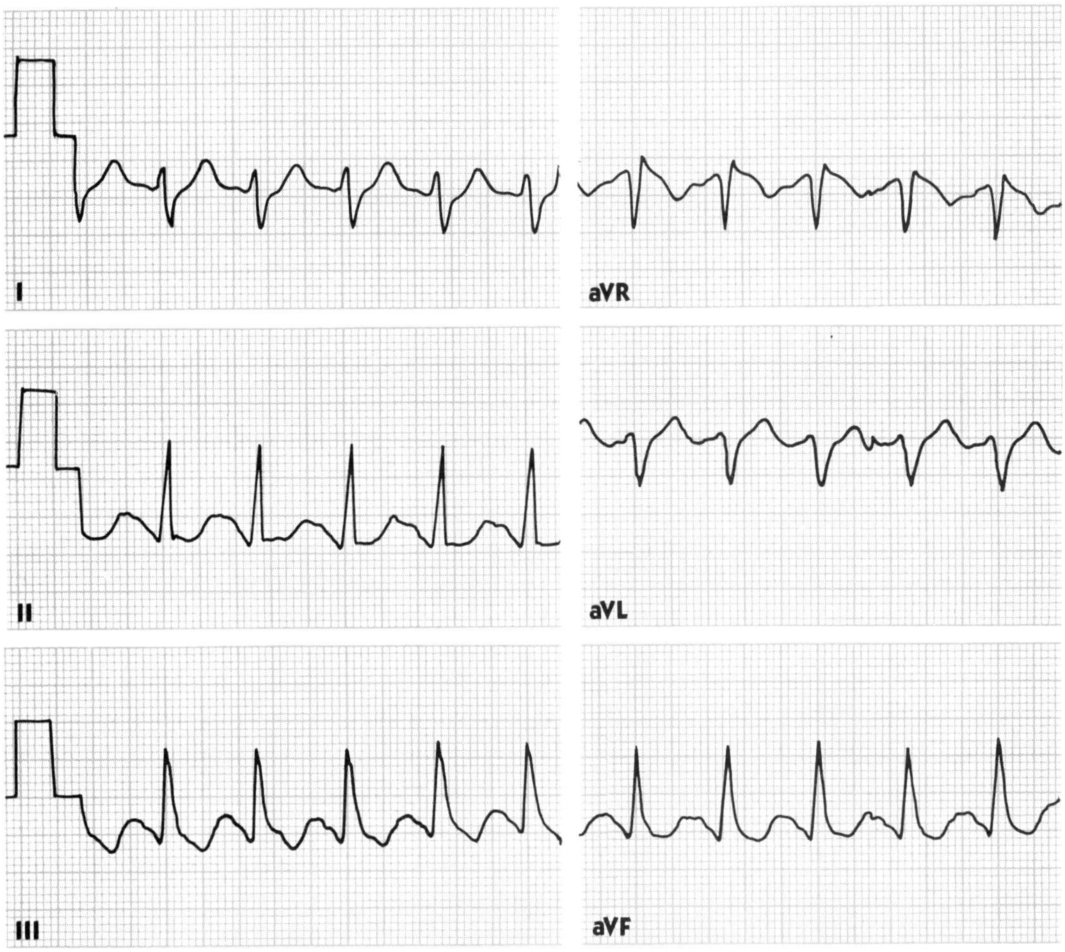

This ECG was recorded from a 23-year-old man who attempted suicide by taking an overdose of tricyclic antidepressant medication. The rhythm is sinus tachycardia. The PR interval is normal, but the QRS and QT intervals are prolonged (0.16 and 0.38 second, respectively). The mean frontal plane QRS axis of +110° and the qR pattern in leads II, III, and aVF suggest the possibility of conduction delay in the left posterior fascicle of the left bundle branch. The rSr′ pattern in lead aVR and the broad S waves in the lateral leads suggest right bundle branch block (RBBB), but in lead V1, the prominent anterior forces (R = S) without a terminal R′ wave do not meet RBBB criteria. The QRS prolongation indicates intraventricular conduction delay, but the pattern is not specific for RBBB. Thus the conduction delay is of undetermined type (see Case 21).

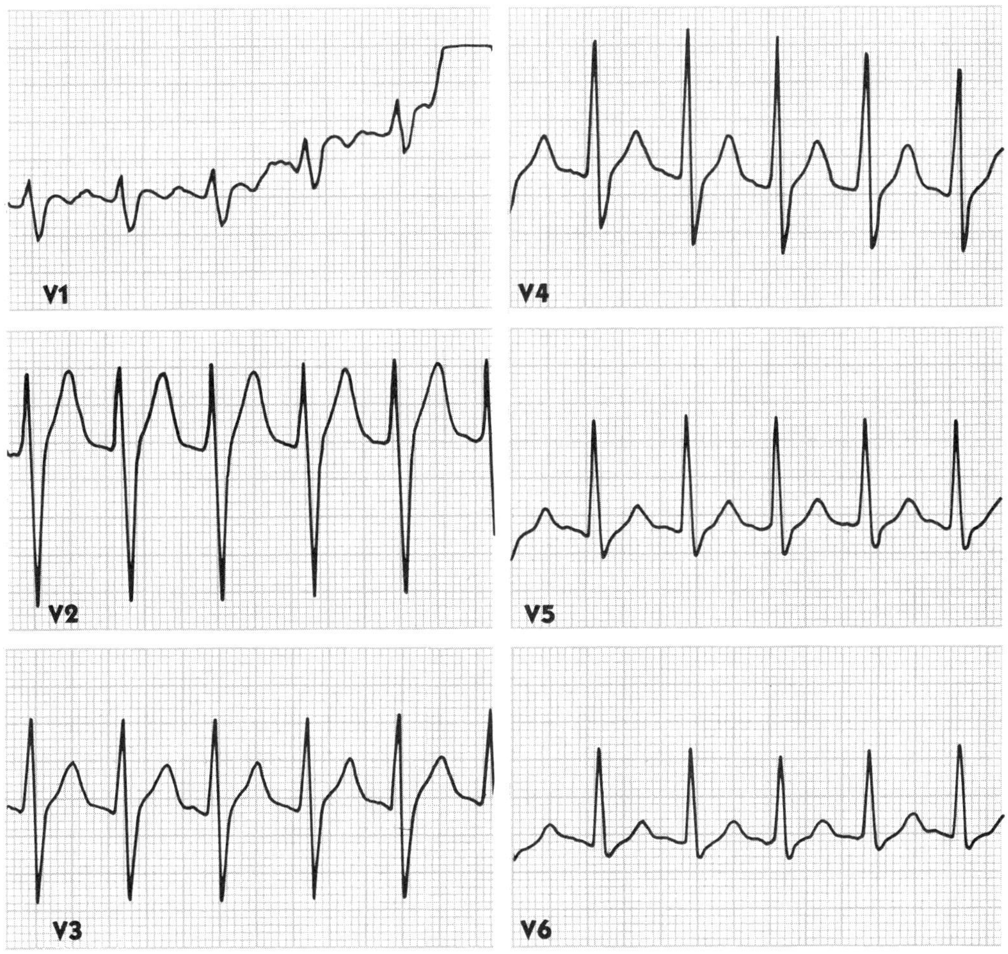

This ECG illustrates the expected abnormalities in tricyclic antidepressant toxicity—sinus tachycardia and prolonged QRS and QT intervals. Even in therapeutic doses, these agents can cause prolongation of the PR interval and ST-T abnormalities, as well as QT and QRS prolongation. Their effects on the ECG resemble those of the type I antiarrhythmic agents (see Cases 57-59).

SECTION X

Normal and Positional Variants

CASE 61

Early Repolarization

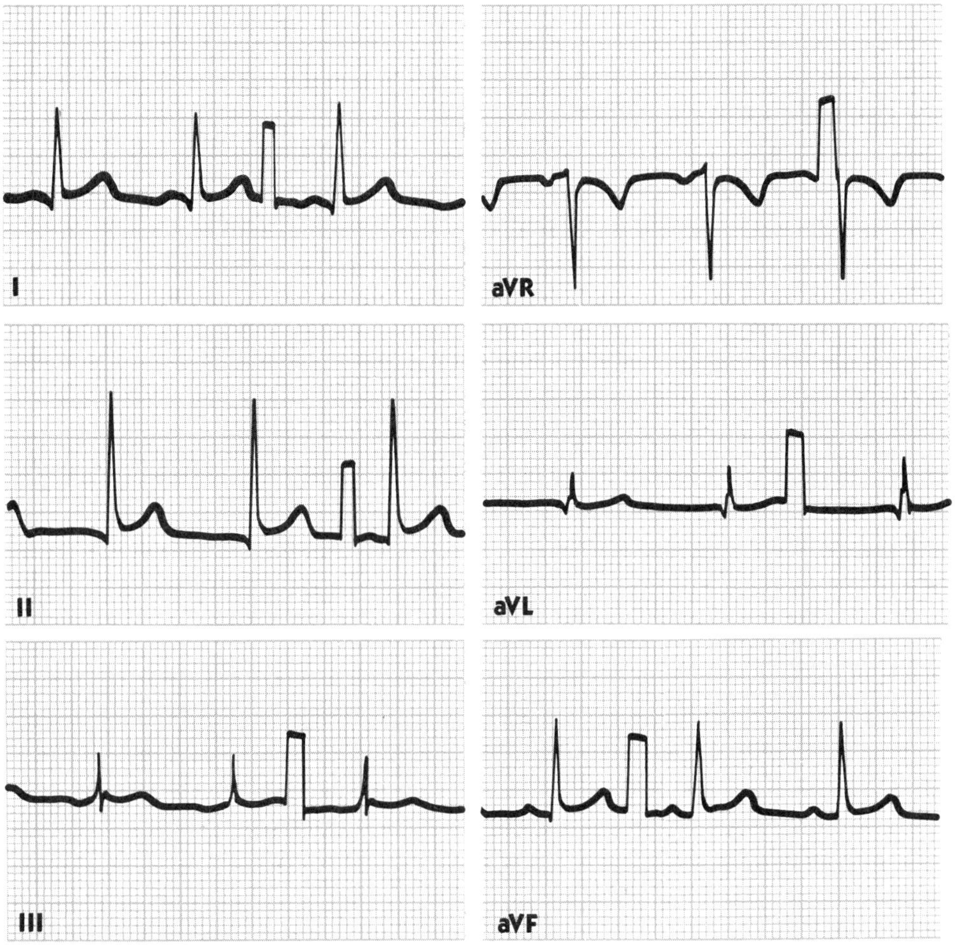

This ECG, recorded from a healthy 31-year-old man, shows sinus rhythm, normal intervals, and a normal mean frontal plane QRS axis. The S wave in lead V1 is 27 mm, and the R wave in V5 is 26 mm. There is J point elevation and concave-upward ST segment elevation in leads II, aVF, and V2-6. The T waves are normal, and small U waves are present in leads V2-4.

Although the precordial leads show pronounced QRS voltage suggesting left ventricular hypertrophy (LVH), the expected ST-T abnormalities are lacking. High precordial voltage alone is not an adequate criterion for the ECG diagnosis of LVH (see Case 1), as it occurs in normal young persons and in those with thin chests.

The ST segment is the most noteworthy feature of this ECG. Myocardial infarction generally causes ST segment elevation that is *convex* upward and less diffuse than in this case. Widespread ST segment elevation that is *concave* upward should raise the suspicion of pericarditis in the appropriate clinical situation. But in this normal individual, the ST segment represents the phenomenon of early repolarization.

It is sometimes difficult to differentiate early repolarization from the changes of pericarditis. The following four guidelines can be helpful: (1) Pericarditis is generally associated with ST segment changes in both limb and precordial leads; in early repolarization, the ST changes involve limb leads in only about 50% of cases. (2) The ST changes in pericarditis evolve and resolve with time; they remain unchanged in early repolarization. (3) PR segment depression occurs often in pericarditis. It occurs much less often

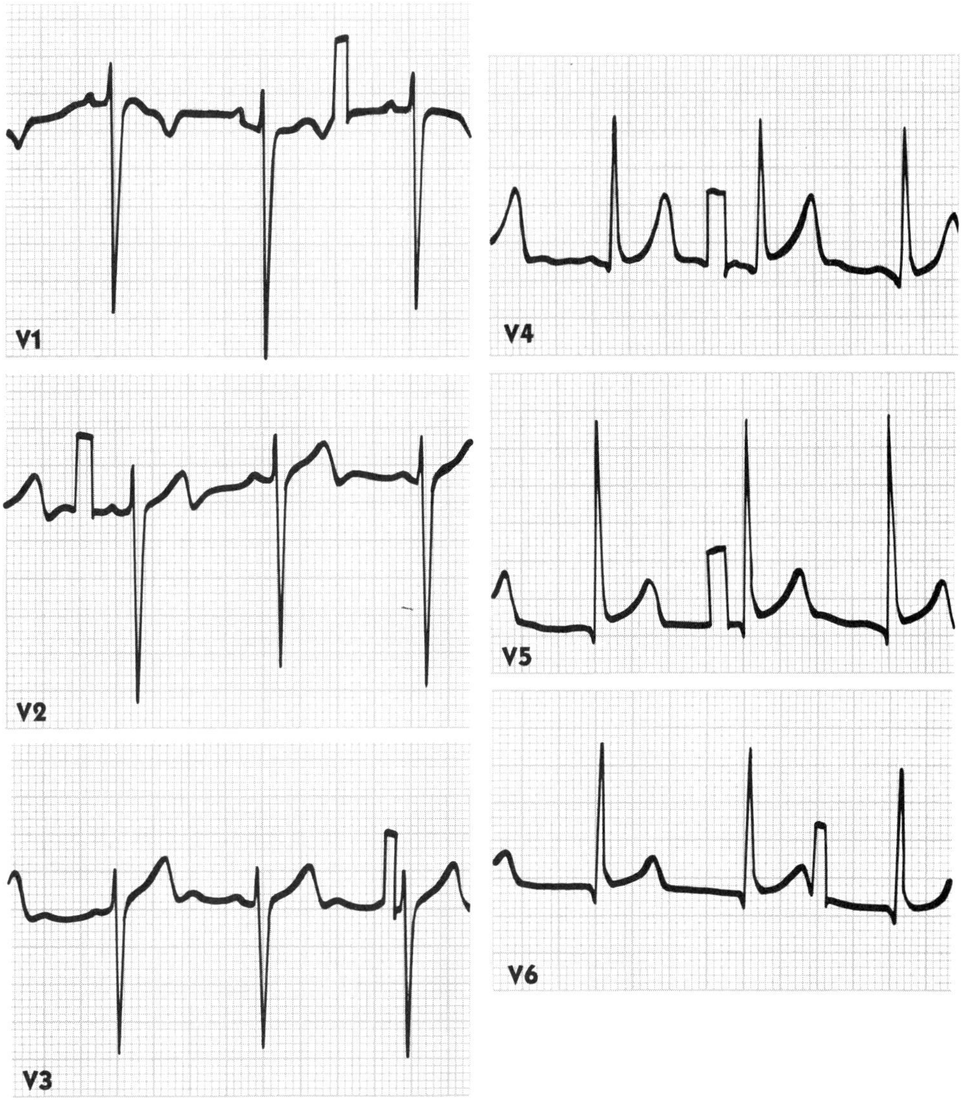

in early repolarization, but when it does, it is generally confined to either limb or precordial leads—not both. (4) ST changes representing early repolarization become less obvious and may disappear with exercise; those of pericarditis do not change.

CASE 62

Juvenile Pattern

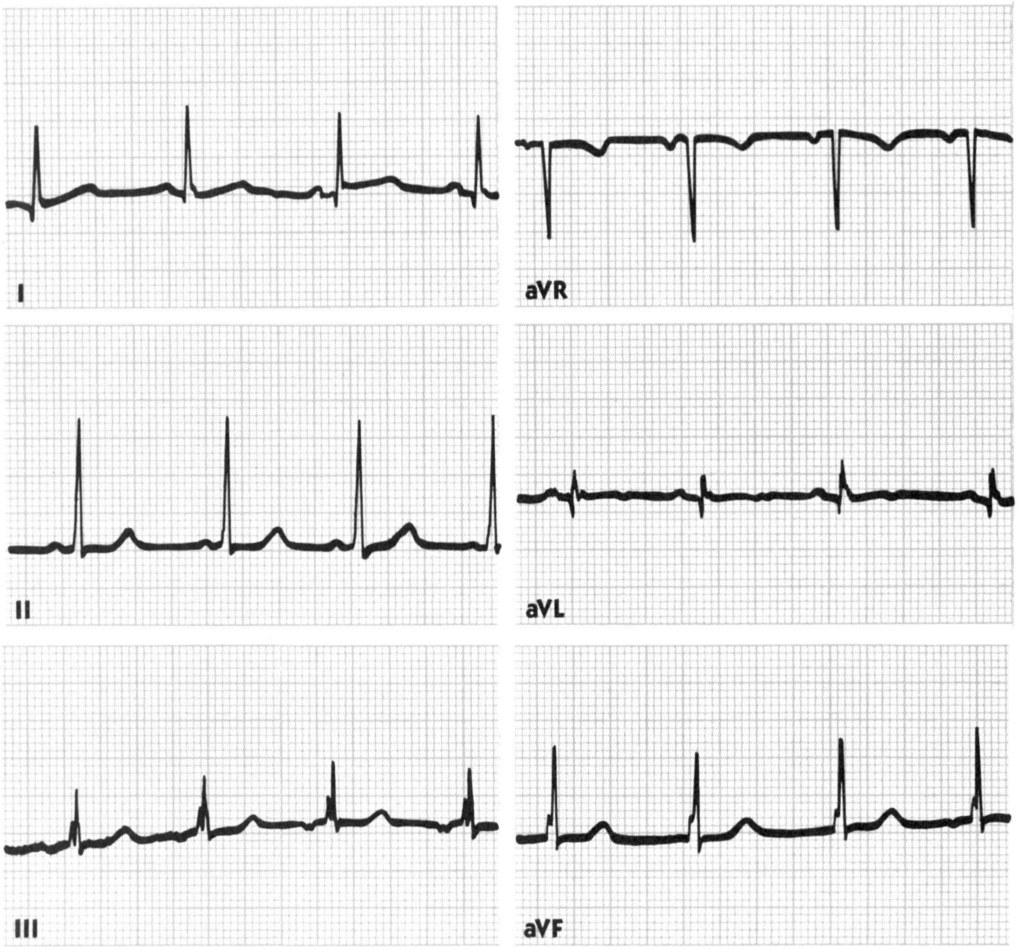

This 10-year-old boy had a routine ECG during hospitalization for orthopedic problems. His ECG shows sinus arrhythmia, normal intervals, and a normal mean frontal plane QRS axis of +60°. The QRS morphology is notable for deep S waves in lead V2 and tall R waves (52 mm) in lead V5 (note the half-standard setting in leads V2-6). Also noteworthy are the deep T wave inversion and slight ST segment elevation in the anterior precordial leads.

This young, healthy patient without heart disease is expected to have a normal ECG. His ECG is, indeed, a variant of normal, not uncommonly seen in young children. The pronounced precordial voltage meets the voltage criteria for left ventricular hypertrophy (LVH) in adults (see Case 1), but the criteria do not apply in children. The distance between the precordial leads and the heart is smaller in children due to the thinner chest wall, resulting in larger generated potentials and deflections of greater amplitude.

The T wave inversion in the anterior precordial leads might suggest ischemia, myocardial infarction, or pericarditis under different clinical circumstances. However, repolarization changes with mildly elevated ST segments and biphasic or inverted T waves in the anterior precordial leads are also common normal variants. These findings are frequently referred to as a "juvenile pattern." The T wave changes generally do

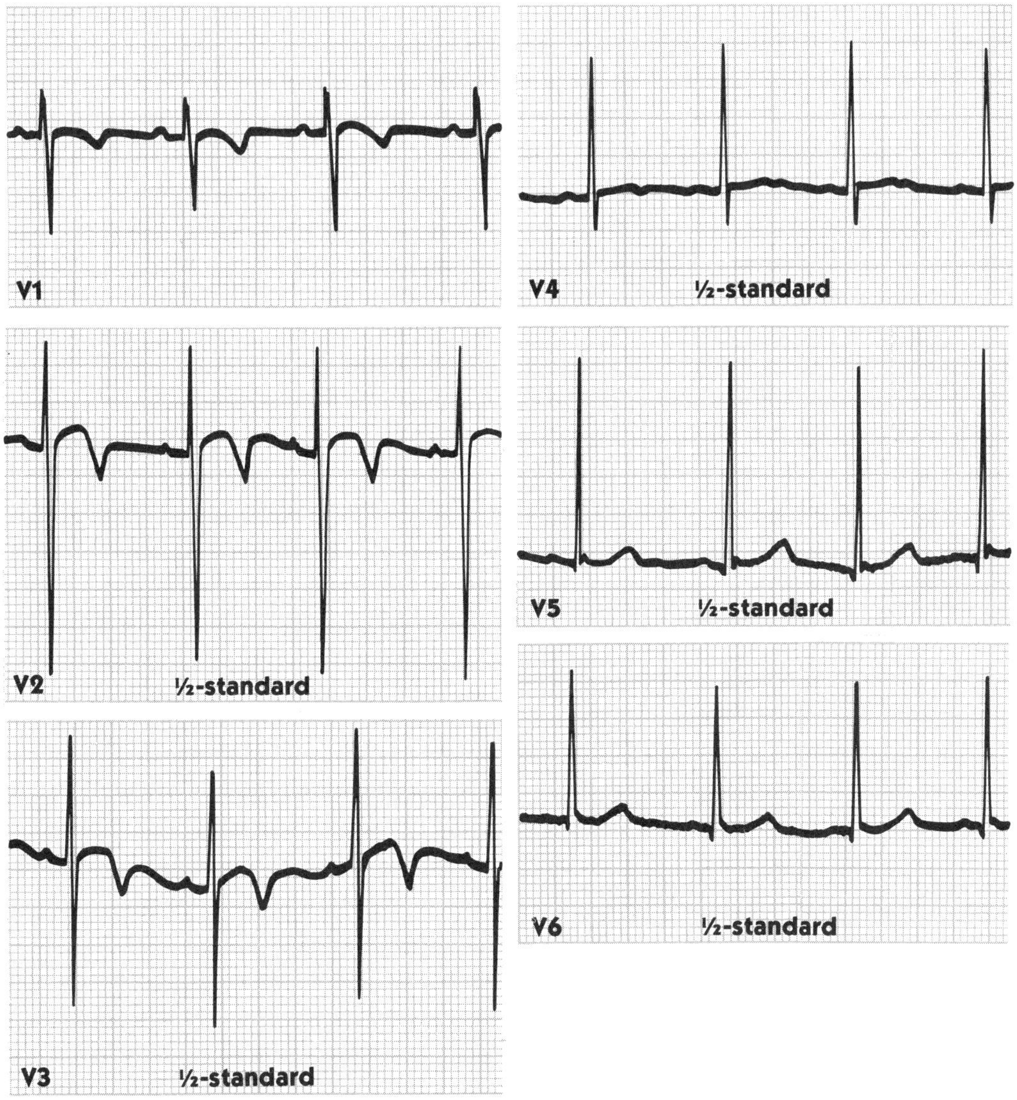

not extend beyond lead V4; lateral T wave inversion with prominent voltage might be more suggestive of LVH. It is not known with certainty why ST-T changes occur in young healthy persons, but it has been shown that the frequency decreases with age.

CASE 63

Poor Precordial R Wave Progression Due to Pectus Excavatum

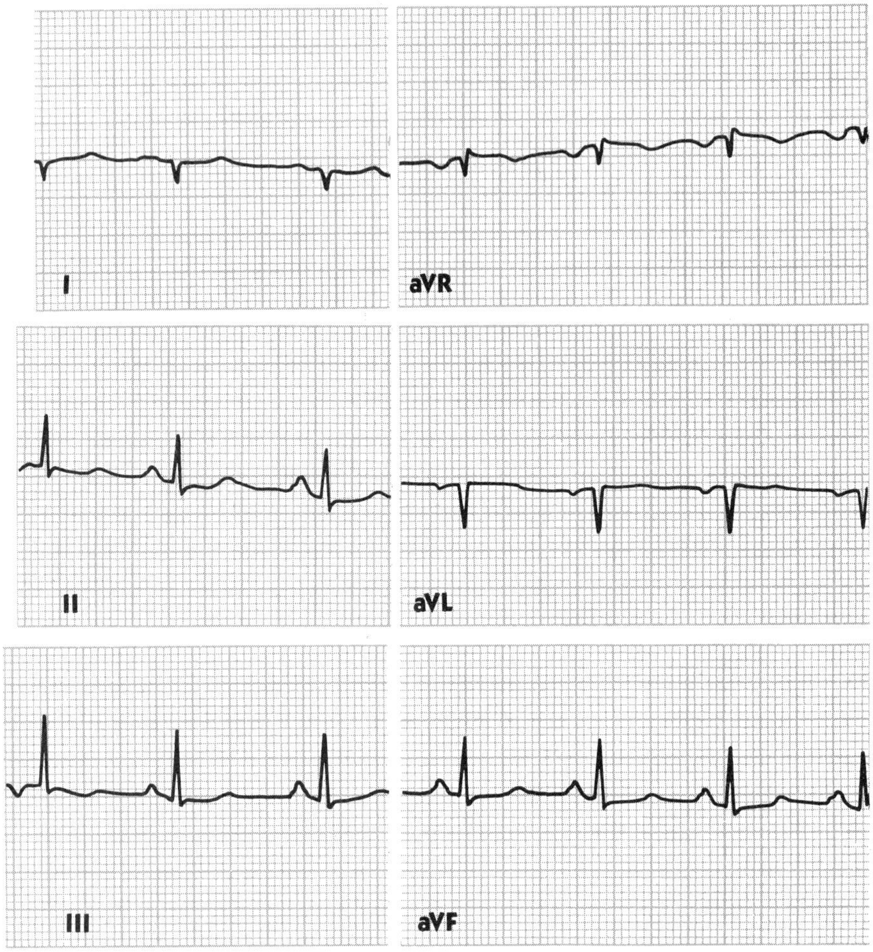

This woman has severe pectus excavatum, multiple nonejection clicks, a family history of "heart attacks," and an abnormal ECG. The ECG shows sinus rhythm and normal intervals. The mean frontal plane QRS axis is rightward at +110°. There is a QS pattern in leads I, aVL, and V1; a Qr pattern in lead V2; and an rS pattern across the rest of the precordium. The minor ST segment elevation and T wave inversion in leads V1-2 are nonspecific.

The patient's marked pectus excavatum explains her ECG. In this condition, the anteroposterior dimension of the mediastinum is decreased, and the heart is pushed leftward and occasionally inferiorly, rotating the left ventricle posteriorly. The mean QRS vector is therefore directed posteriorly (and occasionally inferiorly). Consequently, R waves develop ampli-

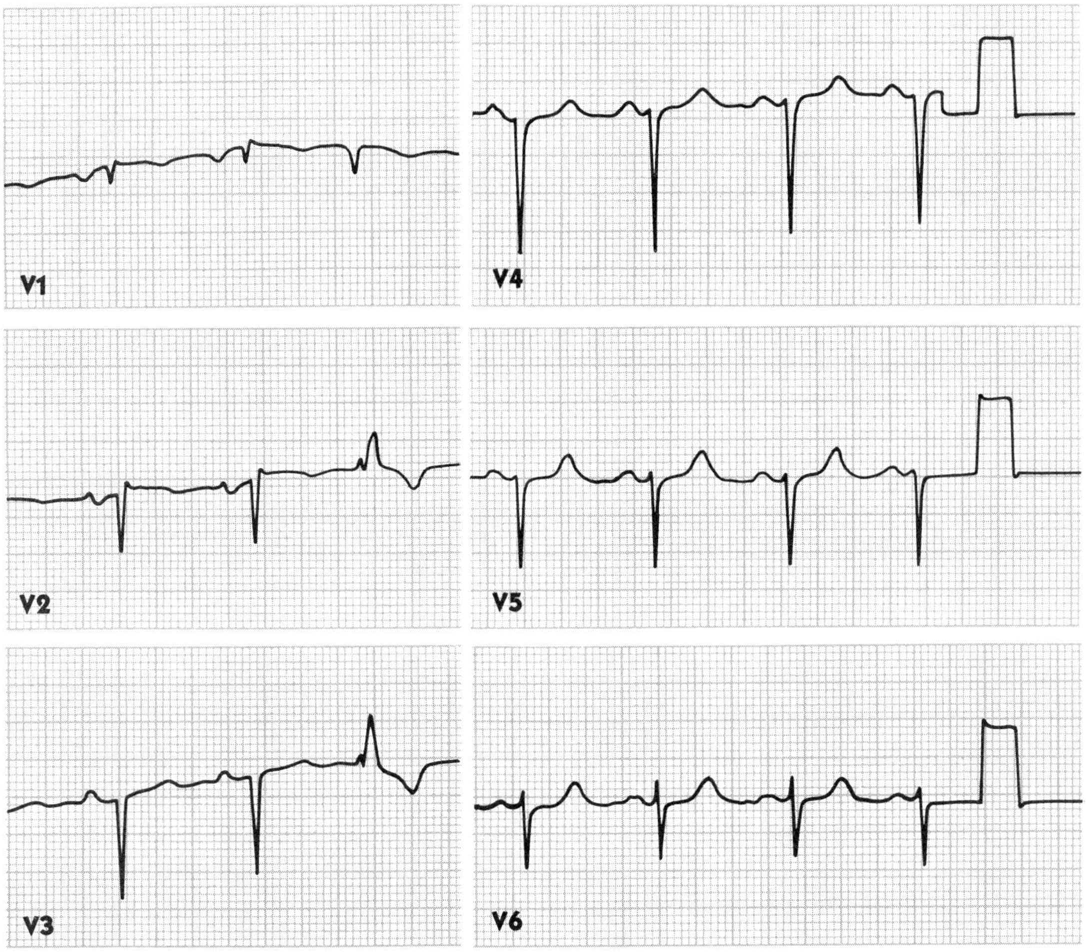

tude poorly across the precordium, and occasionally the mean frontal plane QRS axis is inferior and rightward. Even with normal myocardium, this posterior redirection of ventricular forces can mimic anterior or high lateral myocardial infarction, as in this case. The process is similar to the genesis of poor R wave progression in left ventricular hypertrophy (see Case 3).

The straight back syndrome is another chest cage abnormality in which this ECG pattern may be seen. But this pattern is not specific for chest cage deformities and may occur in a number of other types of conditions (see Table 2 in the Appendix).

CASE 64—A and B

Poor Precordial R Wave Progression Due to High Precordial Lead Placement

CASE 64A

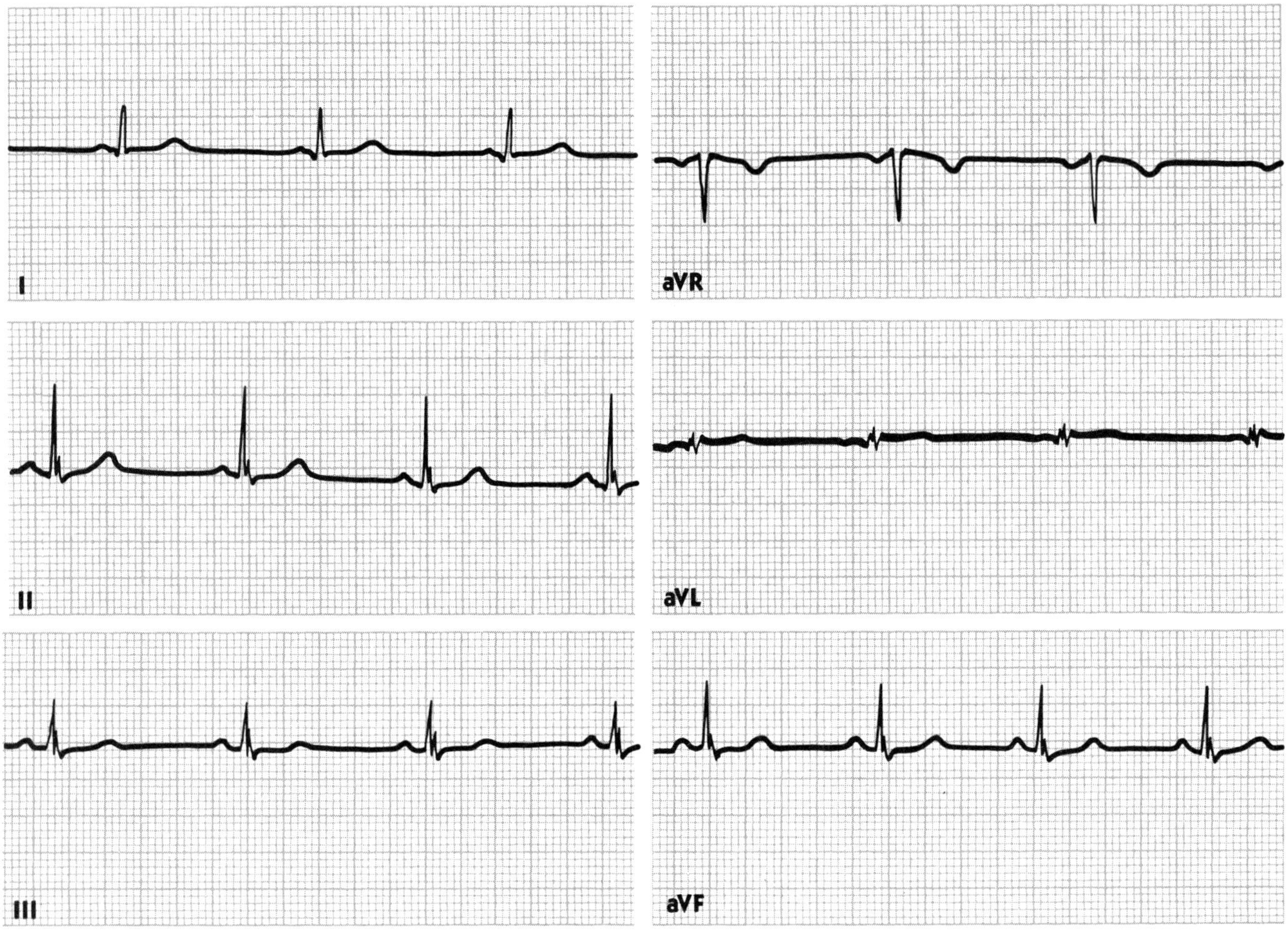

The first ECG (A) was recorded from a healthy 28-year-old medical resident during a routine examination. It shows sinus rhythm, normal intervals, and a normal mean frontal plane QRS axis. There are notched Rs complexes in leads II, III, and aVF; Qr complexes in leads V1-2; and rSr′ complexes in lead V3. The T waves are inverted in leads V1-2.

The poor precordial R wave development raises the possibility of cardiac or pulmonary disease or chest cage abnormalities (see Table 2 in the Appendix). However, this healthy subject had neither history nor evidence of underlying disease. On close questioning, it was discovered that the right precordial leads had been placed at about the second intercostal space on the chest wall. The second ECG (B)

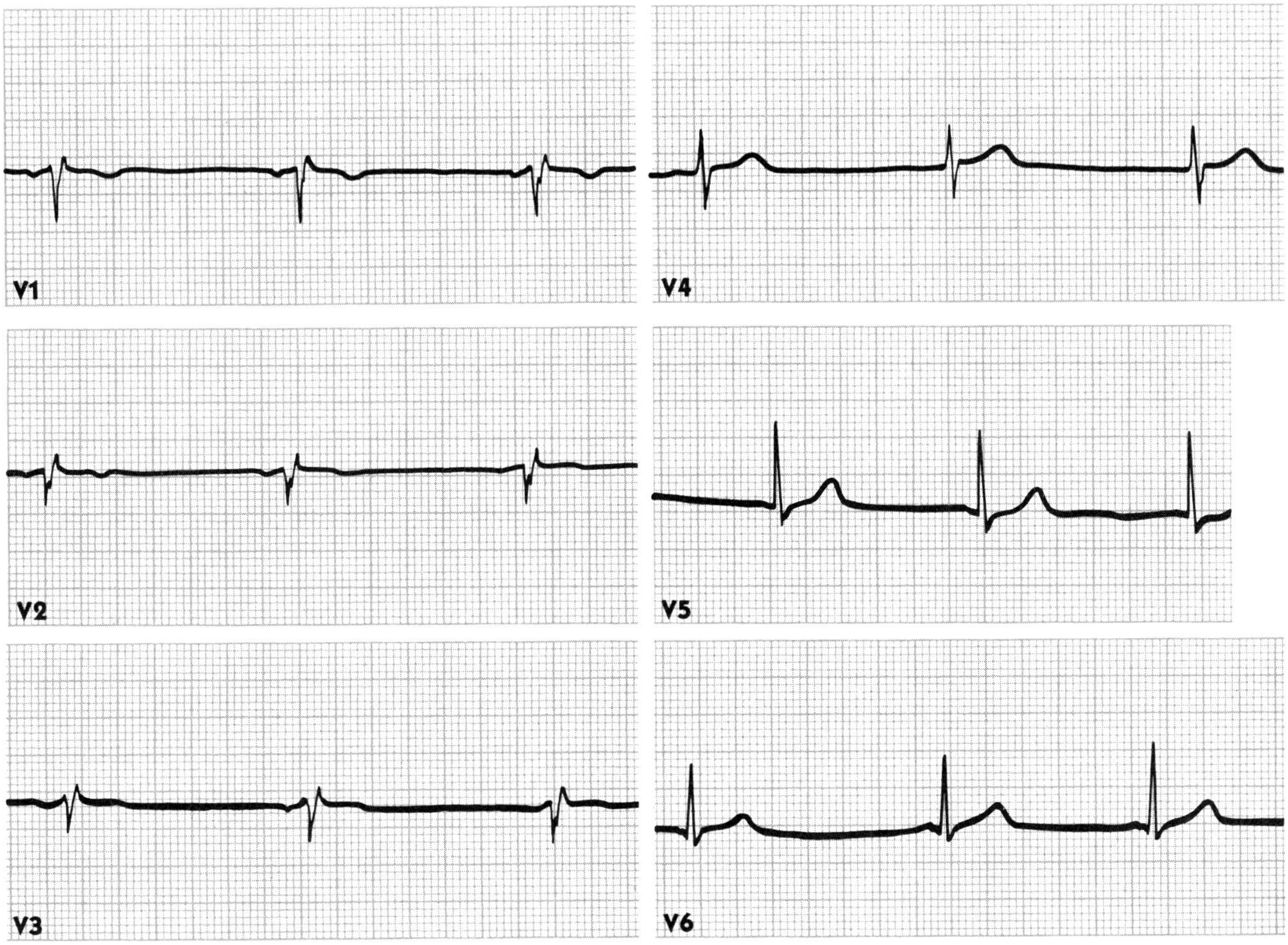

continued

was recorded with special attention to correct placement of the right precordial leads at the fourth intercostal space. It was normal.

If the precordial leads are placed too high or the heart is displaced inferiorly relative to the chest wall, the precordial leads will record potentials above the mean QRS vector and, thus, poor progression of R waves. Poor R wave progression can also be a normal variant—even with correct lead placement—if the mean QRS vector is directed sufficiently inferiorly. Placement of the electrodes one interspace lower will usually record normal R wave progression in such cases. These normal and positional variants must be recognized to avoid erroneous diagnoses of cardiopulmonary disease.

CASE 64B

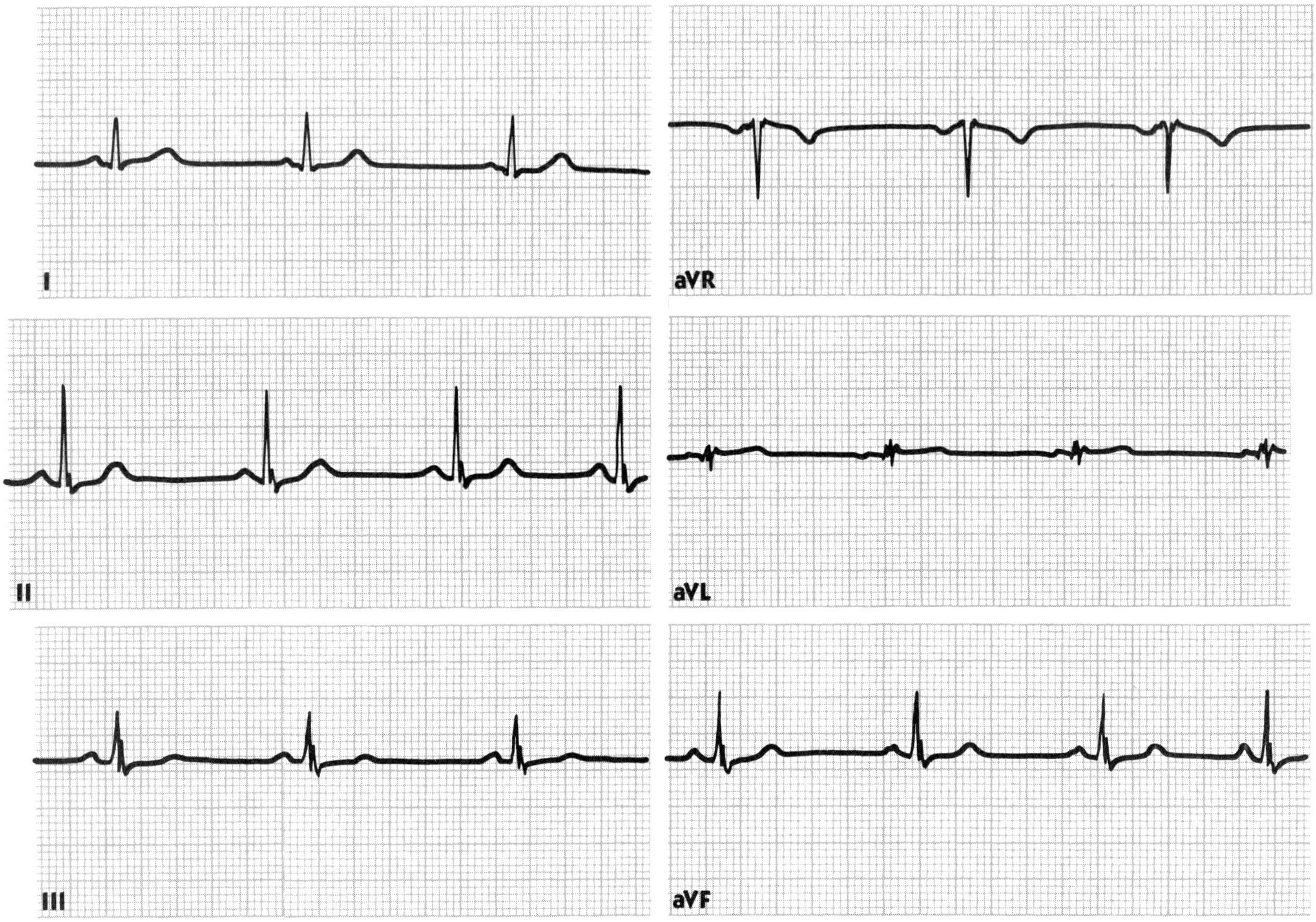

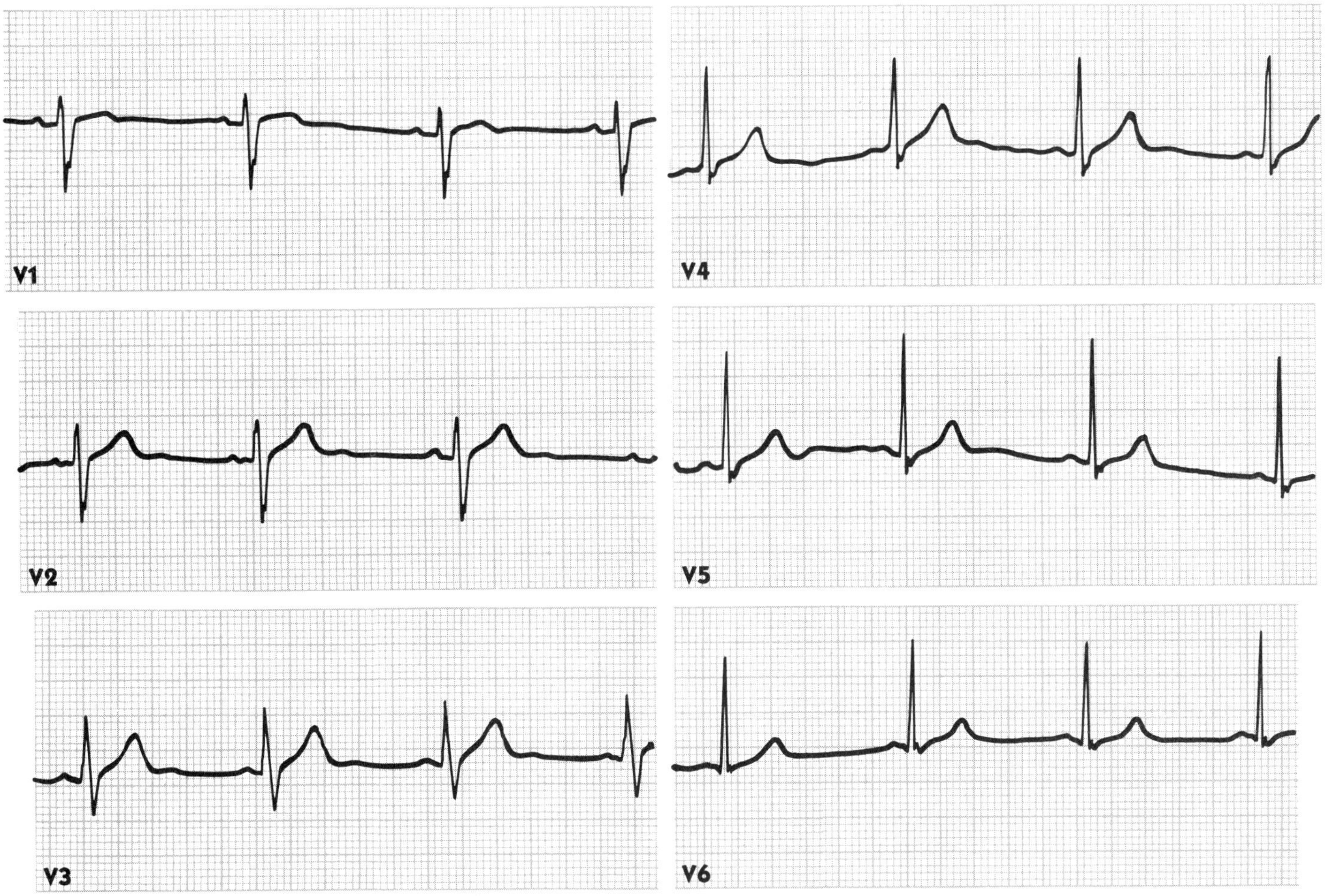
V1
V2
V3
V4
V5
V6

CASE 65—A, B, and C

Limb Lead Misplacement Mimicking Lateral Myocardial Infarction

CASE 65A

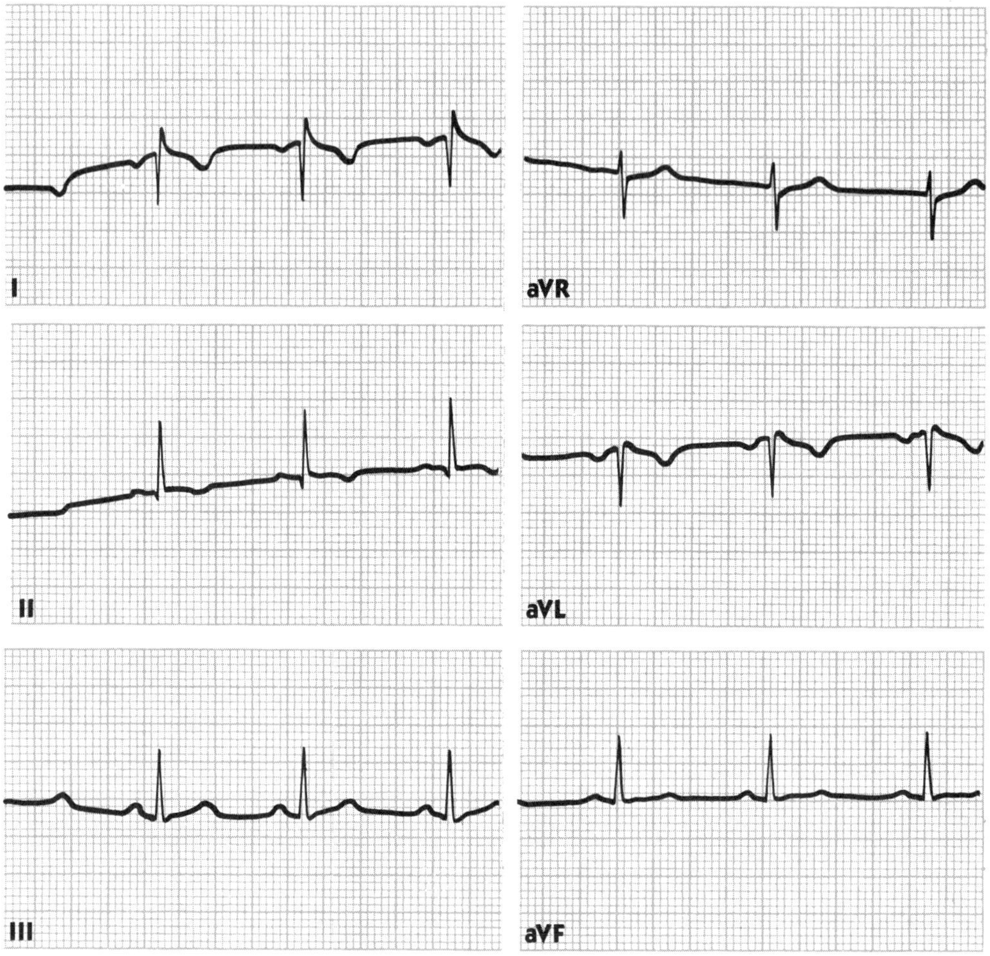

These three ECGs were recorded from a healthy 23-year-old medical student. In the first (A), the PR, QRS, and QT intervals are normal, and the mean frontal plane QRS axis is rightward at +110°. There are deep Q waves with symmetrical T wave inversion in leads I and aVL. Particularly notable are the inverted P waves in leads I and aVL, resulting in a rightward P wave axis.

The subject might appear to have had a high lateral myocardial infarction in the past. But closer inspection reveals two important points: First, the mirror image of the lead I tracing shows normal P-QRS-T morphology. Second, aVL looks like a normal aVR, and *vice versa*. These clues point to an obvious explanation of the observed abnormalities: The right and left arm leads were inadvertently reversed when the ECG was recorded, resulting in inversion of right and left P-QRS-T complexes. The ECG was repeated with the limb leads placed correctly (B). This second tracing is within normal limits.

Arm lead reversal should be suspected when the mean vectors of *both* the P wave and the QRS complex are redirected while normal precordial QRS patterns are preserved. When ECG findings are difficult to explain on pathological grounds, the possibility of technical errors should be considered. Otherwise, normal subjects may receive erroneous diagnoses.

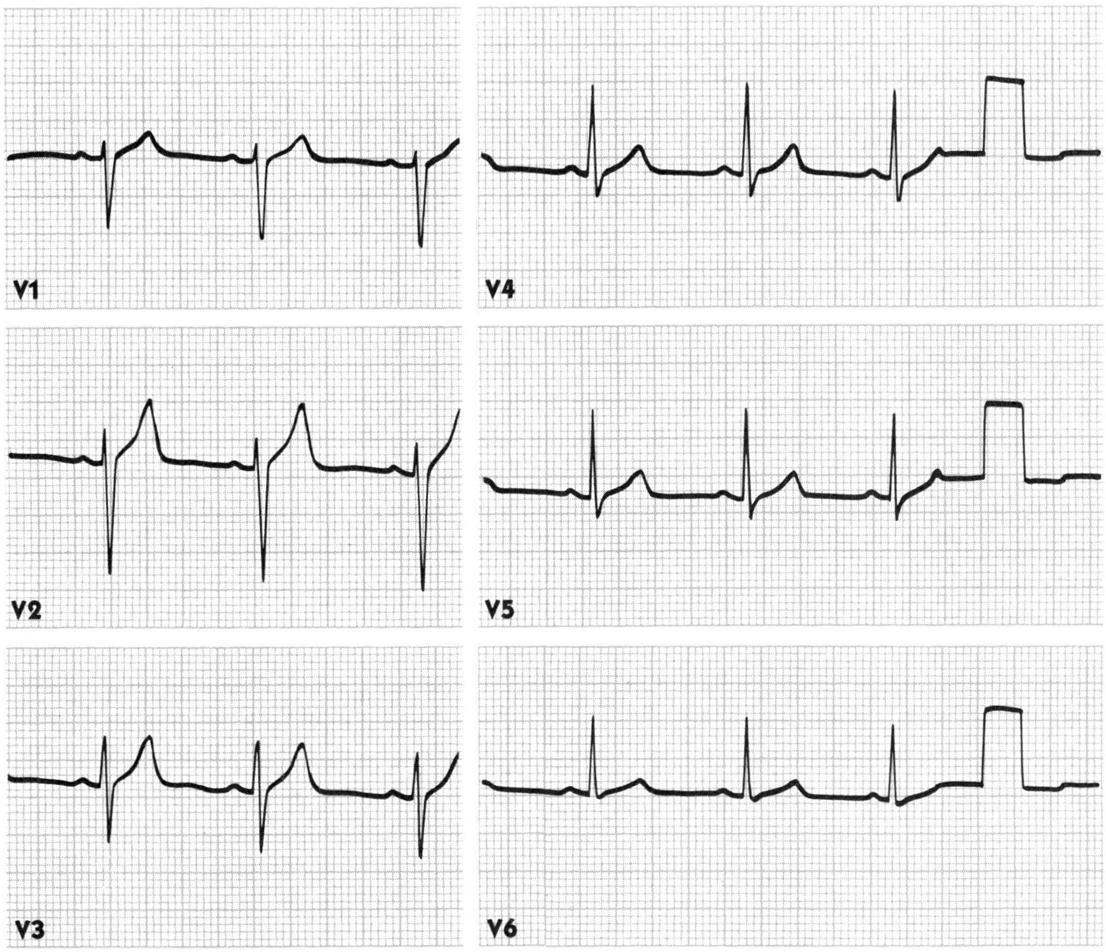

continued

In the third ECG (C), leads from the right and left leg were deliberately reversed; since there has been only a modest change in the vector of the recording electrodes, there is minimal, if any, change from the true ECG.

CASE 65B

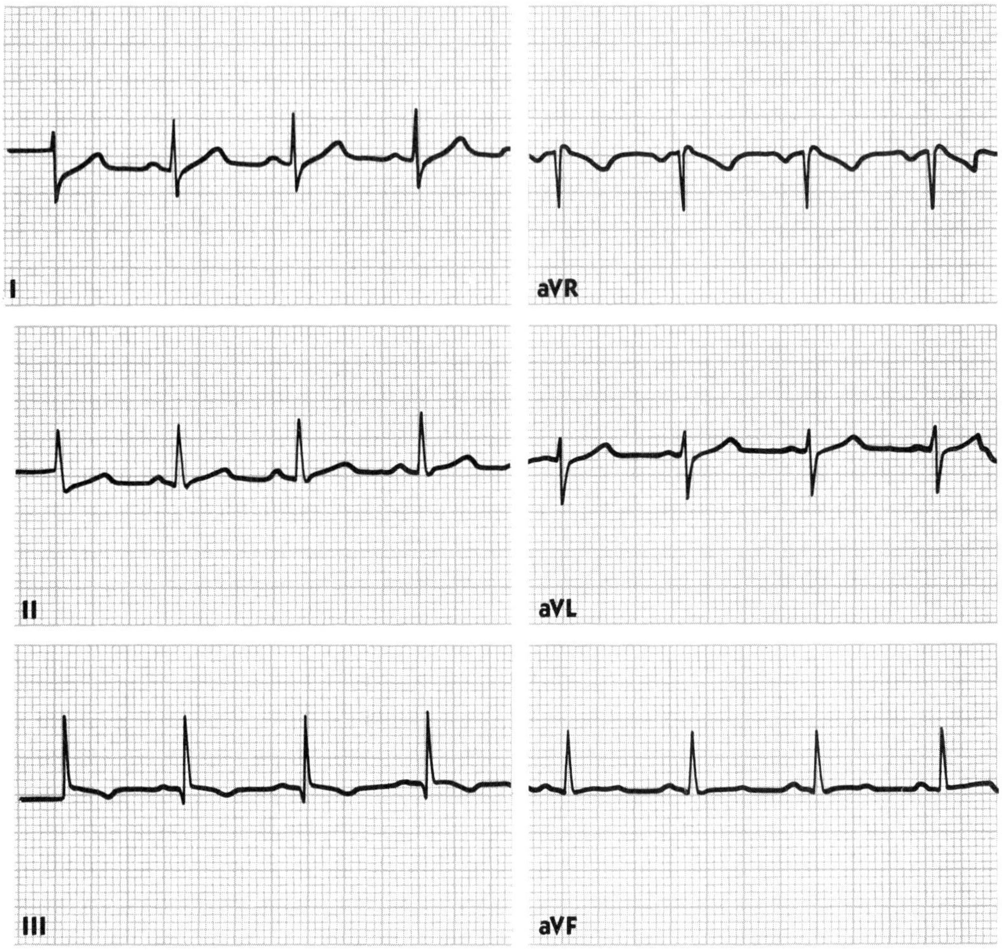

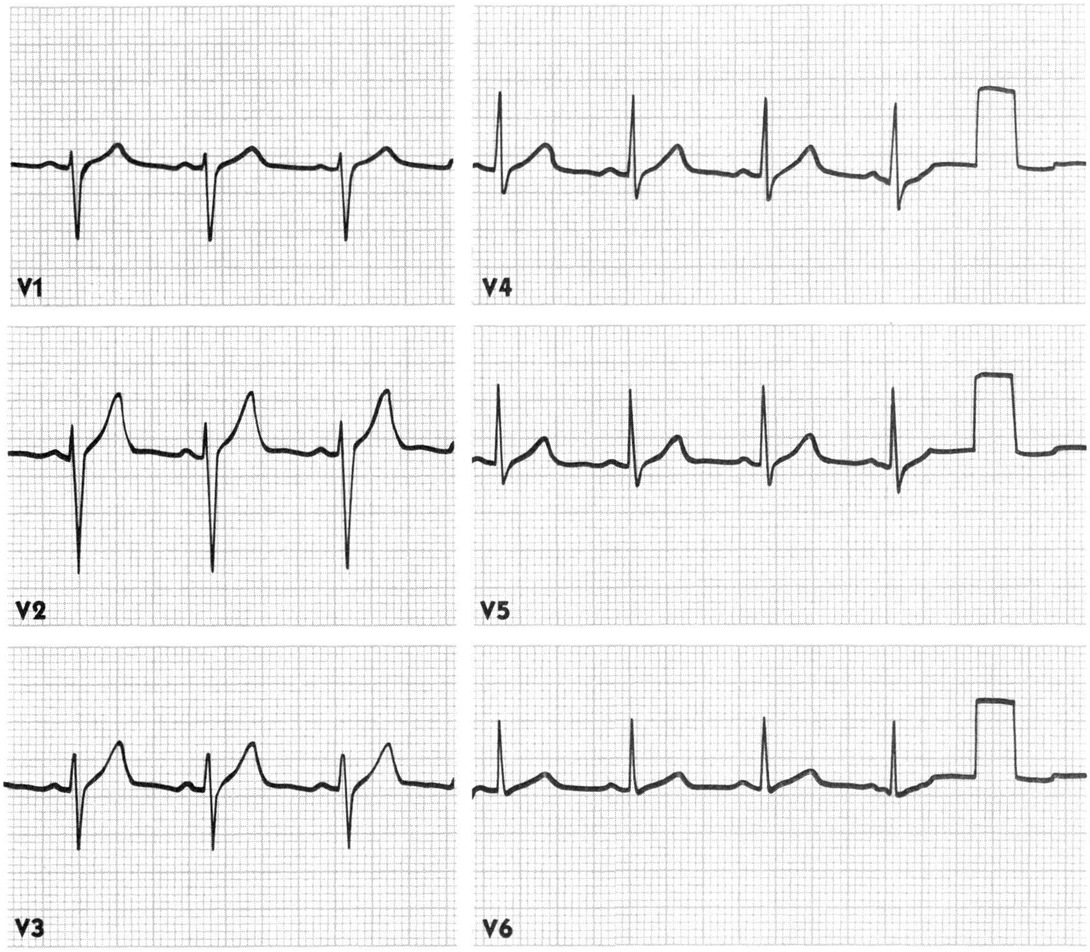

continued

CASE 65C

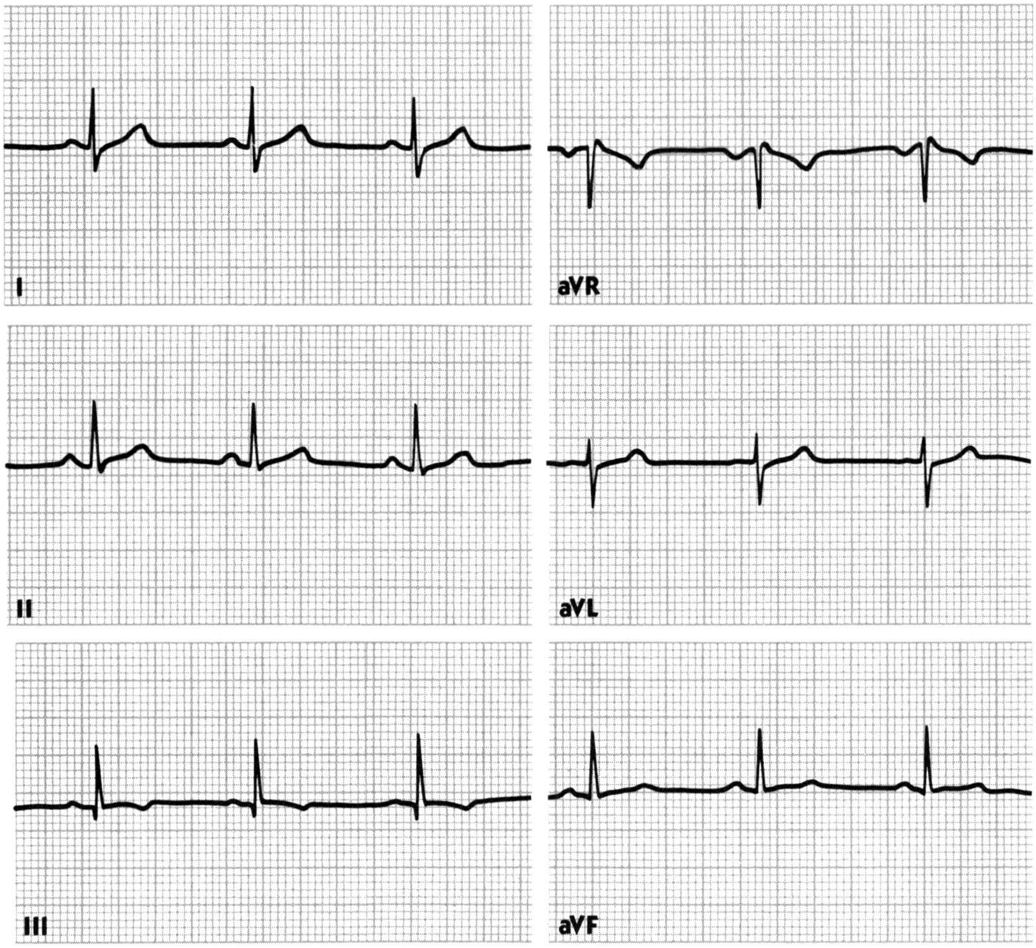

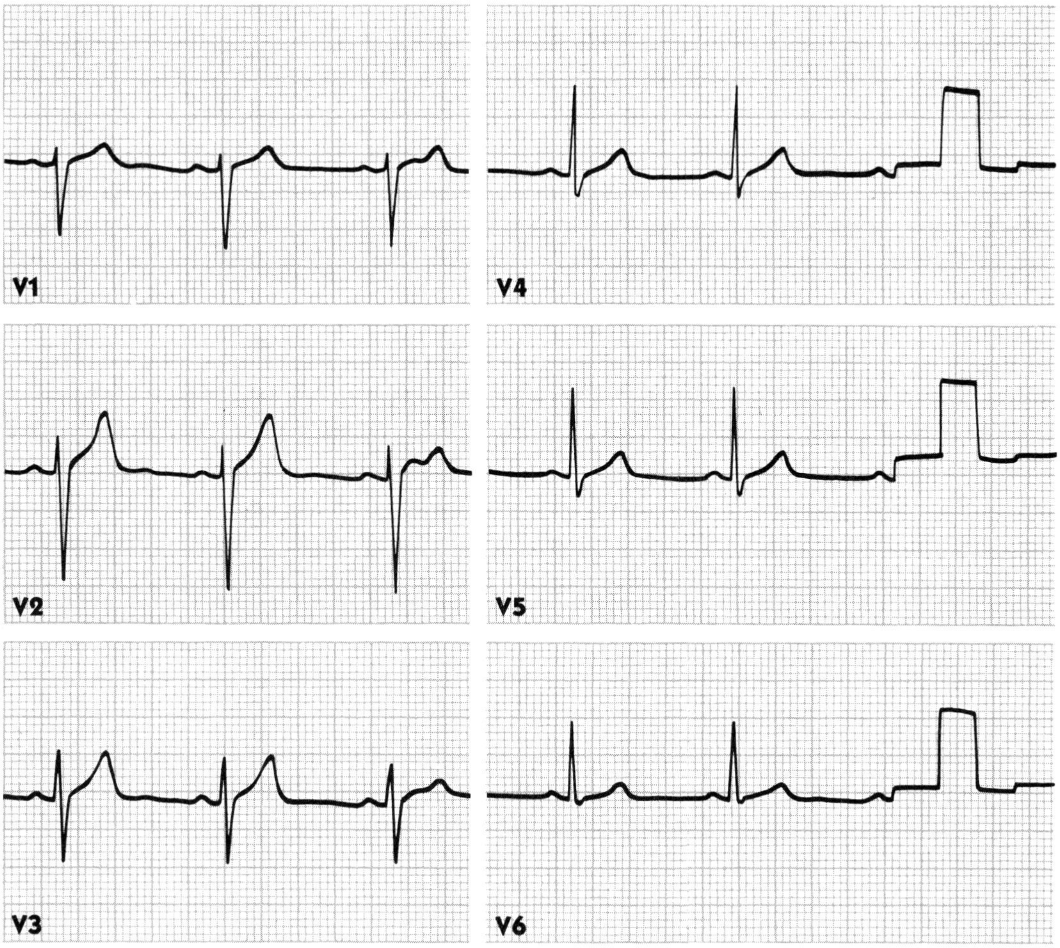
V1
V4
V2
V5
V3
V6

CASE 66—A and B

Dextrocardia With Situs Inversus

CASE 66A

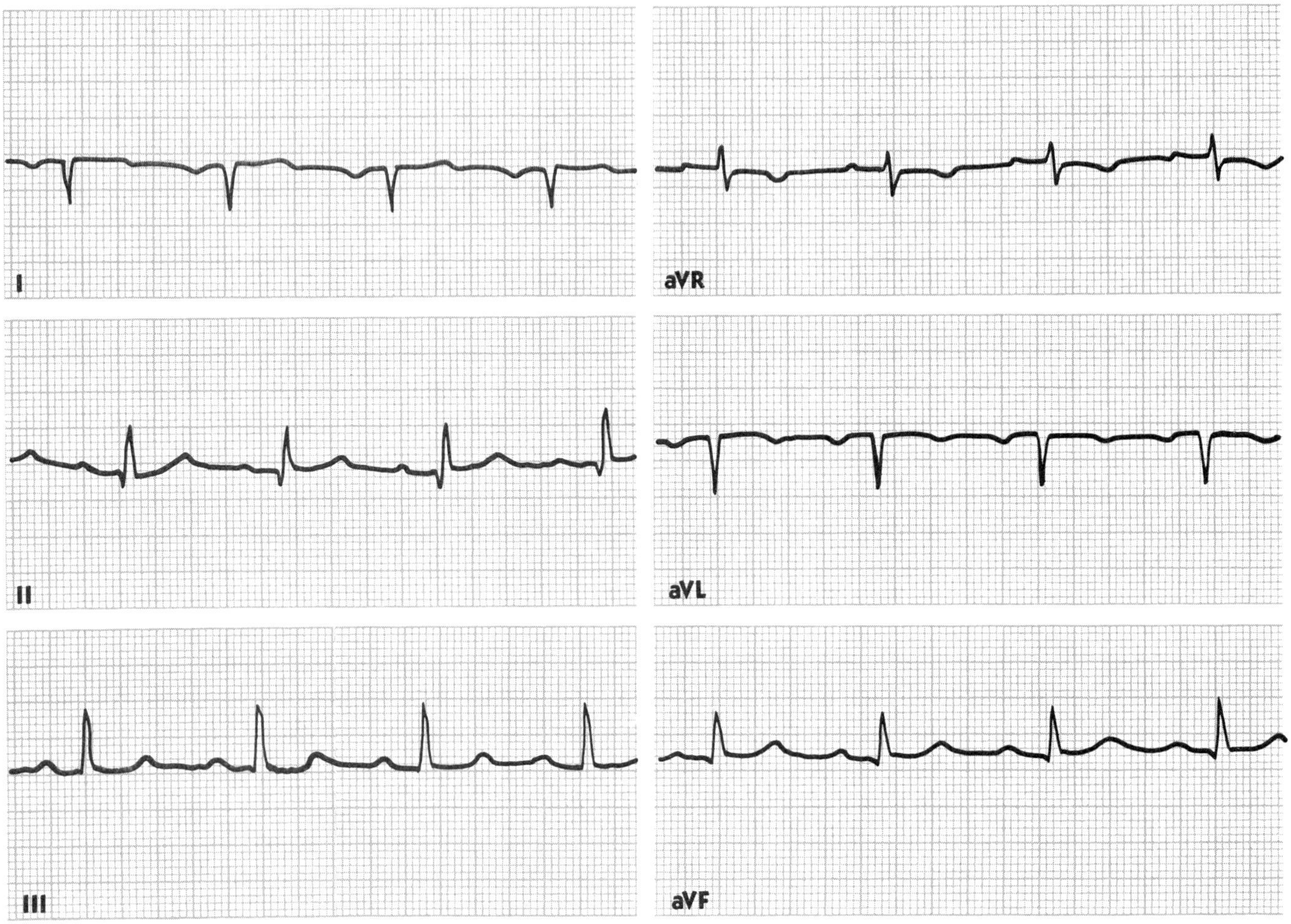

This case involves a 58-year-old man with no history of heart disease. The first ECG (A) shows sinus rhythm, first degree AV block (PR interval = 0.24 second), and normal QRS and QT intervals. The mean frontal plane QRS axis is markedly rightward at +120°. The P wave is inverted in leads I and aVL. There are QS complexes in leads I, aVL, and V2-6, with decreasing depth of the QS complexes laterally. The T waves are inverted in leads aVL and V1-6.

This patient has dextrocardia with situs inversus, a mirror-image reversal of the right and left sides of the body. Thus, the left ventricle is located to the right of the right ventricle. The electrical patterns inscribed in dextrocardia are the reverse of normal; the limb lead tracings are similar to those produced by reversal of the right and left arm leads in a normal subject (see Case 65). In dextrocardia, lead I is expected to show inversion of the P wave, QRS complex, and T wave. The upright T wave in this case suggests a second process. The normal patterns of leads aVR and aVL and of leads II and III are transposed. Intentionally reversing the right and left arm leads would normalize the limb lead pattern in this case, except for the nonspecific T wave abnormality in lead I.

Simple reversal of arm leads will not, however, change the precordial pattern (compare Case 65), since forces in the transverse (anteroposterior) plane will not be altered. In dextrocardia, the cardiac apex is located in the right chest, and the QRS axis is directed to the right. The left precordial leads regis-

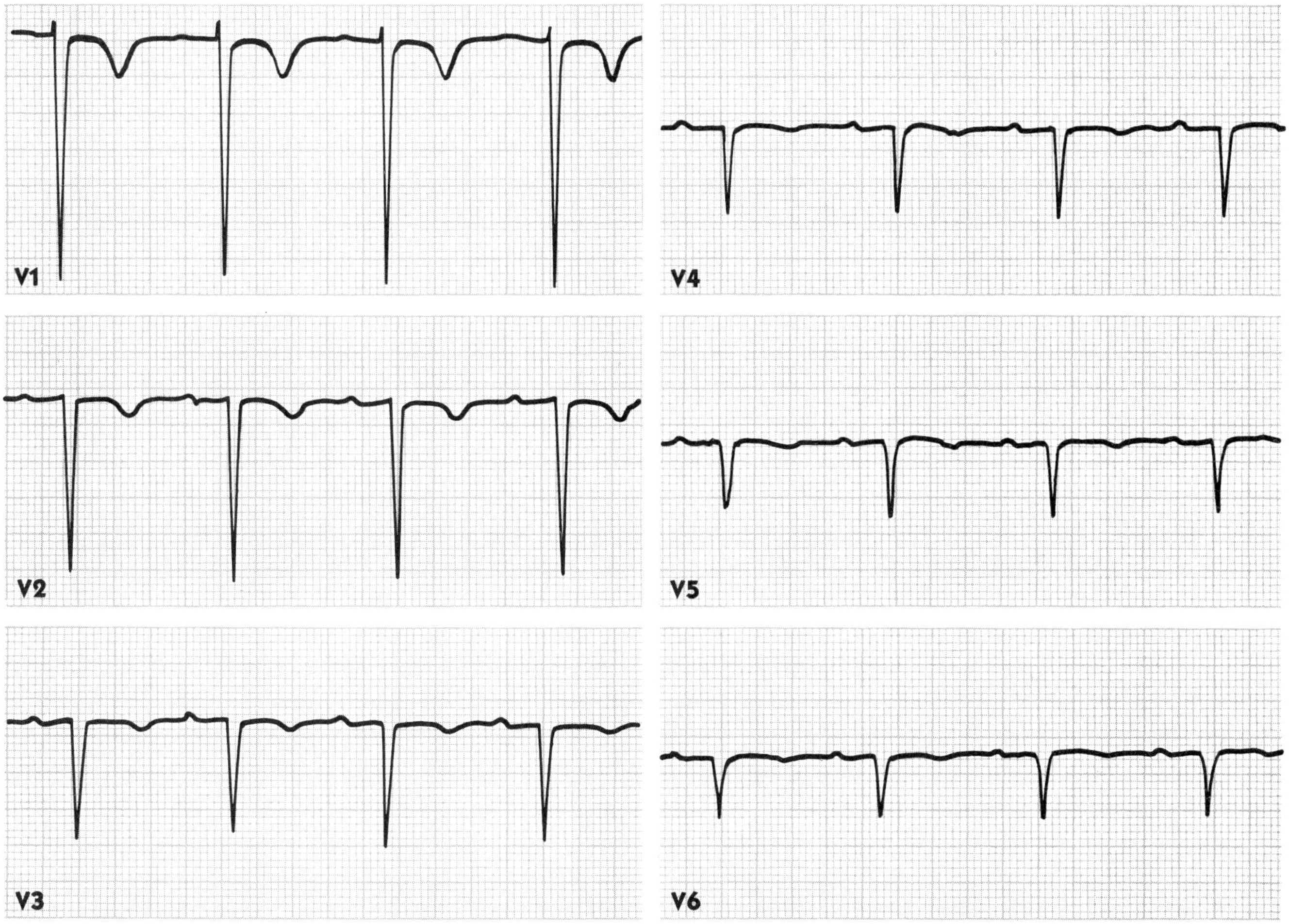

continued

ter these rightward forces as deep S waves or QS waves. Septal depolarization is directed to the left, superiorly, and anteriorly, occasionally producing small R waves in leads V1-2. Since the ventricles are displaced to the right, the left lateral leads are farther away from them than usual, and the QRS deflections progressively decline from lead V1 to V6.

This pattern—right-left reversal in the limb leads and progressively smaller QS (or rS) complexes in the left lateral precordial leads—is, of course, highly suggestive of dextrocardia. But it also could conceivably be interpreted as anterolateral wall myocardial infarction. Tracings obtained from the right precordial leads (B) will show normal R wave development in dextrocardia, confirming the diagnosis.

The anterior T wave inversion in leads V1-4 (A) persists even in the second tracing (B), with the precordial leads located on the right chest (using leads V1R-V6R). This suggests primary T wave changes (see Table 5 in the Appendix).

CASE 66B

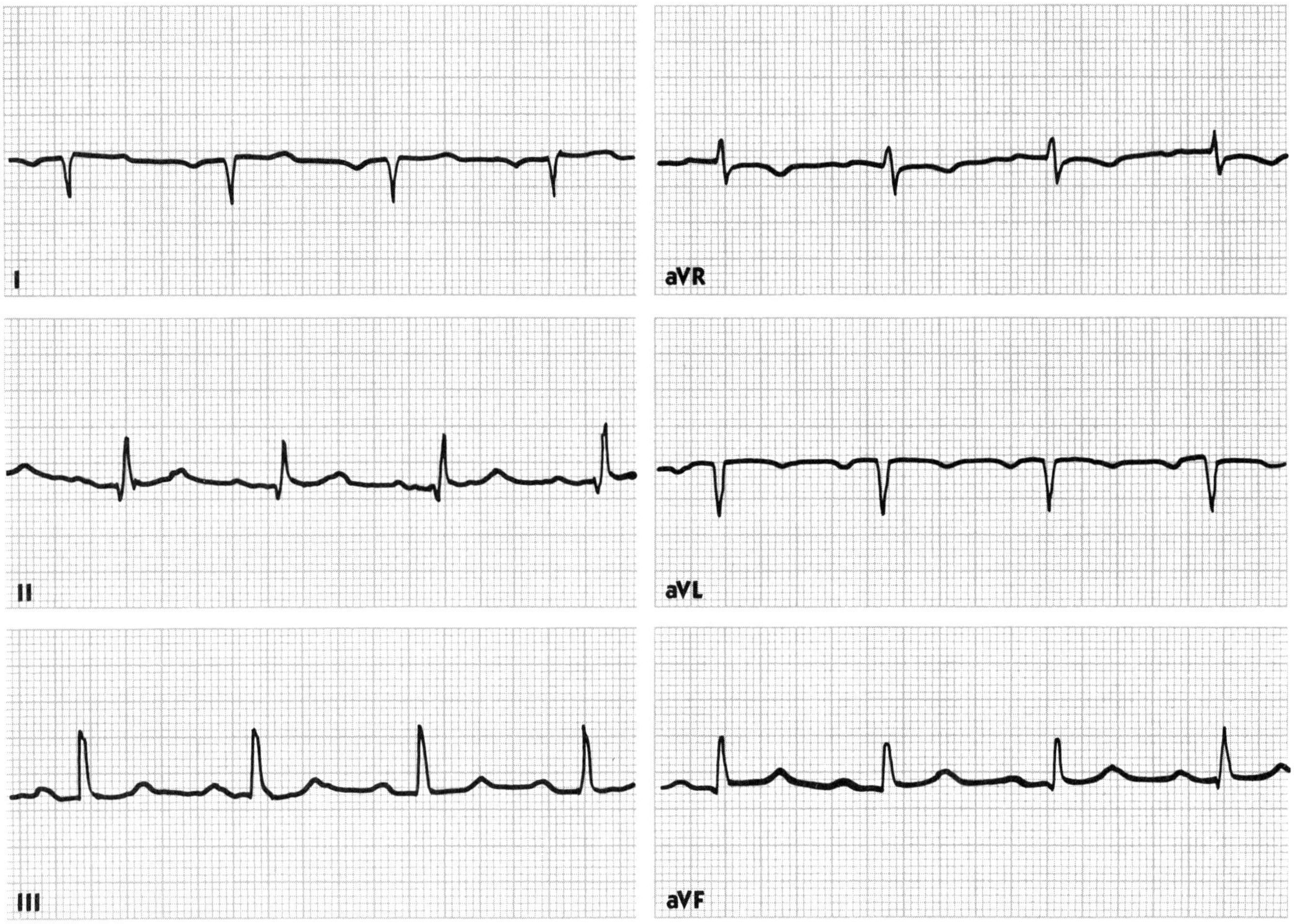

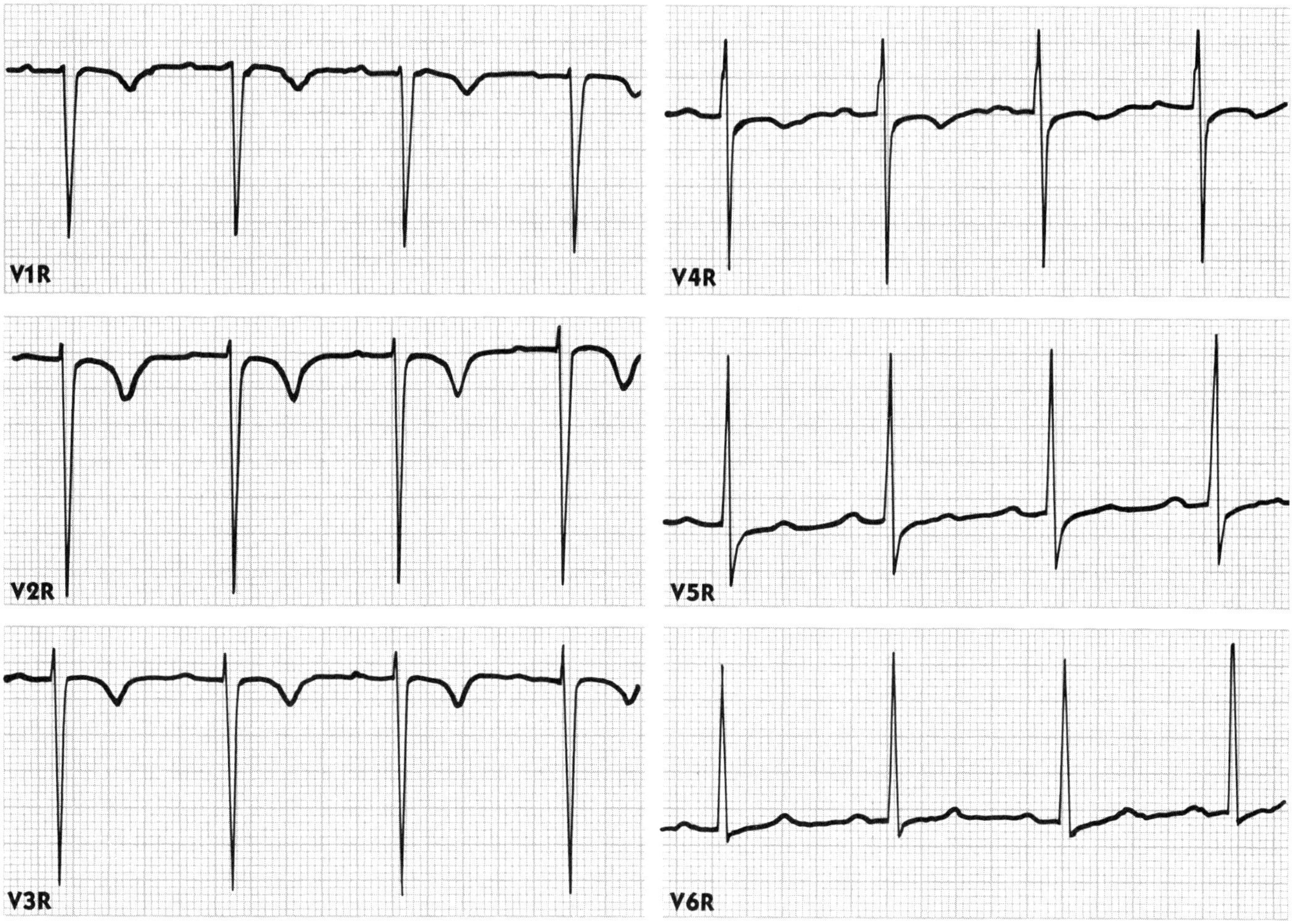
V1R
V4R
V2R
V5R
V3R
V6R

SECTION XI

Unknown Tracings for Interpretation

CASE 67

Unknown 1

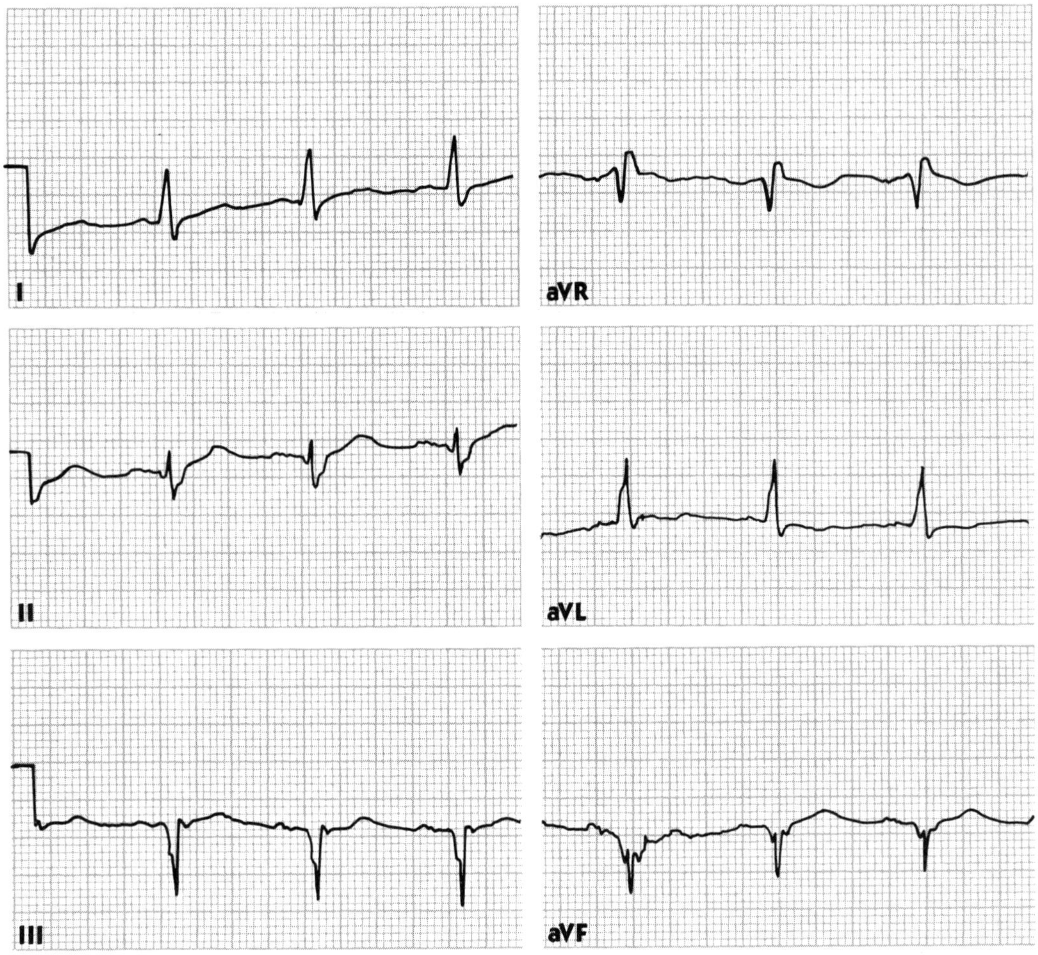

This ECG was recorded from an 80-year-old woman with a history of a previous myocardial infarction. She was admitted for an unrelated problem. *See page 222 for the interpretation.*

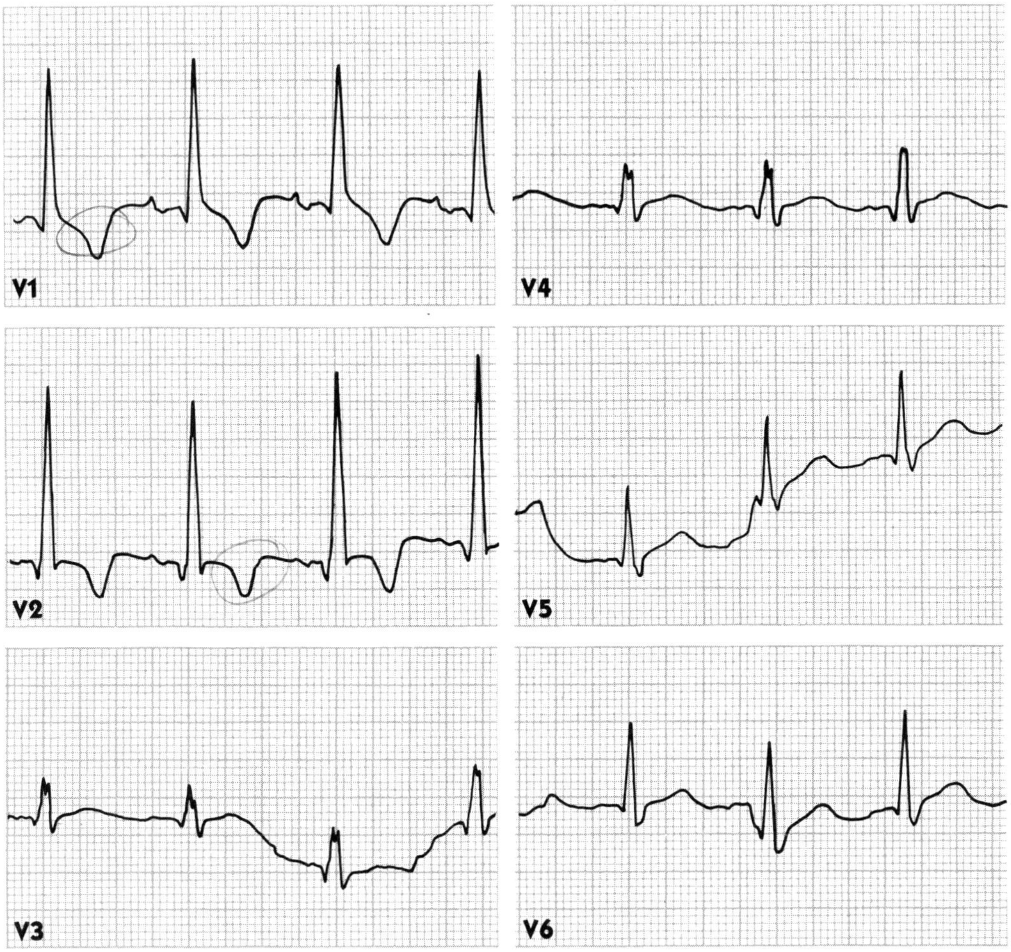
V1
V2
V3
V4
V5
V6

CASE 68

Unknown 2

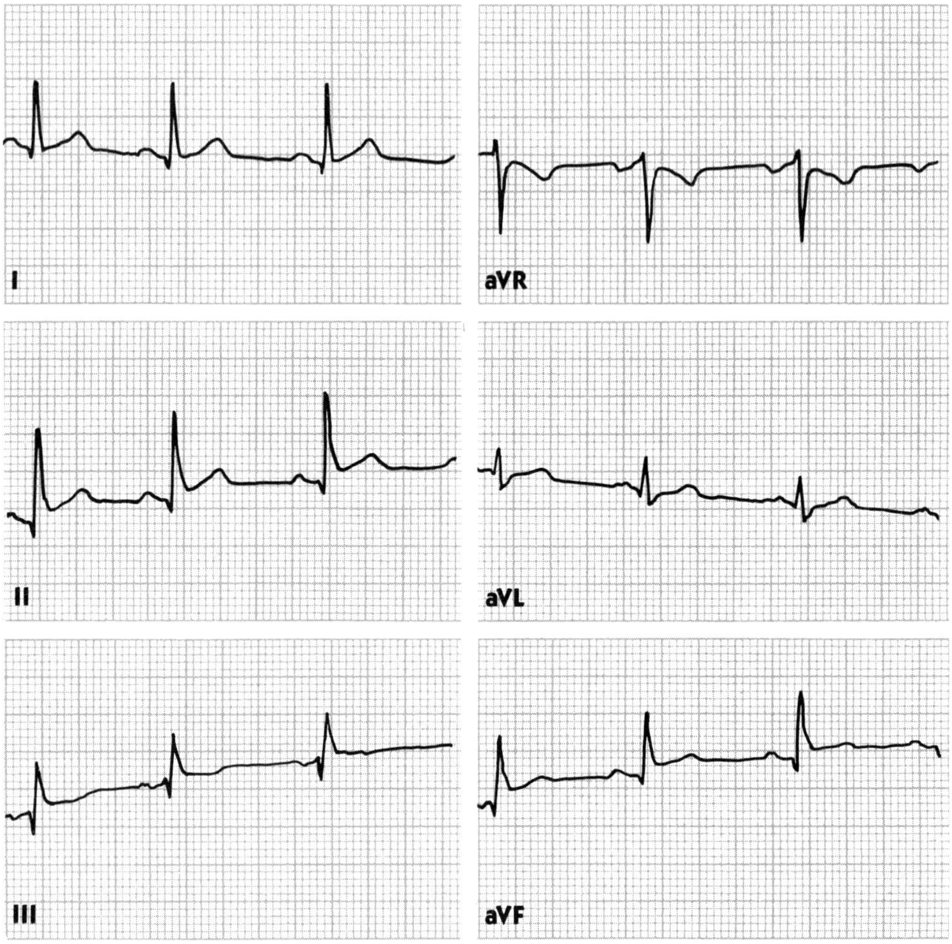

This ECG was recorded from a 23-year-old active, healthy male admitted for a manic-depressive disorder. *See page 222 for the interpretation.*

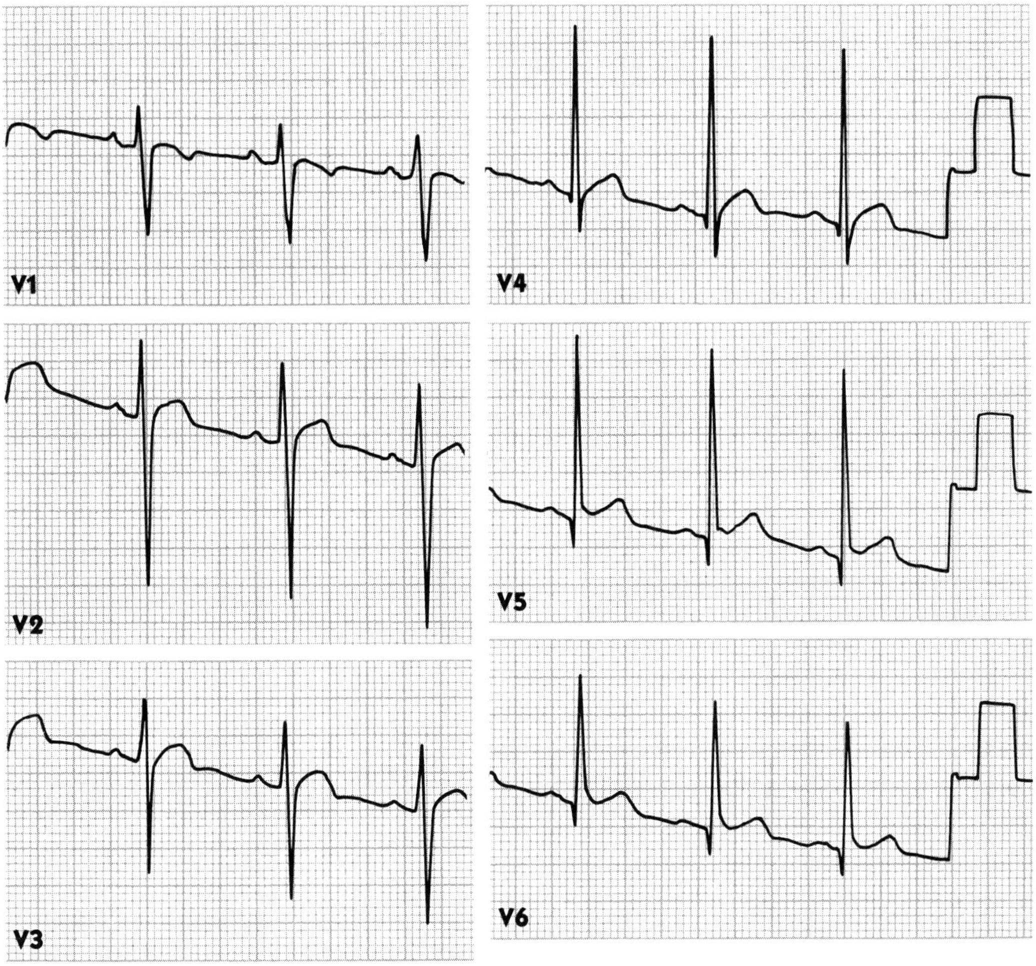
V1
V2
V3
V4
V5
V6

CASE 69

Unknown 3

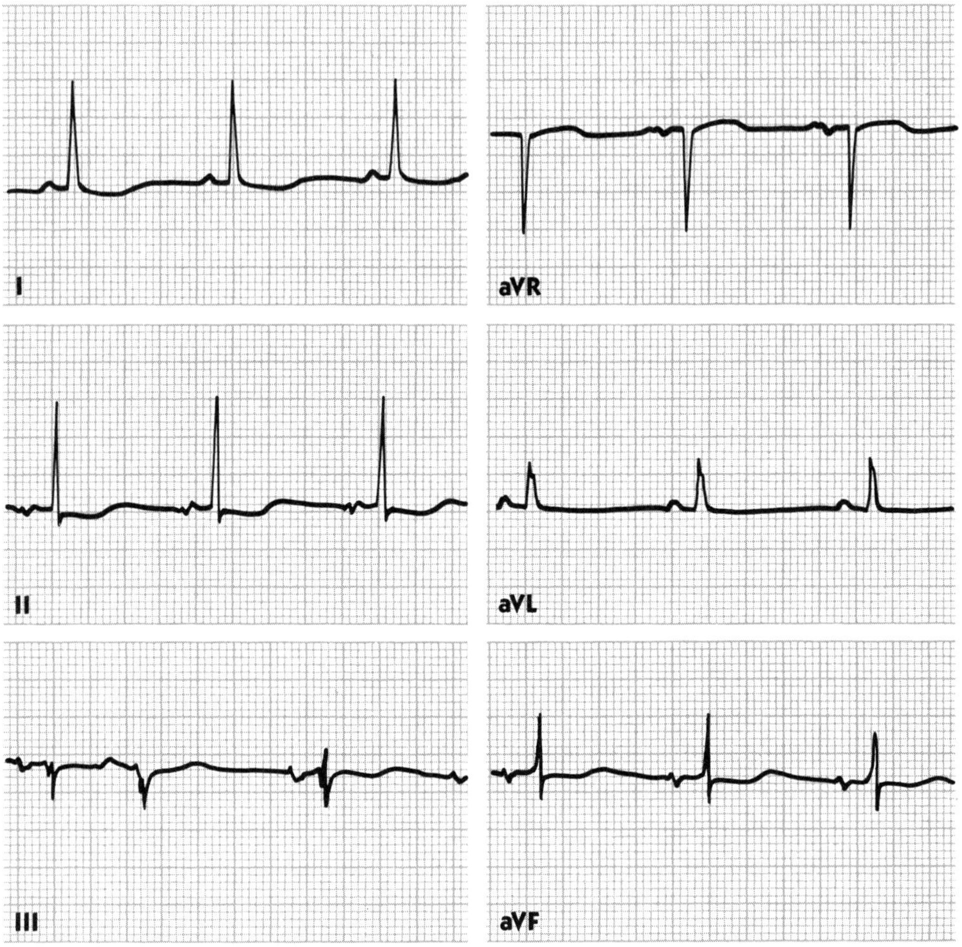

This tracing is from an 85-year-old man with a history of hypertension and intermittent atrial fibrillation treated with digoxin and quinidine. *See page 222 for the interpretation.*

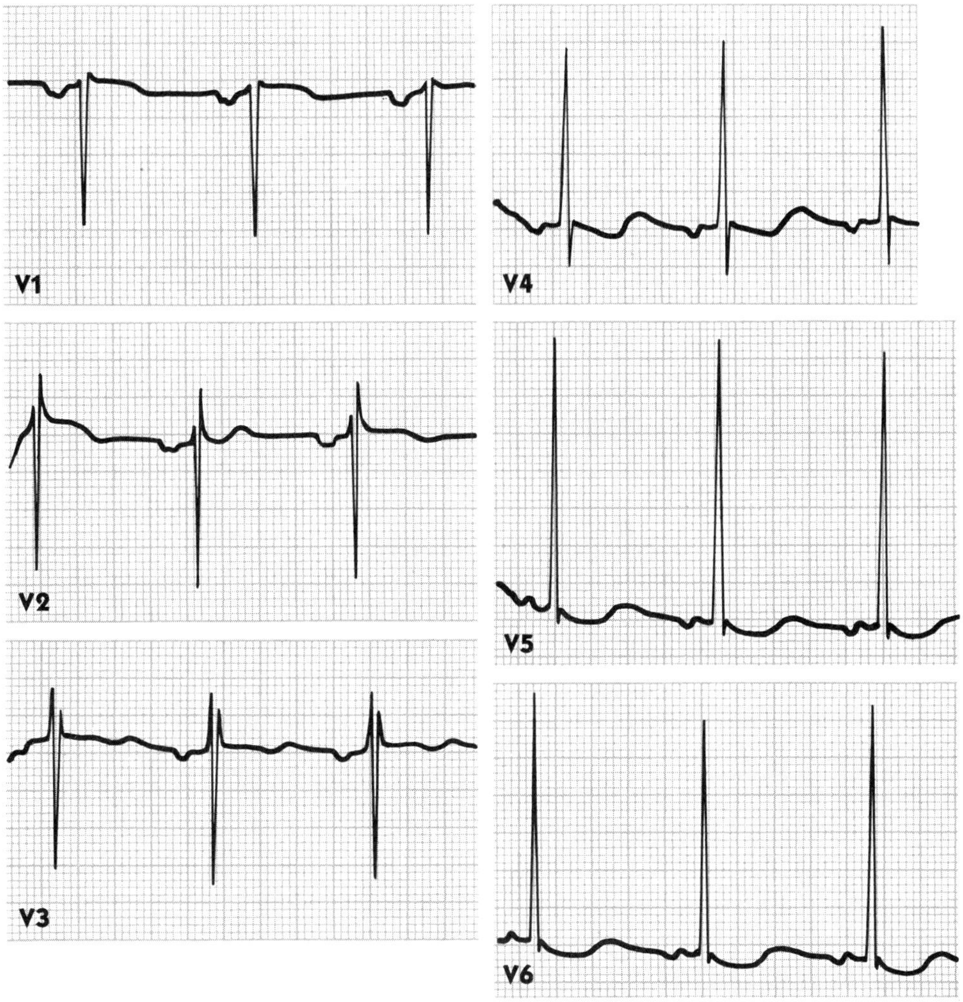
V1
V2
V3
V4
V5
V6

CASE 70

Unknown 4

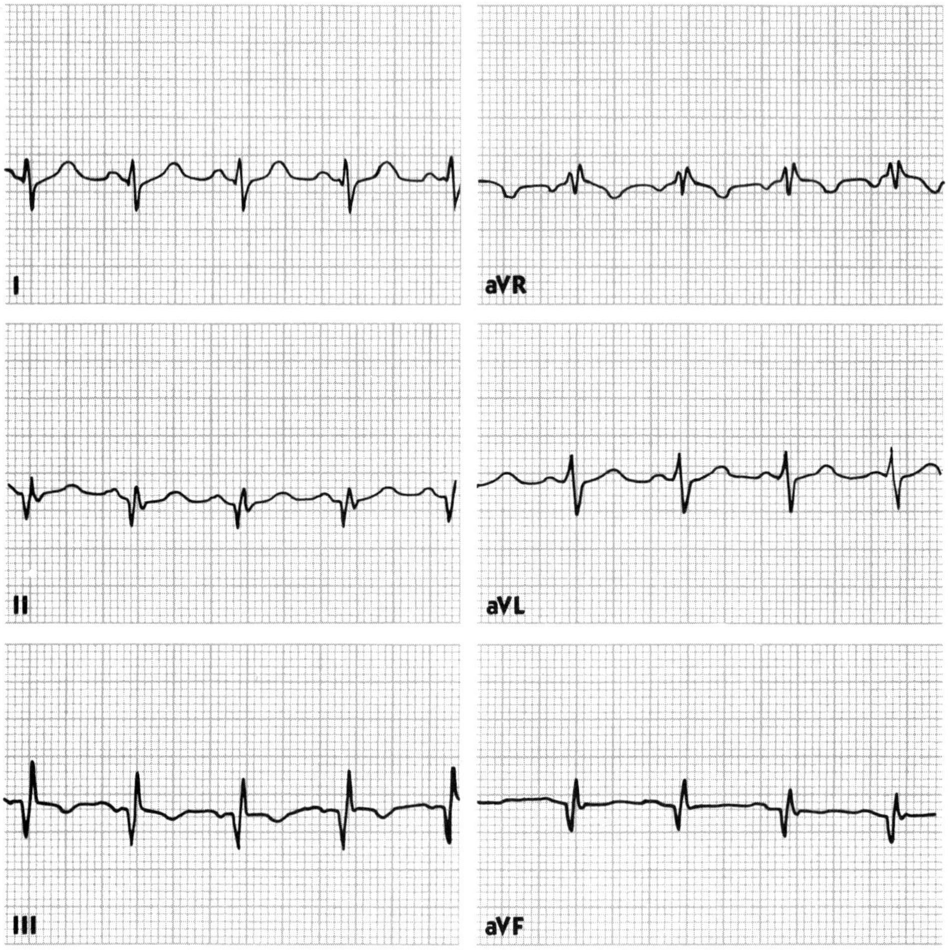

This 51-year-old man has a history of a previous myocardial infarction. *See page 222 for the interpretation.*

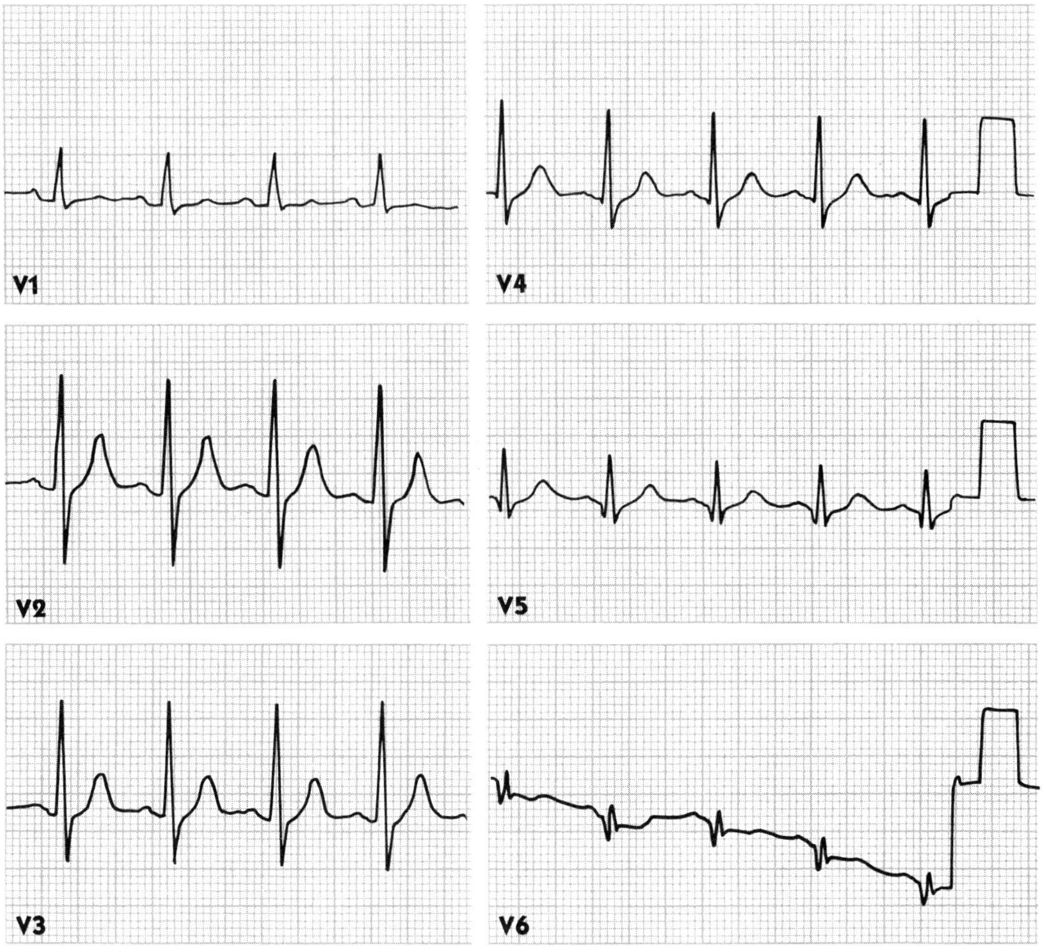
V1
V2
V3
V4
V5
V6

CASE 71

Unknown 5

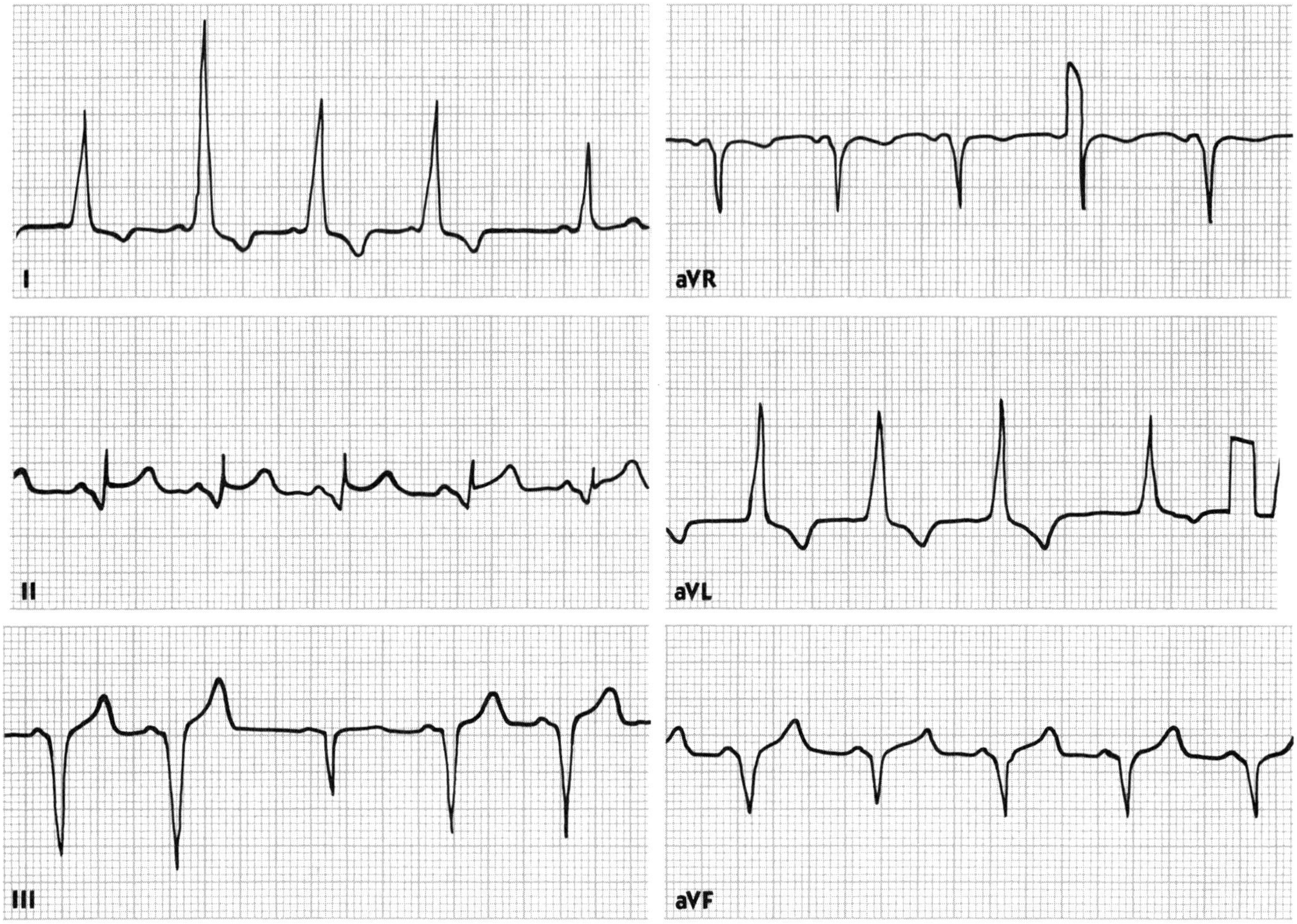

This ECG is from a 24-year-old woman with a history of palpitations. *See page 222 for the interpretation.*

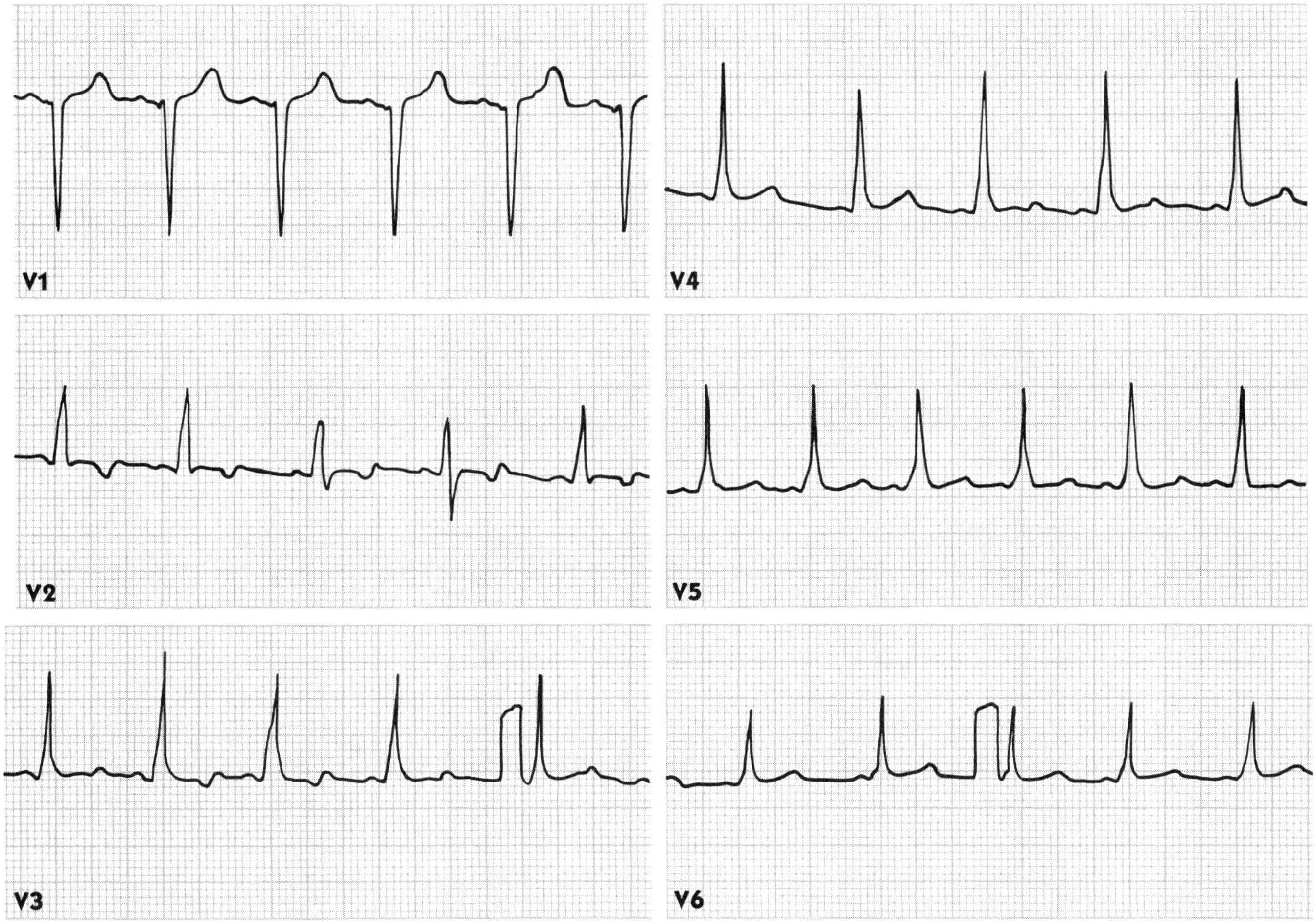
V1
V4
V2
V5
V3
V6

CASE 72

Unknown 6

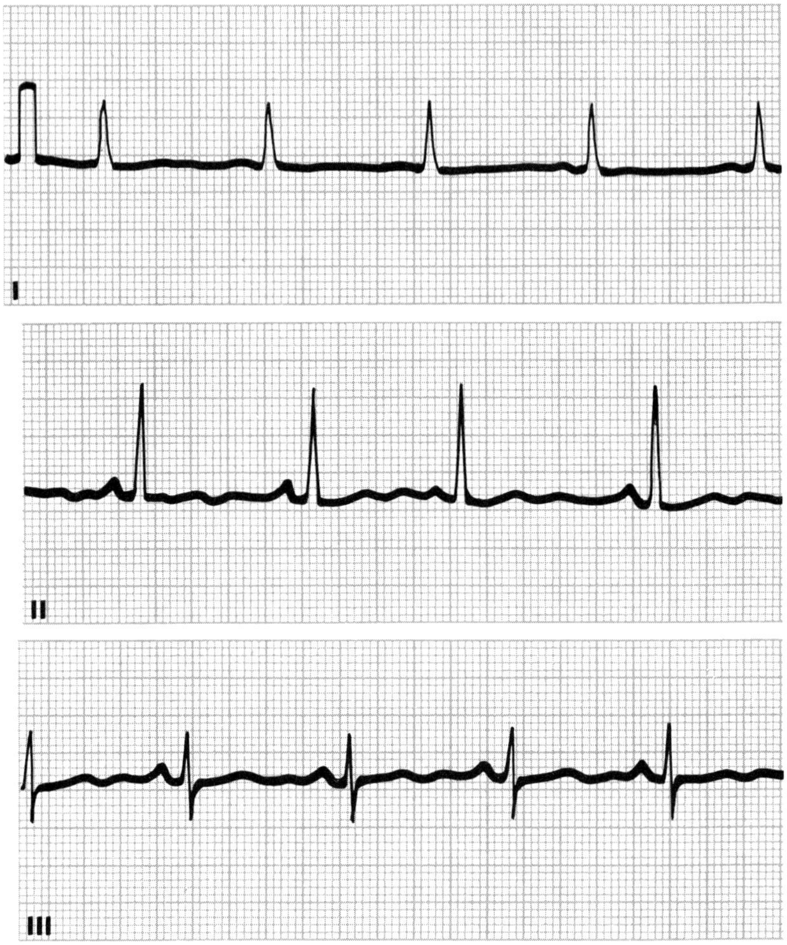

This tracing was recorded from a 42-year-old man with dementia and cachexia receiving no medications. *See page 222 for the interpretation.*

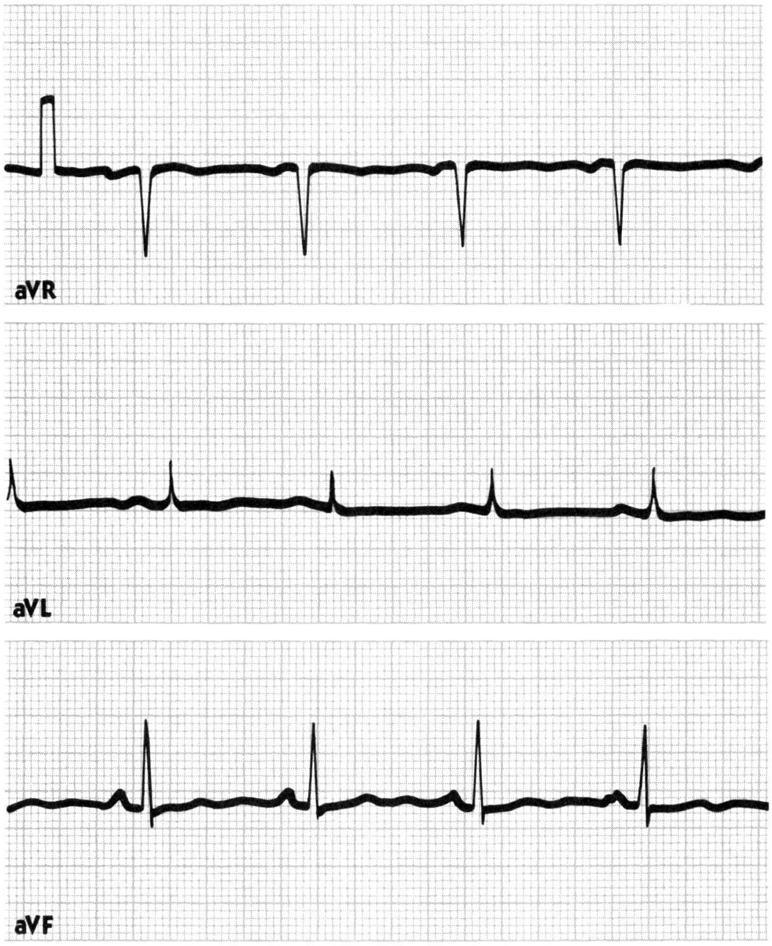

continued

CASE 72 *(continued)*

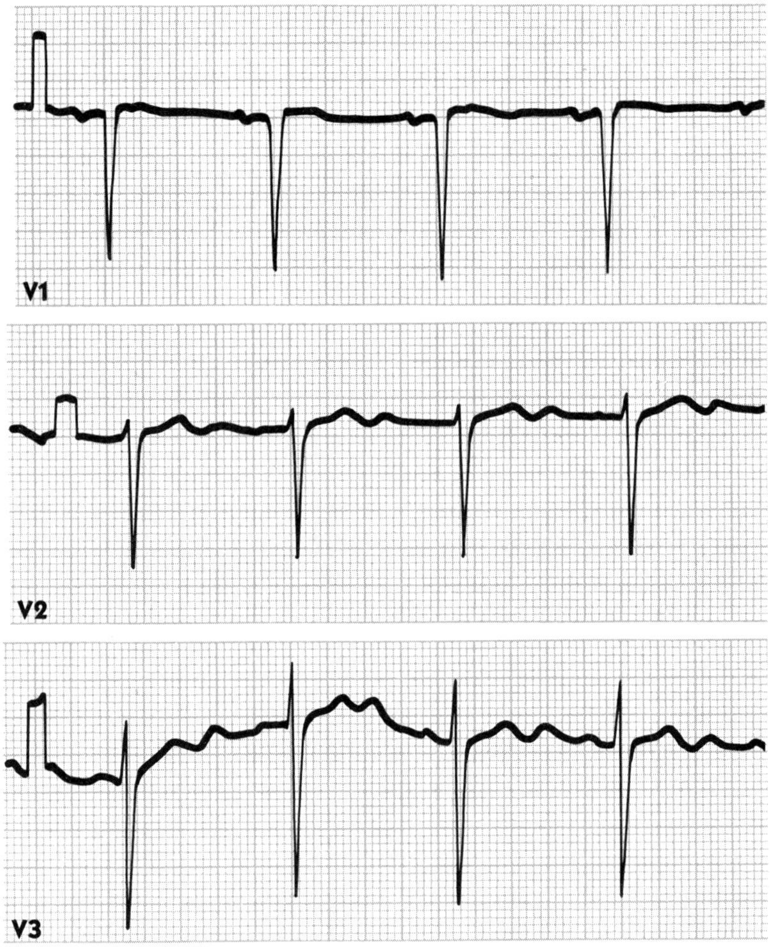

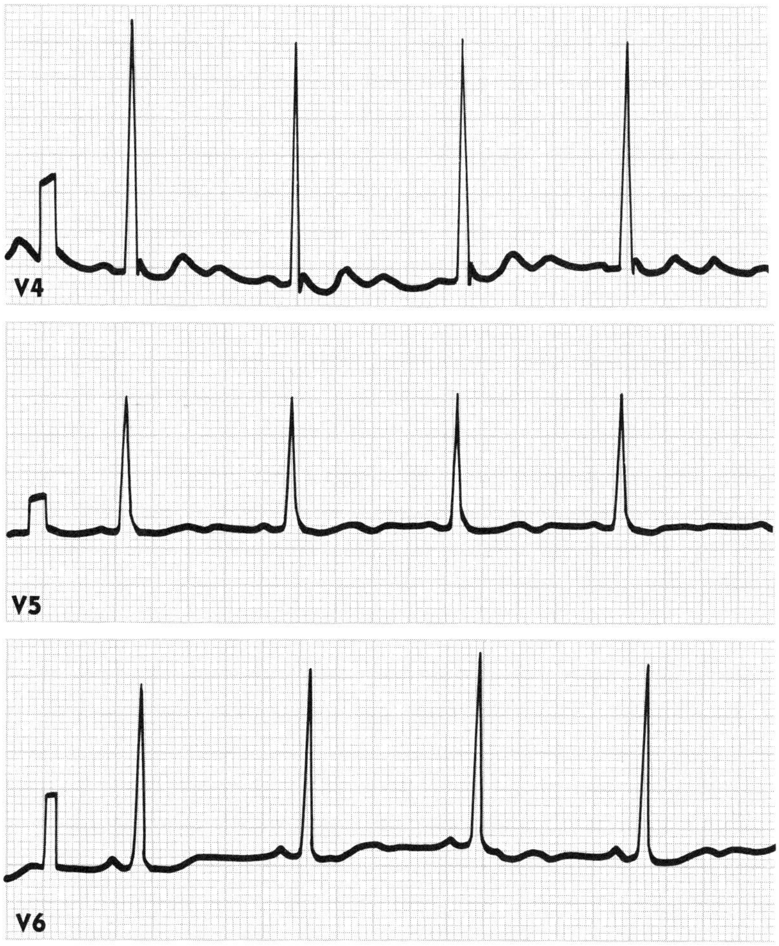
V4
V5
V6

CASE 73

Unknown 7

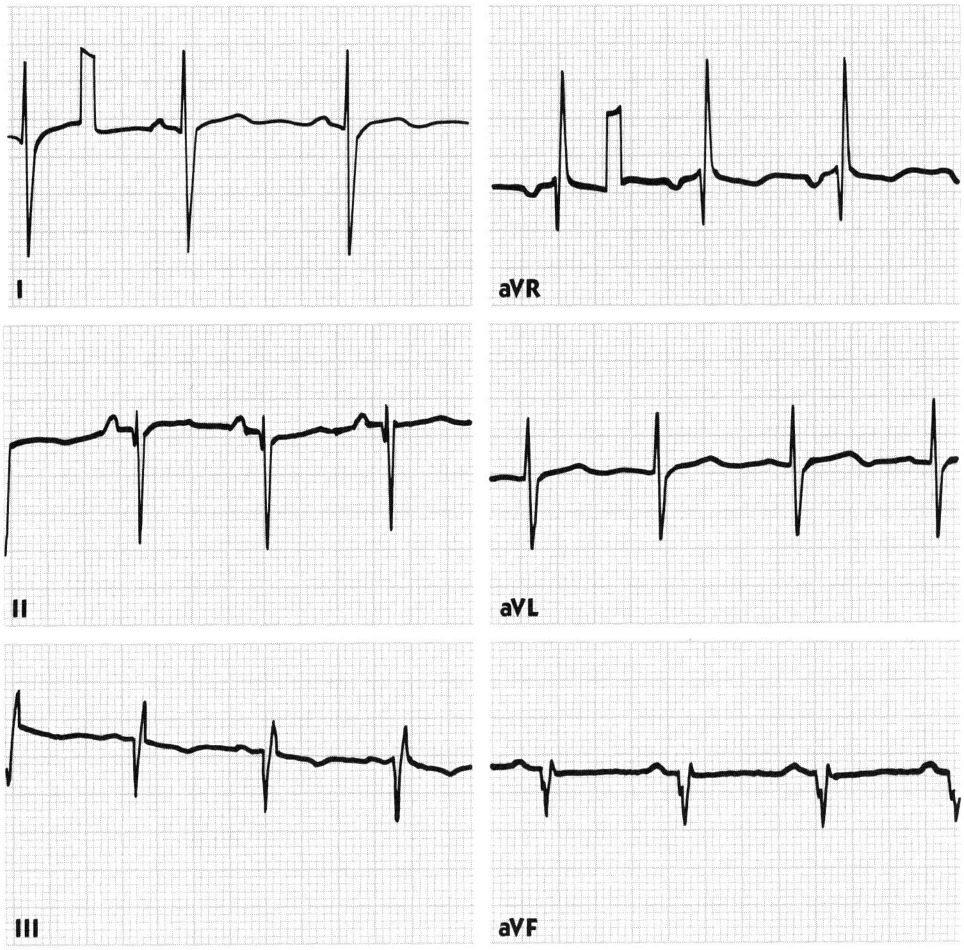

This tracing is from a 17-year-old woman with Down's syndrome and atrioventricular canal. *See page 223 for the interpretation.*

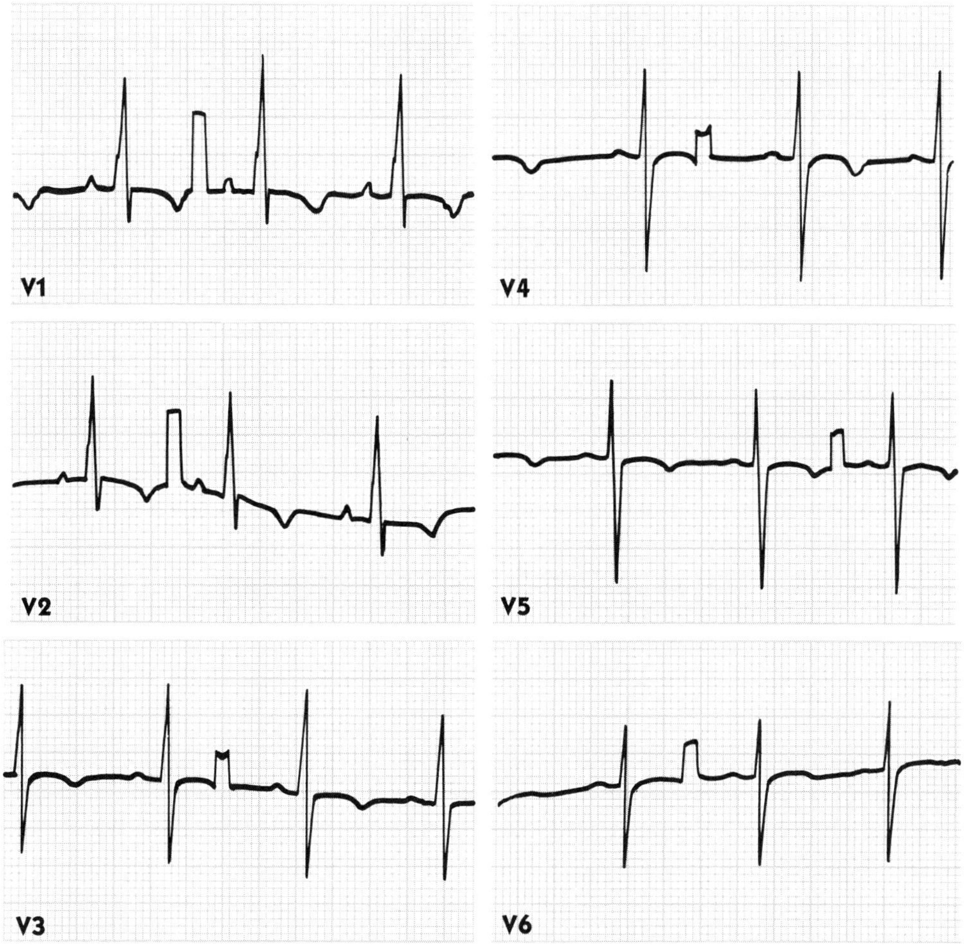
V1
V4
V2
V5
V3
V6

CASE 74

Unknown 8

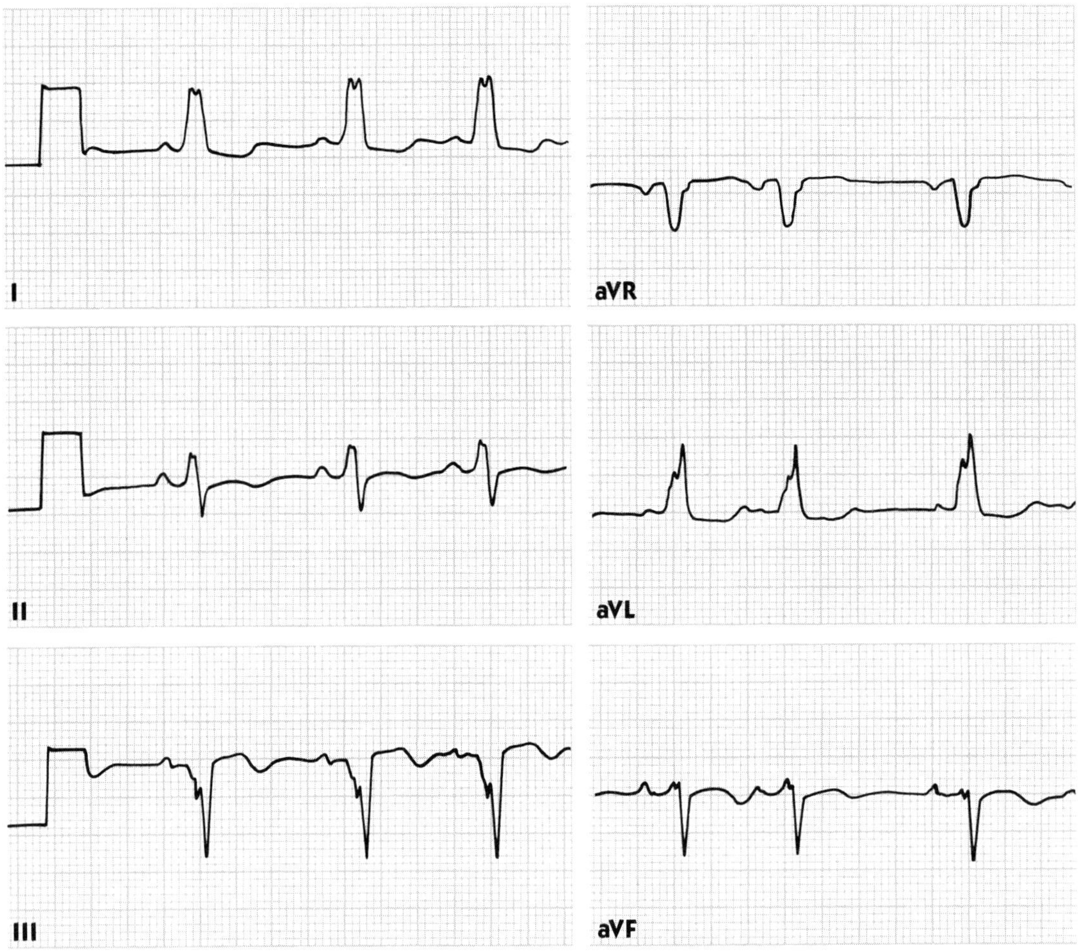

This ECG was recorded from a 79-year-old woman with a history of ischemic heart disease. *See page 223 for the interpretation.*

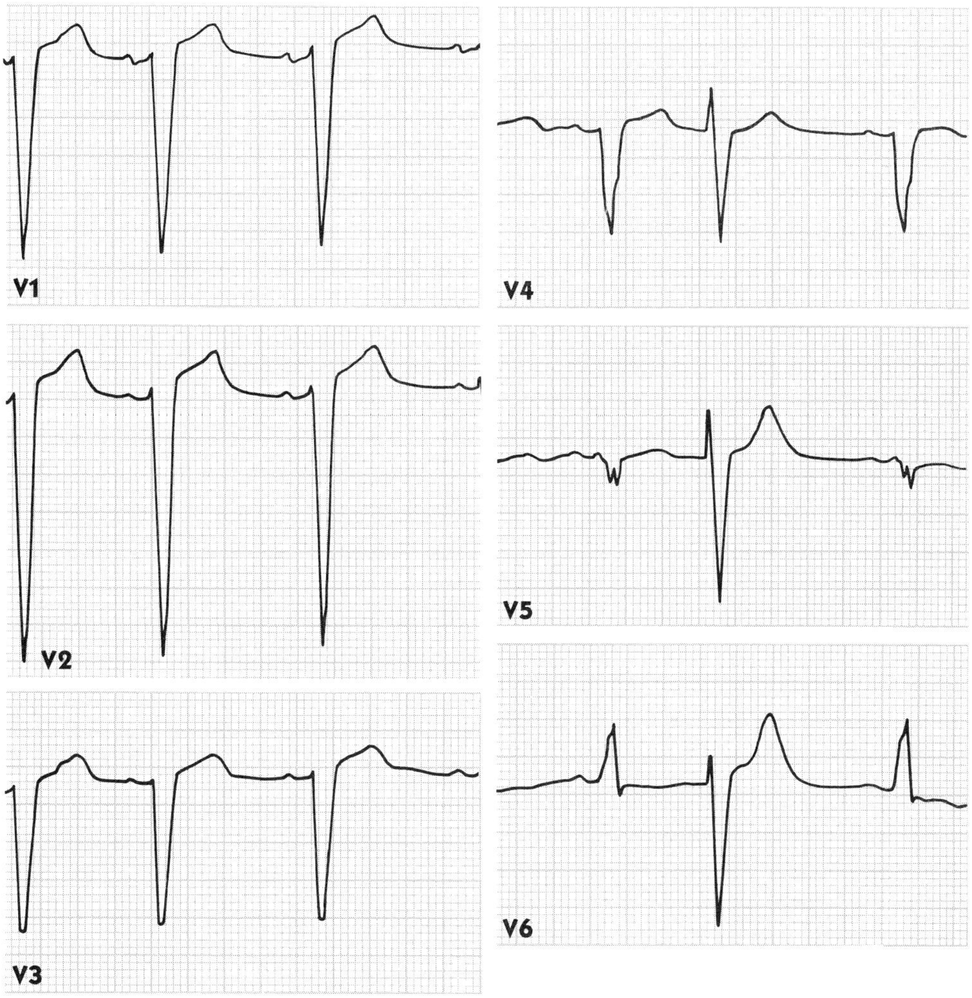
V1
V2
V3
V4
V5
V6

CASE 75

Unknown 9

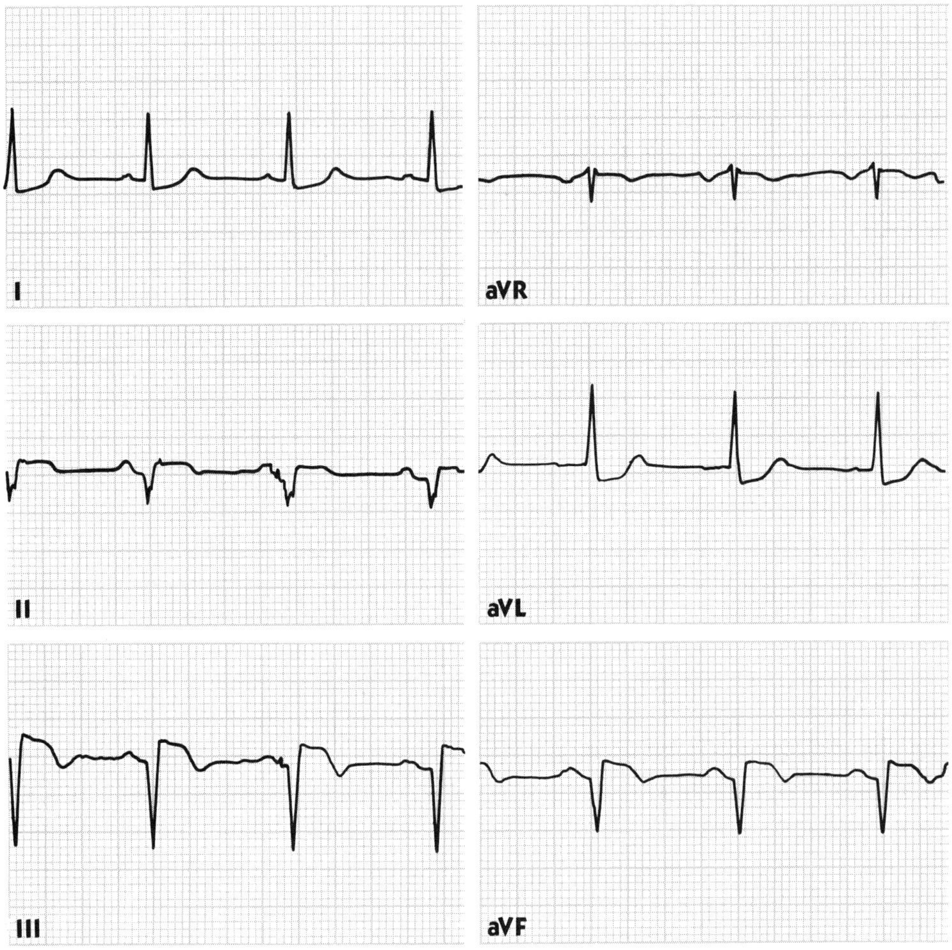

This ECG was recorded in the Emergency Room from a 56-year-old man with severe substernal chest pain. *See page 223 for the interpretation.*

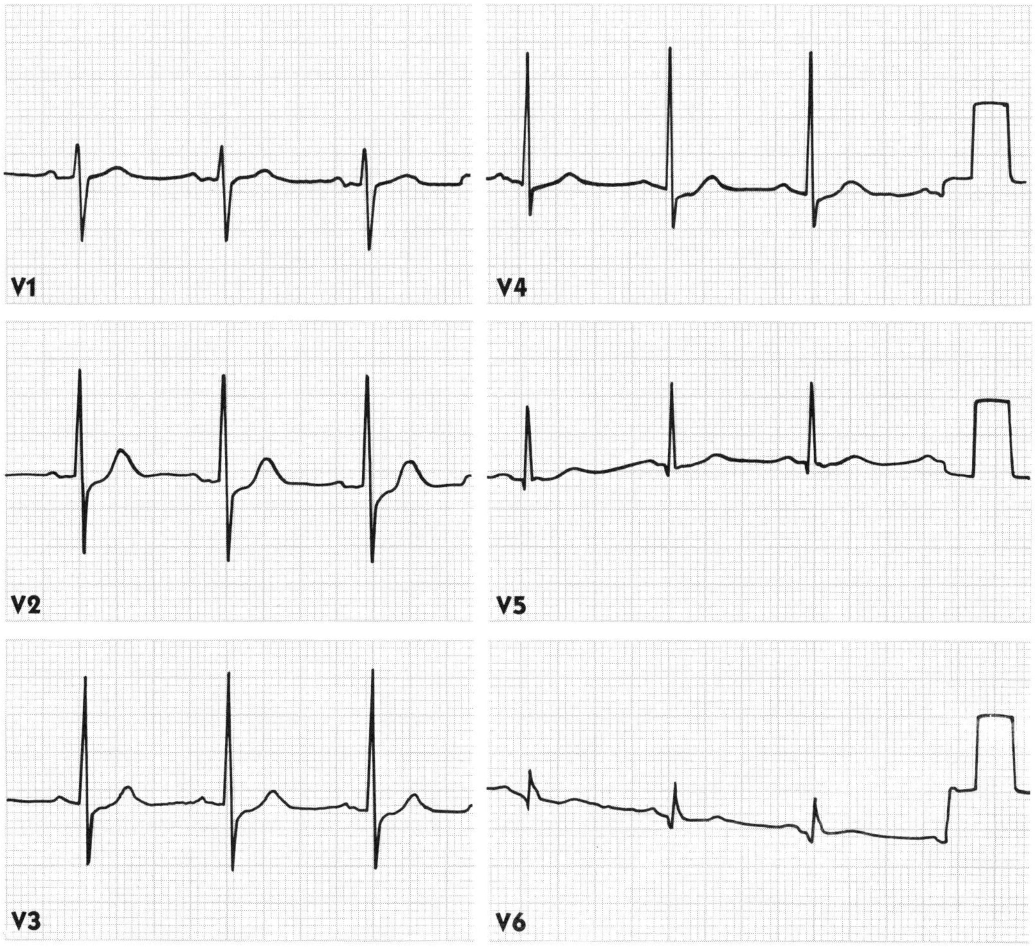
V1
V4
V2
V5
V3
V6

CASE 76

Unknown 10

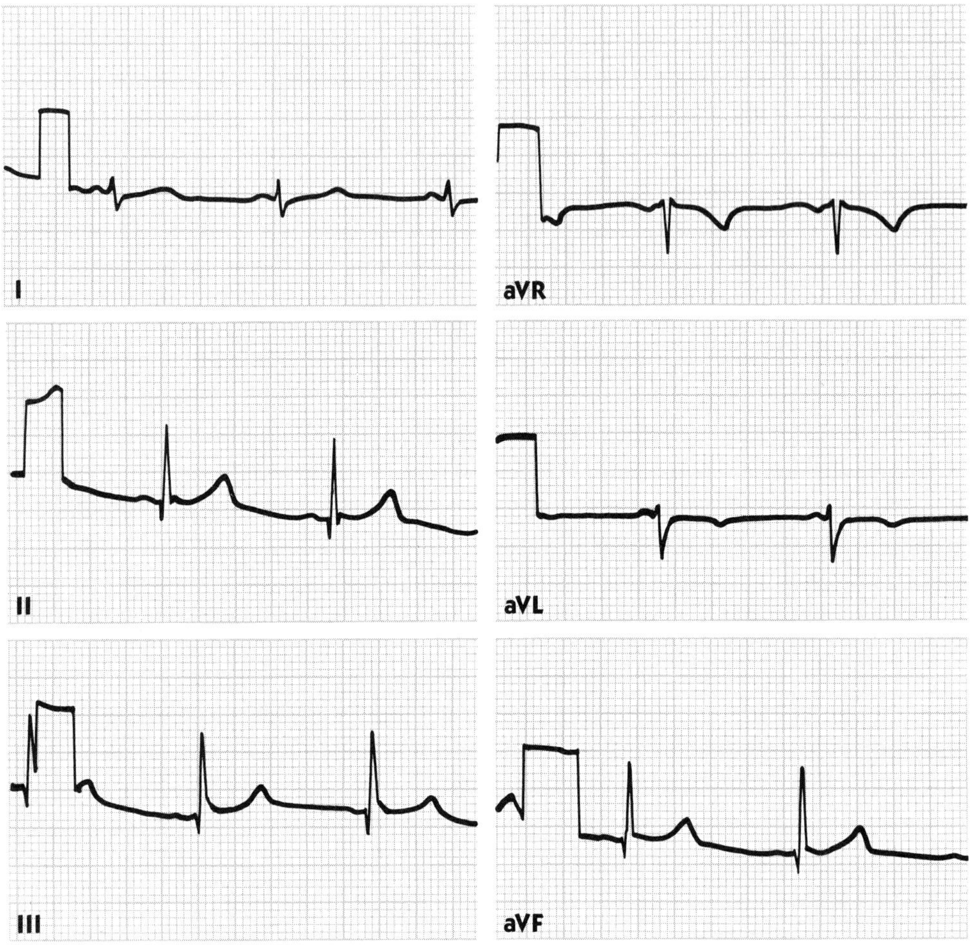

This ECG is from an otherwise healthy 39-year-old woman who developed pancreatitis secondary to cholelithiasis. *See page 223 for the interpretation.*

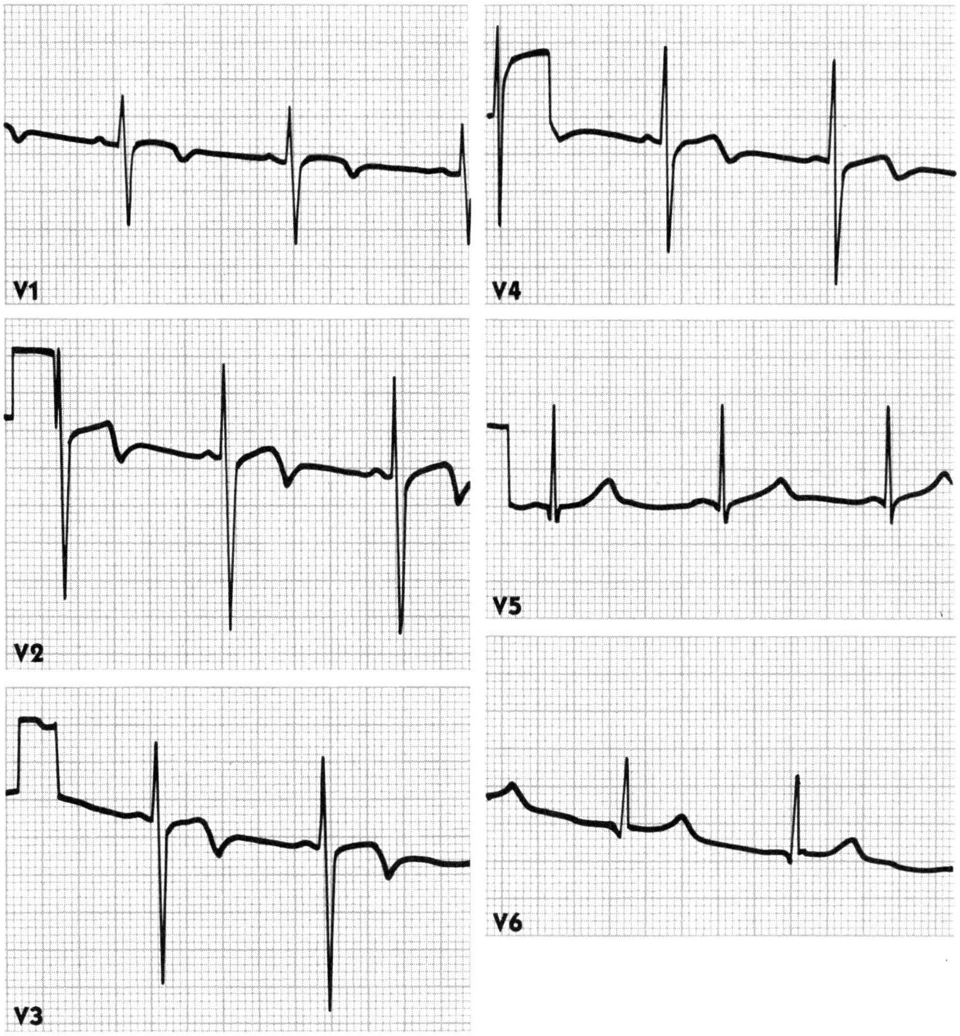
V1
V4
V2
V5
V3
V6

Case 67 Interpretation

Right Bundle Branch Block (RBBB) and Old Anterior and Inferior Wall Myocardial Infarction (MI)

The broad QRS interval, qR complexes in lead V1, broad terminal S waves laterally, and secondary T wave changes all indicate RBBB (see Case 11). The marked left axis deviation may seem to suggest left anterior fascicular block, but the QS complexes in leads III and aVF indicate past inferior wall MI (see Cases 26 and 16). The broad Q waves across the precordium suggest old anterolateral wall MI (see Case 19). There are no primary ST-T changes to suggest ongoing ischemia or infarction (see Case 18).

Case 68 Interpretation

Early Repolarization Changes

This tracing shows diffuse J point and ST segment elevation, presenting a differential diagnosis of pericarditis or early repolarization (see Cases 40, 41, and 61). The distinction must be made on clinical grounds. There is no PR segment depression or electrical alternans consistent with pericarditis (see Cases 42-44). The possibility of myocardial infarction is raised by the lateral and inferior Q waves, but these are neither significantly wide nor deep and probably represent septal Q waves. Moreover, the ST elevation is diffuse and not marked. These features are more likely in early repolarization or pericarditis.

Case 69 Interpretation

Left Ventricular Hypertrophy (LVH), Left Atrial Abnormality (LAA), and Digitalis and Quinidine Effects

The marked lateral R wave voltage (3 points); the deep, terminally negative P waves in lead V1 suggesting LAA (3 points); and the ST-T changes (1 point in the presence of digoxin therapy) provide adequate criteria for the diagnosis of LVH (see Case 1 and Table 1 in the Appendix). The lateral downsloping ST segment is nonspecific; it could represent digitalis effect, the ST-T changes of LVH, or other possibilities (see Cases 1 and 56, and Table 5 in the Appendix). The long QT interval and prominent U waves (best seen in lead V3) suggest the quinidine effect (see Case 57).

Case 70 Interpretation

Inferoposterolateral Wall Myocardial Infarction (MI) of Indeterminate Age

The deep Q waves in the inferolateral leads and the loss of R wave amplitude laterally indicate inferolateral wall MI. The tall monophasic R wave in lead V1 suggests concomitant posterior wall MI (see Case 28). The differential diagnosis should include right ventricular hypertrophy (see Case 6) and asymmetric septal hypertrophy (see Case 4). These cannot be excluded on ECG grounds alone; independent means are necessary.

Case 71 Interpretation

Wolff-Parkinson-White (WPW) Conduction

The short PR interval and the prominent delta waves (best seen in leads I, aVL, and V3-6) confirm the diagnosis (see Cases 34-35). Of note is the occasional narrower, smaller QRS complex (see leads I and III). The differing QRS morphology illustrates the variable degree to which the accessory pathway is contributing to ventricular activation (see Case 37). The ventricles are being depolarized via a varying combination of WPW conduction (with its broad delta wave) and the normal His-Purkinje system (with its narrower QRS complex). The deep Q waves or QS complexes inferiorly represent one of the many pseudoinfarction patterns seen in WPW conduction (see Case 36).

Case 72 Interpretation

Hypokalemia

The very prominent U waves in the anterior precordial leads and the diffuse T wave flattening suggest a number of possible etiologies (see Table 5 in the Appendix). The most common possibilities are hypokalemia and drug effect (see Cases 51 and 57). In this case, hypokalemia was documented by measurement of a very low serum potassium. Though very prominent R waves appear in the precordial leads, there is no other evidence for left ventricular hypertrophy (LVH). Voltage criteria alone are insufficient to make the diagnosis of LVH (see Case 2).

Case 73 Interpretation

Right Ventricular Hypertrophy (RVH) With Markedly Superior Axis

As expected in cases of atrioventricular (AV) canal with resultant pulmonary hypertension, this patient has RVH. The Rs complexes in lead V1, deep lateral S waves (note the half-standard setting in precordial leads V3-6), and right precordial T wave inversion suggest the diagnosis (see Cases 5 and 6). The markedly superior axis may seem paradoxical in RVH, but left axis deviation frequently accompanies RVH in atrial septal defects (ASD) of the ostium primum type (or in patients with AV canals). The axis is normal or rightward in ASDs of the ostium secundum type.

Case 74 Interpretation

Left Bundle Branch Block (LBBB) With Occasional Premature Ventricular Contractions (PVCs)

The prolonged QRS interval with broad terminal S waves in lead V1 and the primarily monophasic R waves in leads I and V6 indicate LBBB (see Case 13). Because the deep QS in lead III is not accompanied by other significant Q waves inferiorly, it is probably secondary to the bundle branch block rather than to previous myocardial infarction (MI). Similarly, the poor anterior R wave development is probably due to LBBB. In both instances, however, previous MI can be definitively excluded only by other clinical means. The inverted T waves in leads III and aVF match the direction of the terminal portion of the QRS complexes, thus representing primary T wave changes. This finding could support the diagnosis of previous MI in the area of the heart represented by those leads (see Case 14). Of incidental interest is the PVC in leads V4-6; its configuration differs from the sinus-initiated LBBB pattern.

Case 75 Interpretation

Acute Inferolateral Wall Myocardial Infarction (MI)

There are QS complexes inferiorly in leads II, III, and aVF; Q waves (probably significant) in lead V6 (approaching one-third of the QRS height); upwardly convex ST segment elevation with inverted T waves inferiorly; and ST segment depression with upright T waves laterally in leads I and aVL. The inferior ST elevation with T wave inversion is typical of an acute infarction that is only minutes to hours old. The lateral ST depression could represent concomitant lateral ischemia and infarction or simply changes reciprocal to the inferior MI seen in distant leads (see Cases 24 and 26). The actual etiology of the lateral changes cannot be determined on ECG grounds alone; additional evaluative means are required.

Case 76 Interpretation

Nonspecific ST-T Changes Secondary to Pancreatitis

This ECG is notable for 1-mm ST segment elevation in leads II, III, aVF, and V1-4; T wave inversion in leads V1-4; and mild QT interval prolongation. Although these ST segment and T wave changes might suggest myocardial ischemia or infarction in another clinical situation, they are very nonspecific by themselves and may occur in a number of disorders (see Table 5 in the Appendix). In this case, they appeared and resolved coincidently with the patient's pancreatitis. Myocardial infarction was ruled out by serial enzymes.

SECTION XII Appendix

TABLE 1

Point score system for left ventricular hypertrophy (LVH)

	Points
1. Amplitude	3
• Largest R or S wave in limb leads ≥ 20 mm	
• S wave in lead V1 or V2 ≥ 30 mm	
• R wave in lead V5 or V6 ≥ 30 mm	
2. ST-T changes	
• Without digitalis	3
• With digitalis	1
3. Left atrial abnormality	3
• P wave duration in lead II ≥ 0.12 second	
• Negative deflection of P wave in lead V1 > 1 mm²	
4. Left axis deviation (axis left of −30°)	2
5. QRS duration > 0.09 second	1
6. Intrinsicoid deflection in left ventricular leads ≥ 0.05 second	1

5 or more points = LVH
4 points = probable LVH

Adapted from Romhilt DW et al: A critical appraisal of the electrocardiographic criteria for the diagnosis of left ventricular hypertrophy. *Circulation* 40:185, 1969, by permission of the American Heart Association, Inc.

TABLE 2

Causes of poor or absent anterior R wave progression

- Anterior wall myocardial infarction
- Lateral wall myocardial infarction
- Left ventricular hypertrophy
- Right ventricular hypertrophy
- Chronic obstructive pulmonary disease
- Pectus excavatum
- Straight back syndrome
- Left anterior fascicular block
- Wolff-Parkinson-White syndrome (type B)
- Normal variant
- High placement of precordial leads
- Pneumothorax
- Pulmonary surgery
- Dextrocardia

TABLE 3

ECG findings suggesting right ventricular hypertrophy*

Strongly suggestive

- R:S in V1 ≥ 1.0
- Right axis deviation > +110°
- qR in V1

Suggestive

- Reverse R wave development (R:S in V5 ÷ R:S in V1 ≤ 0.4)
- R in V1 + S in V5 or V6 > 10.5 mm
- S in V1 < 2 mm
- R in V1 ≥ 7 mm
- S in V5 or V6 ≥ 7 mm, and both ≥ 2 mm
- R:S in V5 or V6 ≤ 1.0

*These criteria are invalid in the presence of conduction abnormalities and posterior or lateral wall myocardial infarction.

TABLE 4

Causes of dominant R wave in lead V1

- Right ventricular hypertrophy
- Idiopathic hypertrophic subaortic stenosis (asymmetric septal hypertrophy)
- Posterior wall myocardial infarction
- Duchenne's muscular dystrophy
- Other focal infiltrative or fibrosing cardiomyopathies
- Wolff-Parkinson-White conduction (type A)
- Normal variant
- Low placement of precordial leads

TABLE 5

Conditions associated with nonspecific ST-T abnormalities

Cardiac conditions
- Ischemia
- Infarction
- Hypertrophy
- Conduction disturbances
- Pre-excitation syndromes
- Myocardial contusion
- Digitalis therapy
- Myocarditis
- Cardiomyopathy
- Myocardial neoplasm
- Mitral valve prolapse
- Post-tachycardia
- Spontaneous complexes in patients with artificial pacemakers

Pericardial conditions
- Pericarditis
- Pericardial effusion
- Pericardial constriction

Pulmonary conditions
- Chronic obstructive pulmonary disease
- Acute pulmonary embolism
- Pulmonary hypertension
- Pneumothorax
- Hyperinflation of lungs

Miscellaneous conditions
- Cerebrovascular accident
- Anxiety
- Hyperventilation
- Acute cholecystitis
- Acute pancreatitis
- Vagotomy
- Vasoregulatory abnormality
- Recent heavy meal
- Hypothyroidism
- Pheochromocytoma
- Addison's disease
- Hypopituitarism
- Body position
- Pectus excavatum
- Straight back syndrome
- Hypothermia
- Dextrocardia
- Prolonged QT interval syndromes
- Type I antiarrhythmic therapy
- Tricyclic antidepressant therapy
- Hypokalemia
- Normal variant

TABLE 6

Syndromes of accessory atrioventricular conduction

Characteristic	Wolff-Parkinson-White	Mahaim	Lown-Ganong-Levine
Accessory pathway	Bundles of Kent	Mahaim fibers	James fibers; intra-AV nodal fibers
PR interval	Short	Normal	Short
Delta wave	Present	Present	Absent
QRS interval	Normal or prolonged	Normal or prolonged	Normal
ST-T abnormalities*	Present	Present	Absent
Pseudoinfarction and hypertrophy patterns	Present	Present	Absent
Pseudo-bundle branch block patterns	Present	Present	Absent
Reciprocating (re-entry) tachycardias	Present	Present	Present

*Secondary to accessory atrioventricular conduction. Primary ST-T abnormalities (from ischemia, infarction, pericarditis, etc.) obviously may occur independently in association with these syndromes.

TABLE 7

Causes of pseudoinfarction patterns

Cardiac conditions
- Left ventricular hypertrophy
- Right ventricular hypertrophy
- Idiopathic hypertrophic subaortic stenosis
- Infiltrative or fibrosing cardiomyopathies
- Myocarditis
- Cardiac contusion
- Pericardial constriction and fibrosis
- Mitral valve prolapse

Conduction disturbances
- Left anterior fascicular block
- Left posterior fascicular block
- Left bundle branch block
- Pre-excitation syndromes (Wolff-Parkinson-White and Mahaim conduction syndromes)

Pulmonary conditions
- Chronic obstructive pulmonary disease
- Acute pulmonary embolism
- Pneumothorax
- Fibrothorax
- Pulmonary surgery

Miscellaneous conditions
- Normal variant
- Lead misplacement
- Pectus excavatum
- Straight back syndrome
- Dextrocardia
- Cerebrovascular accident
- Pancreatitis

TABLE 8

ECG findings in chronic obstructive pulmonary disease

- Tall (2.5 mm or more in lead II), peaked P waves
- Right axis deviation
- Superior axis deviation
- Right ventricular hypertrophy
- Low QRS voltage
- Pseudoinfarction patterns
  —Inferior
  —Anterior
  —Posterior
- Deep precordial S waves and poor R wave progression
- Septal Q waves in the inferior or lateral leads
- Right precordial and/or inferior T wave inversion secondary to right ventricular hypertrophy
- Right ventricular conduction delay
- Sinus tachycardia
- Atrial arrhythmias
  —Atrial premature complexes
  —Multifocal atrial tachycardia
  —Atrial flutter and fibrillation

TABLE 9

Causes of low QRS voltage in limb leads

Cardiac conditions
- Infiltrative cardiomyopathy (e.g., amyloidosis, hemochromatosis, scleroderma, neoplasm)
- Congestive cardiomyopathy (e.g., idiopathic, viral)
- Myocarditis
- Loss of myocardium from myocardial infarction

Pericardial conditions
- Pericarditis with or without effusion
- Pericardial effusion
- Constrictive pericarditis
- Pericardial neoplasm with or without effusion

Pulmonary conditions
- Chronic obstructive pulmonary disease
- Pleural effusion
- Pneumothorax
- Hyperinflation of lungs during respirator therapy
- Acute pulmonary embolism

Miscellaneous conditions
- Obesity
- Anasarca
- Hypothyroidism

TABLE 10

ECG findings in acute pulmonary embolism

- Sinus tachycardia
- Atrial arrhythmias
- Nonspecific ST-T abnormalities
- Acute right or (occasionally) left axis shift
- Acute right ventricular conduction delay
- Acute right atrial abnormality pattern (P pulmonale)
- $S_1Q_3T_3$ pattern
- $S_1S_2S_3$ pattern
- Prolonged QT interval
- Low QRS voltage

TABLE 11

Causes of prolonged QT (or QTU) interval

Cardiac conditions
- Ischemic heart disease
- Myocardial infarction
- Cardiomyopathies
- Myocarditis
- Mitral valve prolapse
- Post-tachycardia

Central nervous system conditions
- Cerebrovascular accident
- Trauma
- Recent surgery
- Infection
- Vagotomy

Acute pulmonary embolism

Electrolyte disturbances
- Hypocalcemia
- Hypokalemia
- Hypomagnesemia

Pharmacologic agents
- Type I antiarrhythmic agents
  - —Quinidine
  - —Procainamide
  - —Disopyramide
- Psychotropic agents
  - —Phenothiazines
  - —Tricyclic antidepressants

Hypothermia

Endocrinopathies
- Pheochromocytoma
- Adrenal insufficiency

Hereditary surdocardiac syndromes
- Jervell-Lange-Nielsen syndrome (with deafness)
- Romano-Ward syndrome (without deafness)

Bradycardia

TABLE 12

Normal ranges for QT intervals

Heart rate (beats per minute)	Age (years) 18–29	30–39	40–49	50–60
45–55	.39–.45	.39–.45	.39–.46	.39–.46
56–62	.36–.42	.36–.43	.37–.43	.37–.43
63–71	.34–.41	.35–.41	.35–.41	.35–.42
72–83	.32–.39	.33–.39	.33–.40	.33–.40
84–115	.30–.37	.30–.37	.31–.37	.31–.37

Adapted from Simonson E et al: The normal Q-T interval. *Am Heart J* 63:747, 1962.

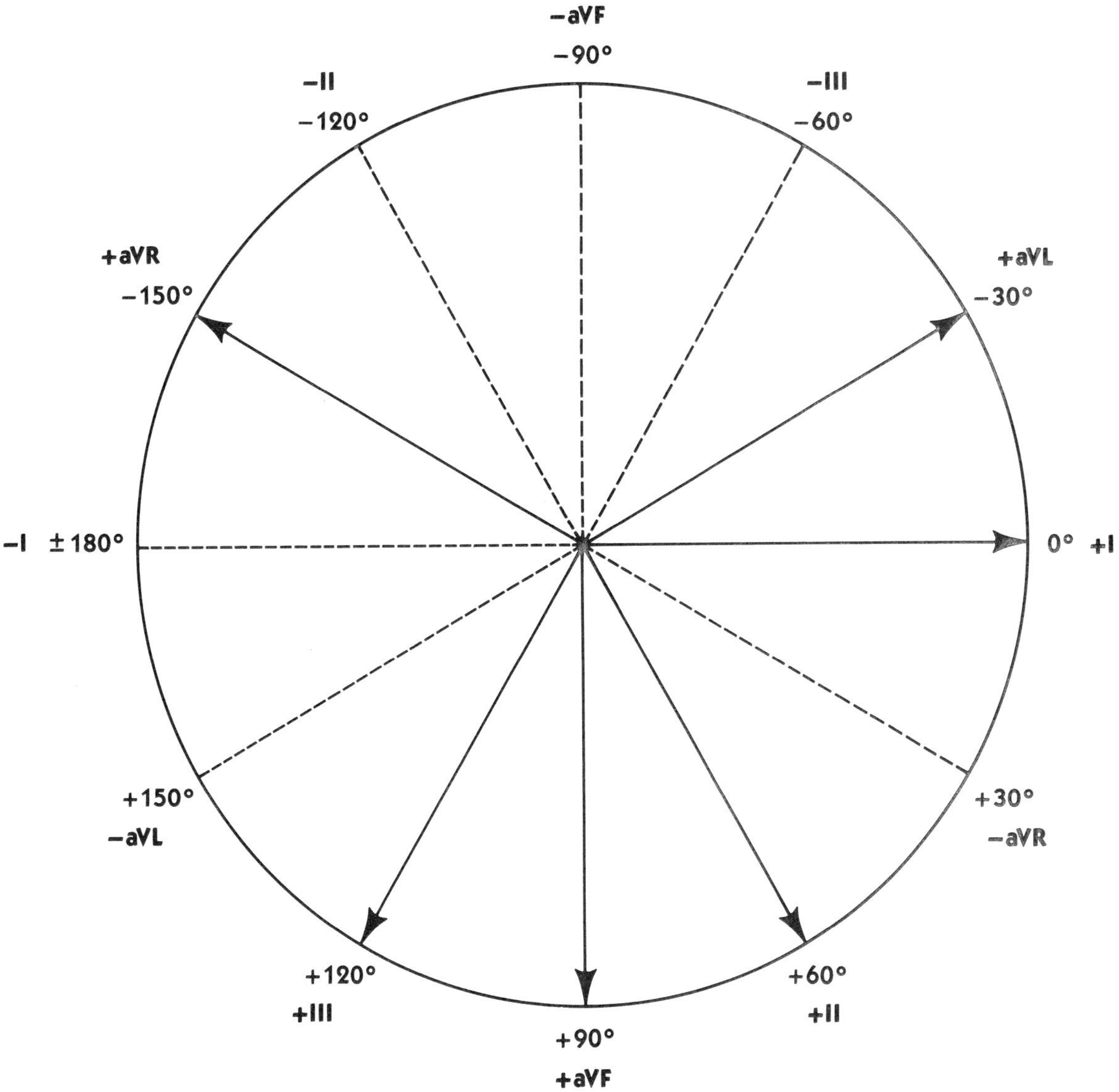

Figure 1
The hexaxial reference system for determining mean frontal plane QRS axis (see Section I). The arrows point toward the positive poles of the six limb leads. A ventricular depolarization wave that spreads toward a positive pole produces an upright deflection on the ECG tracing for that lead; a wave spreading in the opposite direction (toward a negative pole) produces a downward deflection. The mean frontal plane QRS axis is directed at a right angle to the most isoelectric (neither positive nor negative) or biphasic (equally positive and negative) lead, and toward the leads showing the tallest upright QRS deflections.

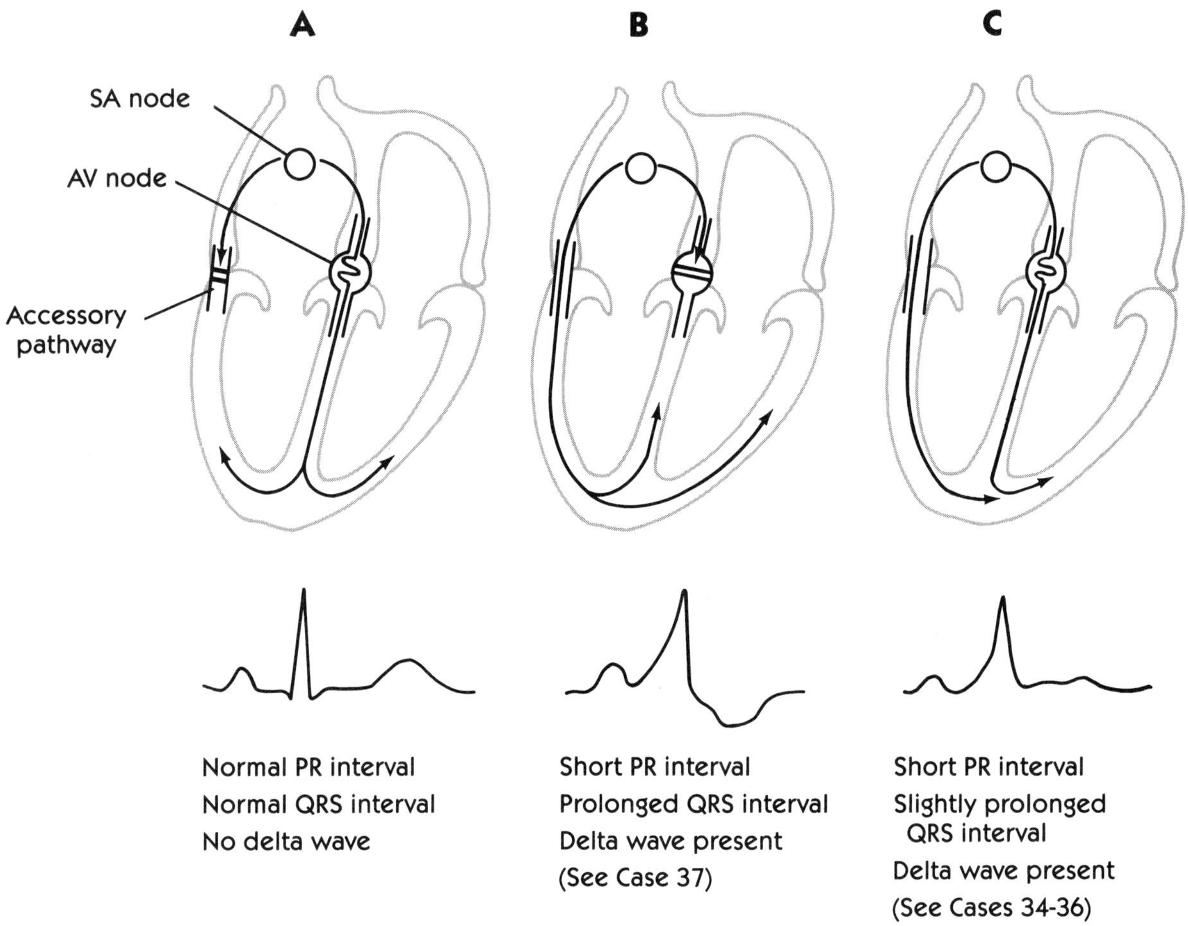

Figure 2
In Wolff-Parkinson-White and other ventricular pre-excitation syndromes, patients often exhibit varying degrees of pre-excitation. Conduction may proceed entirely through the normal AV node-His-Purkinje system (Fig. A); entirely through the accessory pathway (Fig. B); or through both pathways (Fig. C). When both pathways contribute to ventricular activation, the ECG will record a fusion complex.

Bibliography

I. An Approach to the Interpretation of 12-lead ECGs

Chou TC: *Electrocardiography in Clinical Practice.* New York: Grune & Stratton, 1979

Goldman MJ: *Principles of Clinical Electrocardiography.* Los Altos, CA: Lange, 1982

Hurst JW, Myerburg RJ: The electrocardiogram. In Walker HK, Hall WD, Hurst JW: *Clinical Methods. The History, Physical and Laboratory Examinations,* pp 945–1016. Boston: Butterworth, 1976

Marriott HJL: *Workshop in Electrocardiography.* Oldsmar, FL: Tampa Tracings, 1972

II. Ventricular and Atrial Hypertrophy

Chou TC et al: Specificity of the current electrocardiographic criteria for the diagnosis of left ventricular hypertrophy. *Am Heart J* 60:371, 1960

Chou TC: The pseudo P pulmonale. *Circulation* 32:96, 1965

Cosio FG et al: The Q waves of hypertrophic cardiomyopathy. *N Engl J Med* 302:96, 1980

Josephson ME: Electrocardiographic left atrial enlargement. *Am J Cardiol* 39:967, 1977

Lipsett MB: Anatomic and electrocardiographic correlation in combined ventricular hypertrophy. *Am Heart J* 45:86, 1953

Romhilt DW et al: A critical appraisal of the electrocardiographic criteria for the diagnosis of left ventricular hypertrophy. *Circulation* 40:185, 1969

Scott RC: Correlation between the electrocardiographic patterns of ventricular hypertrophy and anatomic findings. *Circulation* 21:256, 1960

Scott RC: The electrocardiographic diagnosis of right ventricular hypertrophy: Correlation with the anatomic findings. *Am Heart J* 60:659, 1960

Zema MJ, Kligfield P: ECG poor R-wave progression. Review and synthesis. *Arch Intern Med* 142:1145, 1982

III. Bundle Branch Blocks

Dodge HT, Grant RP: Mechanisms of QRS complex prolongation in man. Right ventricular conduction defects. *Am J Med* 21:534, 1956

Gardberg M, Rosen IL: Electrocardiogram and vectorcardiogram in various degrees of left bundle branch block. *Am J Cardiol* 1:592, 1958

Hecht HH, Kossmann CE: Atrioventricular and intraventricular conduction. *Am J Cardiol* 31:232, 1973

Lev M et al: Pathology of the conduction system in acquired heart disease. Complete right bundle branch block. *Am Heart J* 61:593, 1961

Lev M: The anatomic substrate of complete left bundle branch block. *Circulation* 50:479, 1974

Rosenbaum MB: The hemiblocks. Diagnostic criteria and clinical significance. *Mod Concepts Cardiovasc Dis* 39:141, 1970

IV. Myocardial Infarction and Ischemia

Besoain-Santander M, Gomez-Ebensperguer G: Electrocardiographic diagnosis of myocardial infarction in cases of complete left bundle branch block. *Am Heart J* 60:886, 1960

Chou TC: Pseudo-infarction (non-infarction Q waves). *Cardiovasc Clin* 5:199, 1973

Grossman JI, Delman AJ: Serial P wave changes in acute myocardial infarction. *Am Heart J* 77:336, 1969

Horace LG et al: Significance of the diagnostic Q wave of myocardial infarction. *Circulation* 43:428, 1971

Meller J et al: Transient Q waves in Prinzmetal's angina. *Am J Cardiol* 35:691, 1975

Schick EC et al: Increase in R-wave amplitude during transient epicardial injury (Prinzmetal's type). *J Electrocardiol* 49:259, 1980

Watson JH, Bartholomae WM: Cardiac injury due to non-penetrating chest trauma. *Ann Intern Med* 52:871, 1960

V. Accessory AV Conduction Syndromes

Chung EK: Wolff-Parkinson-White syndrome—current views. *Am J Med* 62:252, 1977

Ferrer MI: *Pre-excitation, Including the Wolff-Parkinson-White and Other Related Syndromes.* Mt. Kisco, NY: Futura, 1976

Lev M et al: Mahaim and James fibers as a basis for a unique variety of ventricular preexcitation. *Am J Cardiol* 36:880, 1975

Lown B, Ganong WF, Levine SA: The syndrome of short PR interval, normal QRS complex and paroxysmal rapid heart action. *Circulation* 5:693, 1952

VI. Pericarditis

Charles MA et al: Atrial injury current in pericarditis. *Arch Intern Med* 131:657, 1973

Fowler NO: The electrocardiogram in pericarditis. *Cardiovasc Clin* 5:256, 1973

Spodick DH: Differential characteristics of the electrocardiogram in early repolarization and acute pericarditis. *N Engl J Med* 295:523, 1976

Usher BW, Popp RL: Electrical alternans: Mechanism in pericardial effusion. *Am Heart J* 83:459, 1972

VII. The ECG in Lung Disease

Calatayud JB et al: P-wave changes in chronic obstructive pulmonary disease. *Am Heart J* 79:444, 1970

Fowler NO et al: The electrocardiogram in cor pulmonale with and without emphysema. *Am J Cardiol* 16:500, 1965

Spodick DH et al: The electrocardiogram in pulmonary emphysema; relationship of characteristic electrocardiographic findings to severity of disease measured by degree of airway obstruction. *Am Rev Respir Dis* 88:14, 1963

Stein PD et al: The electrocardiogram in acute pulmonary embolism. *Prog Cardiovasc Dis* 17:247, 1975

Wasserburger RH et al: The electrocardiographic pentalogy of pulmonary emphysema. *Circulation* 20:831, 1959

VIII. The ECG in Electrolyte and Metabolic Disturbances

Dimant J, Grob D: Electrocardiographic changes and myocardial damage in patients with acute cerebrovascular accidents. *Stroke* 8:448, 1977

DeGroot LJ: Thyroid and the heart. *Mayo Clin Proc* 47:864, 1972

Lepeschkin E: The U wave of the electrocardiogram. *Mod Concepts Cardiovasc Dis* 38:39, 1969

Schwartz PJ et al: The long Q-T syndrome. *Am Heart J* 89:378, 1975

Surawicz B: Relationship between electrocardiogram and electrolytes. *Am Heart J* 73:814, 1967

VanderArk CR et al: Electrolytes and the electrocardiogram. *Cardiovasc Clin* 5:270, 1973

Weintraub BM, McHenry LC: Cardiac abnormalities in subarachnoid hemorrhage: A résumé. *Stroke* 5:384, 1974

IX. The ECG and Drug Toxicity

Castellanos A, Salhanick L: The electrocardiographic patterns of procaine amide cardiotoxicity. *Am J Med Sci* 253:82/52, 1967

Elkayam U, Frishman W: Cardiovascular effects of phenothiazines. *Am Heart J* 100:397, 1980

Hoffman BF et al: Electrophysiology and pharmacology of cardiac arrhythmias: VII. Cardiac effects of quinidine and procaine amide. *Am Heart J* 89:804, 1975

Marshall JB, Forker AD: Cardiovascular effects of tricyclic antidepressant drugs: Therapeutic usage, overdose, and management of complications. *Am Heart J* 103:401, 1982

Pick A: Digitalis and the electrocardiogram. *Circulation* 15:603, 1957

Surawicz B, Lassiter KC: Effect of drugs on the electrocardiogram. *Prog Cardiovasc Dis* 13:26, 1970

X. Normal and Positional Variants

DeOliveira JM et al: The electrocardiogram in pectus excavatum. *Br Heart J* 20:495, 1958

Goldman MJ: Normal variants in the electrocardiogram leading to cardiac invalidism. *Am Heart J* 59:71, 1960

Goldman MJ: RS-T segment elevation in mid and left precordial leads as normal variant. *Am Heart J* 46:817, 1953

Simonson E et al: The normal Q-T interval. *Am Heart J* 63:747, 1962

Wasserburger RH et al: The normal RS-T segment elevation variant. *Am J Cardiol* 8:184, 1961

Zeppilli P et al: T wave abnormalities in top-ranking athletes: Effect of isoproterenol, atropine, and physical exercise. *Am Heart J* 100:213, 1980